PHARMACO EPIDEMIOLOGY

An Introduction

2nd Edition

EDITED BY

Abraham G. Hartzema, Miquel S. Porta, and Hugh H. Tilson

HARVEY WHITNEY BOOKS

Table of Contents

Foreword

Epidemics distribute suffering as part of the natural tragedy of life, but the tragedy is all the more poignant when the disease results from drugs designed to benefit rather than to harm. Drugs are developed and taken intentionally to avoid disease and pain, and our continued reliance on them is a testament to their wondrous efficacy and safety. But agents that have the power to alter some biological processes to our benefit can alter other biological processes to our detriment, sometimes in occult and surprising ways. To live up to the dictum that we should first of all do no harm, or at least less harm than good, we must bring our best evaluative methods to bear on the measurement of drug effects, both beneficial and adverse.

Pharmacoepidemiology is a natural crossing of scientific paths. Epidemiology is the study of disease occurrence, and pharmacology aims to reduce disease incidence and prevalence through biochemical intervention. The heavy reliance on epidemiologic methods—I include among these the clinical trial—in modern drug development has been instrumental in producing a pharmacopoeia of highly effective and reliable medicines that are among the major contributors to a better quality of life. Epidemiologic methods also have provided crucial insights into modern iatrogenic epidemics, such as adenocarcinoma of the vagina caused by diethylstilbestrol, endometrial cancer caused by exogenous estrogens, and toxic shock caused by the use of tampons.

The escalating health consciousness of our society guarantees an even broader role in the future for pharmacoepidemiologic research. Drug trials for efficacy usually have been clinical trials, aimed at improving the prognosis or symptoms of patients with active disease. Field trials, which evaluate the efficacy of primary preventives, are much more ambitious undertakings. They ordinarily require many thousands of subjects to be followed for long periods, presenting difficult logistical problems. Because these subjects are not ill, recruiting them and maintaining contact is more of a problem than in clinical trials, in which the clinic can be used for both recruitment and follow-up. For these reasons field trials of pharmaceutical agents for primary prevention have been conducted only rarely, usually for vaccines. With growing interest in the primary prevention of disease, however, field trials of disease preventives may become more common. Indeed, a large field trial that examines prevention of cancer with beta-carotene has been underway, using physicians as subjects. [Another component of this study examined the primary prevention of cardiovascular disease with aspirin. It was terminated in December 1987.]

We shall also see more studies that evaluate adverse drug effects, most of which will be case-control studies. Unintended drug effects (UDEs) that occur soon after administration, if they are frequent or severe enough, are usually discovered early in clinical testing. When UDEs are rare or occur only with a lengthy induction time, however, they may easily go undetected. Case-control studies provide an opportunity to investigate rare or delayed UDEs without undertaking cumbersome follow-up studies of awesome cost and logistical complexity. One big obstacle to case-control studies of drug use has been ascertaining the drug history. Information about drug use recorded in medical records varies in quality and completeness, often being little better or even worse than the information about drug use stored in the cerebral cortex of users. Obtaining valid information on drug use is aided greatly by systems that automatically record drug information in computer-readable form as it is prescribed or dispensed. (Of course, even this information differs from actual use.) Automated databases that include drug information and the capability to link it with medical records are increasing in number, and with passing time and accumulating data become more valuable as resources for pharmacoepidemiologic research.

Even with the best data resources, there remains a crucial epidemiologic problem in the study of many UDEs: confounding stemming from the indication for drug use. The causal association between illness and drugs employed to treat the illness can make it difficult or impossible to distinguish whether it is the drug or its therapeutic indication that is responsible for subsequent disease occurrence. Even when some people are treated with different therapies, there are usually important biologic differences among these groups. Confounding from other drugs and the possibility of drug interactions further complicate research of this type. Except in randomized trials, these problems will challenge pharmacoepidemiologists to the limits of their ingenuity and knowledge, making pharmacoepidemiology a proving ground for advances in epidemiologic methods.

Nevertheless, the basic tools to deal with these problems exist; they will inevitably become more refined as researchers gain experience, but the application of currently accepted epidemiologic principles could improve the understanding of many drug effects. For example, a disease such as analgesic nephropathy, the topic of a National Institutes of Health Consensus Development Conference, might cease to exist under the scrutiny of epidemiologic principles.This disease is defined as kidney disease following analgesic use. Because the definition includes the presence of the hypothesized cause, it is impossible to determine whether analgesic use is associated with kidney disease, much less whether a causal relation exists that would merit the term analgesic nephropathy. Even if an association were shown to exist using a proper disease definition that was independent of exposure, confounding by the indication for the analgesic use might account for it. To address such questions requires an epidemiologic perspective. This book is a welcome step toward introducing this perspective to all researchers concerned with the evaluation of drug effects.

Kenneth J. Rothman

Preface to the First Edition

The reasons for this book will be immediately clear to readers who, like us, have been waiting for an overview of pharmacoepidemiology to be compiled in a single place. Such a single source of information can serve different purposes: personal or professional reference; a textbook in pharmacy, pharmacology, or epidemiology; a reference for operating pharmacoepidemiology programs in academia, government, and industry; for drug information units or product surveillance programs; or for rigorous structured pharmacoepidemiologic study.

We became keenly aware of the need for a compendium on pharmacoepidemiology because, wearing one hat or another, we were searching for a reference to accomplish one or more purposes when this happy collaboration began in 1985. At that time, we were developing a short course in pharmacoepidemiology to be offered in the Department of Epidemiology at the School of Public Health at the University of North Carolina. Having canvassed the educational opportunities in and around the area, we found no course offerings suitable for the audience needing to know more about the rapidly evolving field of pharmacoepidemiology. Therefore, we undertook to implement the course designs of Audrey Smith Rogers, a postdoctoral fellow at that time; a contribution of hers appears in this book.

In preparing the syllabus for the course in May 1985, we once again became aware of the lack of good teaching materials, especially those capturing the progress in the field during the 1980s. This was a time period in which new questions were formulated, new approaches taken, new technologies developed, new policies set, and new expectations raised providing for a state of flux in pharmacoepidemiology.

We were somewhat daunted by the complexity of the tasks of designing the course, compiling the materials, and providing expertise in a complex and multidisciplinary area, and particularly by the realization that we—like most workers in this relatively new field—lacked the experience (and, some of our friends even observed, the skills) to do it all ourselves. How did we start?

One of us (H.T.) had recently put together a set of "house rules" for the practicing epidemiologist at a workshop on pharmacoepidemiology, in Minister Lovell, England, sponsored by Dr. Hershel Jick, distinguished pharmacoepidemiologist and one of the founders of the field. Among these "house rules" the cardinal principle was: "In this complex field, don't wait for something to go wrong before you get help!" As the reader can surely judge, the editors succeeded in following this golden rule and established happy and fruitful collaboration with a series of first-rate colleagues who clearly do have claim to expertise, competence, and accomplishment in their chosen disciplinary areas and are highly motivated to contribute to the further development of pharmacoepidemiology.

The materials we have elected to include derive from that early course outline but were, in fact, solicited as a nine-part series in the journal *Drug Intelligence and*

Clinical Pharmacy. Those materials were solicited to follow in a logical sequence that now works as this textbook. Still, no journal series, however complete, can cover the entire length and breadth of a field, much less its depth. Therefore, this book includes significant new material.

This new material includes a chapter on risk assessment providing an international perspective, and an extensive glossary on terms used in the field. The new chapter addresses the international dimensions in pharmacoepidemiology that relate to risk assessment. Further, we determined that, as in any specialized field, the field of pharmacoepidemiology had developed both a jargon and a lore of its own. This language was often needlessly confusing to the neophyte, even to the extent of discouraging excellent scientists with specialty in one, but not the other, of the disciplines that form the basis of pharmacoepidemiology from undertaking work for which they are well qualified. Therefore, we have appended the requisite glossary.

Perhaps it goes without saying (except in a preface like this) that the real reason for this endeavor is the conviction of the three of us that the activities of pharmacoepidemiology are important. It is important for therapeutics, for medicine, for public health, and, hopefully, for the public's health. It is probably necessary to underscore that verity here, because there will be readers or their superiors who date back to the era before the watershed report of the Melmon Commission in January 1980 and remember a time when the contributions of the field were less respected because they were less respectable. Long-term follow-up of large numbers of people is neither easy or cheap; controlling the multiple biases of observational methodology, without knowing the tricks of the trade of the experimentalist, is likewise no easy task. Also, performing the sleuthing tasks of the epidemiologist in an arena dominated by clinicians—nurses, pharmacists, and physicians—is not always either understood or appreciated! Further, some of our predecessors have used manipulative approaches and unobtrusive methods motivated by a desire to co-opt collaborators in the quest for promotion or to distort data in the search for a good image for a drug product. Nor would we assert that the field has wholly purged itself of technical problems, attitudinal barriers, or ethical dilemmas. Most importantly, we suspect that while the potential contributions of epidemiology to pharmacology, and vice versa, are reasonably well established, a proper scientific evaluation of the actual contributions and accomplishments has been only partially undertaken. The valuable trends in the field are presented throughout the book. Chapters 7, 8, and 10 describe the emergence of affordable and powerful technologies using automated data sets. Chapters 1, 14, and 16 describe the development of meaningful products to improve medical practice and public policy and, in the process, protect people who are taking medications.

Finally, we have many people to thank for bringing this book into reality. Each of the contributors will be known by his or her works, but we would like to thank them for the energy and enthusiasm which they brought to these labors. We also thank Barbara Hulka, and the students of "Methods and Issues in Pharmacoepidemiology" for their valuable comments. Most especially, we thank Burroughs Wellcome Co. and the University of North Carolina, whose generosity of spirit provided encouragement to undertake this task and the setting in which this endeavor can grow. Finally, we thank friends and families for understanding the importance of this effort and supporting our preoccupation with it.

Abraham G. Hartzema

Miquel S. Porta

Hugh H. Tilson

Preface to the Second Edition

Pharmacoepidemiology: An Introduction enjoyed a splendid reception: the first edition sold out in one year's time. We have heard from colleagues from Australia to Zimbabwe who are using the book to increase their knowledge in the field; in classes as the primary or sole text, or in combination with reprints; and as the basis for continuing education and professional seminars. That the book partly filled a need in the profession became instantly clear. We are grateful for the comments, suggestions, and encouragement we received to enhance and update the book and are pleased now to offer this second edition.

We have taken all the suggestions we received to heart and, with the help of our prior collaborators and more authors, have compiled a more complete, somewhat more didactic, and up-to-date textbook on pharmacoepidemiology without compromising the immediacy and pragmatism of the first edition. Our first book was an attempt to define the boundaries and content of pharmacoepidemiology as a field. Although we were told we were successful through our own work in the field and our experience using the book in our own classes, we have learned a lot in the time period between the publication of the first edition and the start of the preparation of the second edition and have gained a deeper understanding of what pharmacoepidemiology is. The second edition reflects this understanding.

We have expanded the second edition in areas that readers considered important, broadening the scope by providing a more in-depth discussion, for example, of causality assessment; increasing the didactic value of the book by adding chapters about the statistical analyses used in pharmacoepidemiologic studies; and because of the increased political relevance of pharmacoepidemiology, adding chapters that discuss the implications of and standards for pharmacoepidemiologic research. In addition, all chapters of our first edition are included here, and all but two (which have stood the test of time) have been substantially revised and updated. Further, to increase the value as a reference we have added an annotated bibliography of selected pharmacoepidemiologic studies.

In summary, the second edition will provide readers with a detailed overview of pharmacoepidemiology. As always, we are open to suggestions and comments from our readers. Please let us know your needs so they can be incorporated into the next edition.

Abraham G. Hartzema
Miquel S. Porta
Hugh H. Tilson

Contributing Authors

LTC Darrel C. Bjornson, Ph.D.
Clinical Research Pharmacist, Walter Reed Retrovirus Research Group
Walter Reed Army Medical Center, Washington, DC 20307
Chapter 7

J. Gregory Boyer
Pharmacoeconomic Research, Glaxo Inc.
Five Moore Drive, Research Triangle Park, NC 27709
Chapter 11

Thomas J. Craig, M.D., M.P.H.
Clinical Director, Rockland Psychiatric Center, Orangeburg, NY
Professor of Psychiatry and Behavioral Science, State University of New York
Health Science Center at Brooklyn, Stony Brook, NY 11794
Chapter 14

Stanley A. Edlavitch, Ph.D.
Senior Research Associate, Director of Pharmacoepidemiology Studies
University of Minnesota, Minneapolis, MN 55455
Chapter 8

Thomas R. Einarson, Ph.D.
Faculty of Pharmacy, University of Toronto
Toronto, Ontario, Canada M5S 2S2
Chapter 13

Denis M. Grant, Ph.D.
Assistant Professor of Pediatrics and Pharmacology, University of Toronto
Division of Clinical Pharmacology and Toxicology, Hospital for Sick Children
Toronto, Ontario, Canada M5G 1X8
Chapter 2

Harry Guess, M.D., Ph.D.
Senior Director, Epidemiology
Merck Sharp & Dohme, West Point, PA 19486
Chapter 17

Abraham G. Hartzema, Ph.D., M.S.P.H.
Associate Professor, Division of Pharmacy Administration, School of Pharmacy
Clinical Associate Professor, Health Policy and Administration, School of Public Health
University of North Carolina, Chapel Hill, NC 27599
Preface, Chapters 1, 7, 9, 10, and 20

Gary G. Koch, Ph.D.

Professor of Biostatistics, Department of Biostatistics, School of Public Health
University of North Carolina, Chapel Hill, NC 27599
Chapter 9

David A. Lane, Ph.D.

Professor, School of Statistics, University of Minnesota, Minneapolis, MN 55455
Chapter 6

Donald C. McLeod, M.S.Pharm.

Senior Medical Analyst, Center for Epidemiologic and Medical Studies
Research Triangle Institute, Research Triangle Park, NC 27709
Chapter 20

Steven R. Moore, B.S.Pharm., M.P.H.

Assistant Chief of Staff, Office of the Assistant Surgeon General
U.S. Public Health Service, Rockville, MD 20857
Chapter 4

Ann Myers, B.S.Pharm., M.P.H.

Chief, Document Management and Reporting Branch, Center for Drug Evaluation and
  Research
Food and Drug Administration, Rockville, MD 20857
Chapter 4

Robert C. Nelson, Ph.D.

Director, Office of Professional Development and Staff College, Center for Drug Evaluation
  and Research
Food and Drug Administration, Rockville, MD 20857
Chapter 15

Harry Otway, Ph.D.

Division Office, Health, Safety and Environment Division
Los Alamos National Laboratory, Los Alamos, NM 87545
Chapter 16

Eleanor Perfetto, M.Sc.

Research Associate, Center for Health Promotion and Disease Prevention
University of North Carolina, Chapel Hill, NC 27599
Chapter 10

Miquel S. Porta, M.D., M.P.H.

Adjunct Associate Professor, Department of Epidemiology, School of Public Health
University of North Carolina, Chapel Hill, NC 27599
Associate Professor, Institut Municipal d'Investigació Mèdica
Universitat Autònoma de Barcelona, Barcelona, Spain
Preface, Chapter 1

Kenneth J. Rothman, Dr.P.H.

Senior Epidemiologist, Epidemiology Resources, Inc.
Chestnut Hill, MA 02167
Professor, Department of Family and Community Medicine
University of Massachusetts, Worcester, MA 01655
Foreword

Joaquima Serradell, Ph.D., M.P.H.
Assistant Professor, Pharmacy Administration, School of Pharmacy
Philadelphia College of Pharmacy and Pharmaceutical Sciences, Philadelphia, PA 19104
Chapter 7

Audrey Smith Rogers, Ph.D.
Chief of Epidemiology Special Studies, AIDS Administration
Maryland State Department of Health and Mental Hygiene, Baltimore, MD 21201
Chapter 5

Stephen P. Spielberg, M.D., Ph.D., FRCPC
Professor of Paediatrics and Pharmacology
Director, Centre for Drug Safety Research, University of Toronto
Director, Division of Clinical Pharmacology and Toxicology
Hospital for Sick Children, Toronto, Ontario, Canada M5G 1X8
Chapter 2

Bert Spilker, M.D., Ph.D.
Director of Projects Coordination, Burroughs Wellcome Co.
3030 Cornwallis Rd., Research Triangle Park, NC 27709
Chapters 3 and 18

Andy S. Stergachis, Ph.D.
Associate Professor, Department of Pharmacy, School of Pharmacy and Department of
  Epidemiology
School of Public Health and Community Medicine
Scientific Investigator, Center for Health Studies
Group Health Cooperative of Puget Sound, Seattle, WA 98121
Chapter 12

Hugh H. Tilson, M.D., Dr.P.H.
Director, Division of Epidemiology, Information, and Surveillance
Burroughs Wellcome Co.
Clinical Professor, Department of Family Medicine, School of Medicine
Adjunct Professor, Department of Epidemiology, School of Public Health, Department of
  Pharmacy Administration, School of Pharmacy
University of North Carolina, Chapel Hill, NC 27599
Preface, Chapter 19

Raymond J. Townsend, Pharm.D.
Pharmacoeconomic Research, Glaxo Inc.
Five Moore Drive, Research Triangle Park, NC 27709
Chapter 11

Julie Magno Zito, Ph.D.
Research Scientist, Clinical Division
Nathan S. Kline Institute for Psychiatric Research, Orangeburg, NY 10962
Research Assistant Professor (part-time), Department of Psychiatry
New York University School of Medicine, New York, NY 10003
Chapter 14

Introduction to the Field

1

The Contribution of Epidemiology to the Study of Drugs

Miquel S. Porta
Abraham G. Hartzema

Abstract

This first chapter is an introduction to the potential contributions of epidemiology to the study of drugs. Epidemiology is concerned with the distribution of disease and health in human populations. Drugs are one of the factors that influence such a distribution. Pharmacoepidemiology can be defined as the application of epidemiologic knowledge, methods, and reasoning to the study of the effects (beneficial and adverse) and uses of drugs in human populations. Pharmacoepidemiology aims to describe, explain, control, and predict the effects and uses of pharmacologic treatment modalities in a defined time, space, and population. Not only does epidemiology aid pharmacology in better understanding drug uses and effects; pharmacology helps epidemiology by increasing the knowledge about the causes of diseases, the distribution of health, and the functioning of the healthcare system. The actual contribution of epidemiology to the study of drug uses and effects has been only partially assessed. However, because the health of our society benefits from the dynamic interrelationship of pharmacology, epidemiology, and clinical medicine, the authors conclude that the field of pharmacoepidemiology is full of promise and potential.

Outline

M edications have become an increasingly important therapeutic tool in the hands of healthcare professionals. Effective drugs are continuously entering the marketplace, replacing older and less effective drugs. With the aging of Western populations and consequently a higher prevalence of medical problems, increasingly large numbers of people are exposed to multiple drugs for longer periods of time. Pharmacoepidemiology offers a methodology and a body of substantive knowledge both to increase the health benefits of drugs and to reduce their risks.

Although drug studies historically have been the prerogative of biologists, medicinal chemists, pharmacologists, and clinicians, epidemiologic methods also have been applied to study vaccines and drugs.[1] An increasing number of medical, pharmacy, and public health schools already have or are establishing programs in pharmacoepidemiology.[2] Also, major pharmaceutical firms have established medical surveillance programs based on epidemiologic methods. Thus, the value of epidemiology for drug research and development is gaining widespread recognition.

The purpose of this chapter is to provide the reader with an introduction to the potential contributions of pharmacoepidemiology to the study of drug effects and uses, as well as to indicate the common grounds pharmacoepidemiology shares with other disciplines in the healthcare field. In fact, because the relationship between epidemiology and pharmacology is synergistic, as is illustrated in this chapter, the study of drugs with epidemiologic methods will further our understanding of the etiology of human illness. According to this view, pharmacoepidemiology becomes not just a subspecialty in epidemiology, but rather an extension of epidemiology.

Definition and Aims

Pharmacopidemiology can be defined as the application of epidemiologic knowledge, methods, and reasoning to the study of the effects (beneficial and adverse) and uses of drugs in human populations. It aims to describe, explain, control, and predict the effects and uses of pharmacologic treatments in a defined time, space, and population. Its core lies at the intersection of two subspecialties: clinical pharmacology and clinical epidemiology.[1]

Outlining questions that pharmacoepidemiology attempts to answer or which it poses to other disciplines can help define the interests and boundaries of this fledgling field. Examples of problems addressed within the realm of pharmacoepidemiology include:

1. Are there differences in the number of hypertensive people diagnosed and treated among different populations in the U.S.? What is the impact on cardiocerebrovascular morbidity of such differences? How much of the past years' decline in coronary heart disease can be accounted for by the effects of cardiovascular drugs? What are the most common uses of beta-blockers? Why is it that some of those uses do not agree with the academic recommendations and what conclusions can be drawn from these observations? Will the treat-

ment of hypertension be influenced by changes in the healthcare system in the next ten years?

2. What is the effectiveness of psychotropic drugs in defined populations? Does the effectiveness of psychotropic drugs depend on age, gender, and sociocultural level? What changes can we predict in the prevalence of mental illness based on the current drug consumption trends? How can new therapeutic developments improve the long-term outcome of psychiatric patients? Is therapeutic information a determinant of the quality of psychotropic drug prescriptions? What can we learn about our culture from the way mental illness is treated?

These two clusters of questions relate to antihypertensive and psychotropic drugs; however, similar questions can be developed for other therapeutic categories. Pharmacoepidemiology provides the key to many questions that arise in the process of drug development, prescribing, and use. More examples are presented in Table 1 to further illustrate the scope of the discipline and the common research questions epidemiology shares with other disciplines, such as the social sciences, health economics, pharmacy, and medicine.

Three fundamental questions flow from the previous discussion: Can epidemiology help improve the development and use of drugs? Can pharmacology help expand our knowledge of disease etiology? Is the health status of our society going to benefit from the interrelationship of pharmacy, clinical medicine, and epidemiology? Because the answer to these three questions is a resounding "yes," the field of pharmacoepidemiology is full of promise and potential. This potential will be discussed in this book.

Epidemiology studies the distribution of health and disease in human populations; drugs are among the factors that influence such distribution. Thus, from a public health perspective it is of utmost importance that pharmacoepidemiologists assess the impact that vaccines and drugs have on the overall patterns of diseases. However, because of the complexities involved in evaluating pharmacotherapeutic outcomes, specific epidemiologic techniques have to be used in the study of drugs. This chapter briefly discusses the need for specific methodologic considerations in the study of drugs, merely to support the evidence for the development of pharmacoepidemiology as a specific discipline. Quantitative techniques available to the pharmacoepidemiologist are discussed in more detail in Chapter 9. Application of epidemiologic methodologies to drug effects and uses is demonstrated most clearly in postmarketing surveillance (PMS) of drugs.

Methodologic Considerations

The term pharmacoepidemiology emphasizes the use of epidemiologic reasoning and methods, regardless of the phase of drug development. Postmarketing

How can we accelerate the process of discovery of new clinically relevant unintended drug effects?

What is the cost effectiveness of hepatitis B vaccine, oral hypoglycemic agents, cerebrovascular vasodilators, hypolipemiants, estrogens, or cephalosporins for selected indications?

What can be done by the pharmaceutical industry to alleviate the burden of disease in older populations?

What factors in the physician-patient encounter influence treatment compliance and continuity of care?

What is the most appropriate control group for a hospital-based case-control study of drug-related congenital malformations?

How should the validation of large clinical databases be approached?

What factors should guide the decision to conduct formal postmarketing epidemiologic studies?

In what type of clinical trials is it desirable to incorporate economic analysis?

How does cancer chemotherapy interact with the natural course of the disease?

What can be done to prevent the development of resistance to antibiotics in the general population?

What algorithms are most useful to validate unintended drug effect reports?

Is endstage renal disease caused by analgesic abuse?

What is a good design for studying the factors that influence clinical decision making, including prescribing?

Can we use a composite measure of health status in epidemiologic studies to evaluate patient outcomes?

Can we learn something about the prognostic factors for juvenile arthritis from the way it is treated by primary care physicians?

What psychological factors and sociocultural values influence risk perception?

Table 1
Examples of Questions Addressed by Pharmacoepidemiology

surveillance refers to a specific time in the life of a drug: the time span that begins once a drug enters the general market (also known as Phase IV). At present, PMS is the most common activity of pharmacoepidemiologists.[3]

PMS is important because at the time a drug is approved for marketing a number of clinically and epidemiologically important questions are unknown. For example, premarketing studies assess the efficacy of hypoglycemic agents in controlling diabetic symptoms (primary efficacy) but they rarely assess their efficacy in preventing cardiovascular or renal complications of diabetes (secondary efficacy). Hypoglycemic agents were approved solely for their primary effects, but are widely used for both.[4] The long-term effects of drugs in the prevention of disease or its complications is just one of the numerous questions unknown at the time of marketing. These questions must be addressed by postmarketing studies. Table 2 summarizes the basic types of questions addressed in postmarketing studies.[5]

Upon approval of a new drug by the FDA, thousands of individuals become exposed to the drug in a variety of sociocultural and clinical settings. Furthermore, the therapeutic use of drugs is often extended to population subgroups not included in premarketing studies, to new indications emerging in clinical practice, and for periods of time much longer than those covered in most clinical trials (Table 2). Patients present a wide range of diagnoses and risk factors, as well as concomitant exposure to other drugs and environmental agents. In conclusion, drug epidemiology also deals with what Lasagna calls the most important question for therapeutics: How does a drug actually perform in clinical practice?[6]

Table 2
Taxonomy of Main Areas of Inquiry Addressed in Postmarketing Studies[5]

Area of Inquiry	Example
Long-term effects	
manifest after long periods of use	use of exogenous estrogen during menopause and endometrial cancer
manifest after long latency periods	adenocarcinoma of the vagina due to diethylstilbestrol
Low-frequency effects	
can only be detected in large populations	aplastic anemia: phenylbutazone; colitis: clindamycin; jaundice: halothane
Effectiveness in customary practice	
patients	children, pregnant or elderly women
therapeutic situations	with concurrent pathologies and several simultaneous treatments, flexible dosages, tolerance, noncompliance, nonresponse
healthcare settings	emergencies, ambulatory care
healthcare professionals	according to training, specialty information sources
Efficacy in new indications	
discovered after marketing	propranolol as an antihypertensive, captopril in rheumatoid arthritis, amantadine in Parkinson's disease, antihistamines in motion sickness
including secondary effects	antihypertensives to prevent cardiovascular disease, hypoglycemic agents to prevent complications of diabetes
Modifiers of efficacy	
concurrent drugs	a decrease in sodium intake can improve the efficacy of some diuretics in hypertension
disease severity	severe asthmatics do not respond to metaproterenol without supplementary therapy
lifestyle	risk of myocardial infarction in women who use oral contraceptives may be increased by cigarette smoking

Both experimental (i.e., with random allocation of treatments) and nonexperimental (observational) epidemiologic methods are used by drug epidemiologists. As explained in Chapter 8, randomized clinical trials (experimental studies) tend to be more common before a drug is marketed; observational studies (e.g., cross-sectional surveys, follow-up studies, case-control studies) usually are conducted after marketing.

LIMITATIONS OF CLINICAL TRIALS

Clinical evaluation of a drug in the premarketing phase seeks to validate scientific premises of the drug's extensive use in common therapeutic practice.[7] Although the randomized controlled clinical trial is the most powerful tool available to clinical scientists, its limitations, mostly due to ethical, practical, and economic reasons, should be recognized.

As Table 2 shows, the need for PMS arises from the limitations of Phase I, II, and III clinical trials, which study the efficacy and risks of a drug for selected clinical indications before the drug is marketed. Phase III clinical trials include a relatively small number of often nonrepresentative patients (nonrepresentative of the population and indications for which the drug eventually will be used), followed for short periods of time and very strictly defined conditions (e.g., double-blindness, random allocation of treatments, frequent and thorough examinations, placebo treatments, fixed-dose regimens, and tertiary care hospitals).[5,8-14] More recently, the FDA has attempted to remedy these pitfalls in Phase III studies. Consequently, Phase III clinical trials currently mandated by the FDA are usually multicentric and include patient populations representative of the population that would receive the drug. Furthermore, study size is largely determined by the patient population that will be at risk for the drug product. For example, for an antihypertensive drug, a study population between 1000 and 3000 could be required; for an orphan drug, 50–100 patients might be sufficient.

Phase IV clinical trials are defined as those conducted after a drug has been marketed. These are not necessarily mandated by the FDA, but can be negotiated between the manufacturer and the FDA as condition for new drug application approval. In addition, Phase IV clinical trials can be initiated upon signals originating from the FDA's Spontaneous Reporting System. The objectives, design, and sample size are at times similar to those of Phase III clinical trials. In Phase IV (postmarketing) clinical trials, however, larger and more heterogeneous populations usually are available and a stronger emphasis is placed on reproducing the usual clinical care conditions.

Because of their larger sample sizes, Phase IV studies provide additional information on the benefits and risks of drugs. Sample size is a direct determinant of the probability to detect drug effects that occur with a low frequency (see Table 3). The "rule of three" states that to detect an unintended drug effect (UDE) that occurs at a particular frequency, the number of subjects that one needs to follow-up is three times that of the estimated frequency of the event.[15] For example, if a UDE is suspected to occur in 1 of 10 000 drug users, we will have to observe 30 000 users in order to be 95 percent likely to detect it. Lower numbers will be needed if a lower statistical power is chosen. The larger sample sizes employed in Phase IV clinical studies allow for the assessment of drug effects with a low incidence (Table 3).[15]

In the past few years, growing attention has been given in the U.S. and elsewhere to the following question: when is it warranted to undertake a formal postmarketing drug safety study? Table 4 summarizes some suggested guidelines.[16] As can be seen, some of the indications to conduct a pharmacoepidemiologic study stem from the limitations of premarketing research. It is reasoned that:

1. crucial answers to drug safety questions sometimes cannot be provided even by the most valid, complex, and lengthy Phase III studies;
2. it is often more reasonable to expect that such answers be obtained by Phase IV studies; and
3. it may be ethically correct, scientifically sound, and politically wise to allow a drug to be marketed if well-designed pharmacoepidemiologic studies are initiated at the very moment of marketing approval.

When all these assumptions hold, pharmacoepidemiology can help to hasten the drug approval process, and to protect citizens, companies, and governments against unsubstantiated claims of risk. No doubt, beyond the criteria mentioned in Table 4, the decision of why, when, and how to conduct a formal postmarketing safety study also has wide economic and political implications.

Furthermore, it is important to realize the difference in the nature of the question posed in any particular study: premarketing studies usually choose an explanatory or knowledge-oriented question (focusing on the efficacy of the drug under strict experimental conditions); however, postmarketing studies often take a more pragmatic or decision-oriented approach (focusing on the effectiveness of

Table 3 Number of People Exposed to a Drug Necessary to Detect True Frequencies of Unintended Drug Effects[16]		Statistical Power			
	Frequency	95%*	90%*	80%*	63%*
	1/100	300	231	161	100
	1/500	1 500	1 152	805	500
	1/1 000	3 000	2 303	1 610	1 000
	1/5 000	15 000	11 513	8 048	5 000
	1/10 000	30 000	23 026	16 095	10 000
	1/50 000	150 000	115 130	80 472	50 000

*Statistical power: the probability of detecting an unintended drug effect (UDE) if it really occurs in the population under study (e.g., studying 8048 users of the drug will allow eight out of ten times to detect a UDE occurring in 1 out of 5000 exposed people). Most epidemiologists try to achieve sample sizes yielding a statistical power of 80 or 90 percent.

Prevalence of the disease Severity of the medical condition Expected duration of therapy New chemical entity status Chemical class with demonstrated acceptable safety Safety profile of the drug in premarketing trials Formulation of the agent Availability of safe and efficacious alternatives	**Table 4** Factors Influencing the Conduct of Formal Postmarketing Surveillance[7]

the drug under usual clinical circumstances). The explanatory/pragmatic distinction is relevant for both clinical trials and observational studies.[17,18]

It should also be observed that patients admitted to randomized clinical trials must be able to receive any of the study therapies, according to the results of randomization. A consequence of this requirement is that patients with a definitive indication for one of the therapies will be excluded from the trial on ethical grounds (because it would not be ethical to withhold a drug they clearly need). Consequently, therapy is not tested in those most likely to receive it.[19] These patients will have to be observed in PMS.

STRENGTHS OF CLINICAL TRIALS

Randomized controlled clinical trials are generally considered "the most scientifically rigorous method for hypothesis testing available in epidemiology."[20] Clinical trials are a good tool not only to assess the efficacy and safety of pharmaceuticals, but also for general health technology assessment. The impact of clinical studies on medical practice is a subject of increasing interest.[21,22]

Randomization (random allocation of treatments) is what makes clinical trials so powerful. Randomization, the most essential feature of clinical trials, is sometimes the only way to control for a potential confounder, the indication for the drug. Confounding by the indication generally occurs when patients who are prescribed a given drug have a poorer prognosis than those who are not receiving the drug. This is precisely why a health professional often decides that the drug is indicated.

In other words, a set of symptoms or an indication (e.g., lack of response to bronchodilators and sodium cromoglycate, sputum eosinophilia, centrilobular emphysema, and persistent, severe airway obstruction in a patient with asthma), perceived and judged by a health professional, is associated both with the prescription of a drug (prednisolone) and with a higher probability of a particular outcome (asthma attack). In fact, even if prednisolone reduces the risk of an asthma attack, an observational study may show a higher rate of attacks among prednisolone-treated patients than among nontreated patients. The higher rate of attacks among prednisolone-treated patients may be due to their poor prognosis before the drug was prescribed.

Thus, confounding by indication stems from an initial lack of comparability in the prognostic expectations of treated and nontreated subjects. This bias has also been called "susceptibility bias"[23] and "procedure selection bias."[24] Methods other than randomization to control for this confounding effect have been proposed, and at present this particular issue constitutes one of the most interesting methodologic challenges in pharmacoepidemiology.[4,25-30]

Another interesting question was raised during a follow-up study of cimetidine users.[31,32] During this study it was observed that a greater number of patients on cimetidine were admitted to hospital than age- and sex-matched controls from the community. The increased frequency of hospital admission among cimetidine users was largest for patients with diseases of the digestive tract, but also was higher for diseases of the musculoskeletal system, cancers, respiratory tract, and other major systems. Because the study was nonrandomized, the most plausible explanation seemed to be contributory causes to the conditions for which cimetidine is prescribed: smoking is a risk factor for peptic ulcer and respiratory diseases (including lung cancer); nonsteroidal antiinflammatory drugs (NSAIDs) used in musculoskeletal diseases such as rheumatoid arthritis can also produce dyspepsia; a peptic ulcer that bleeds may lead to iron-deficiency anemia; and so on.[31,32] Again, subjects exposed to the drug appeared to have more risk factors for a variety of diseases than subjects not exposed to the drug. This explanation is logically appealing: as the saying goes, "usually people who take drugs are sick."

When looking at a difference between the efficacy and risks of two treatments, two questions should be asked: (1) why was each treatment prescribed? and (2) could those reasons help explain the difference in outcome?

OBSERVATIONAL METHODS

Observational epidemiologic studies are those in which the investigator does not have direct control over the variables of interest (e.g., there is no random allocation of treatments). Observational epidemiologic methods were applied to the study of drug effects and uses well before the terms pharmacoepidemiology or drug epidemiology ever appeared in print.[1] Observational methods include vital and morbidity statistics,[33-35] case-control studies,[36,37] cohort studies,[38,39] descriptive studies of drug utilization,[40-42] and other approaches.[43-52] The strengths and weaknesses of these methods are discussed in detail subsequently in this book.

One of the most promising developments facilitating the use of observational methods is the use of automated databases. Large, automated databases provide follow-up data on drug effects. They allow for relatively fast and cost-effective studies of delayed as well as short-term effects in very large populations.[53-60] However, data quality is a common major limitation, and access to the original clinical records is often crucial for verification purposes.[61] Computerized databases should not replace ad hoc studies when such studies are ethically and logistically feasible.[62,63]

Research Problems and Opportunities

MARKERS OF THE HEALTH SYSTEM'S METABOLISM

A health services issue that is relevant to pharmacoepidemiology is the role of drugs within the healthcare system, the system in which diseases are detected and diagnosed, decisions are made for treatment (or no treatment), and where diseases are modified during their natural course.[64-67] To study the metabolic processes of a particular organism, markers (e.g., radioactive substances) are sometimes administered. Markers allow one to observe unobtrusively the interactions of physical and chemical components in the human body. Metaphorically, drugs may be considered markers for the study of the healthcare system's metabolism. Kunin states that "the therapeutic or prophylactic decisions made by providers or consumers represent the final common pathway of virtually all of the critical factors related to the appropriateness and efficacy of medical care. These decisions represent the synthesis of the mixed ingredients of behavioral, social, cultural, economic, and educational concepts and beliefs about health and diseases in populations."[68]

Drugs not only measure the prevalence of some medical problems,[69] but also reflect how humans experience health and cope with suffering.[66,67] Drug prescribing is one of the most visible indicators of physician practice patterns because it is observable, can be documented, and is rather frequent.[70] Patient compliance with drugs has been found to be a proxy variable for the quality of patient-physician interaction, for the patient's belief in the efficacy of the pharmacotherapeutic treatment, and the effectiveness of patient education.[71] Drugs allow health services researchers to follow the way the medical and lay communities interact in selecting solutions through pharmacologic intervention. Thus, if we study how drugs are developed, promoted, and used, drugs become excellent markers of the functional processes of the healthcare system.[66] The expression "pharmacokinetics in the community" also signifies the tasks of professionals interested in the interaction of drugs and the healthcare system.[72]

NEW CHALLENGES OF BIOTECHNOLOGY

Two genetic engineering techniques, recombinant DNA and the production of monoclonal antibodies via cell fusion, after emerging from basic molecular and cell biology research, have now come of age. Based on these techniques, new products have entered the marketplace, even though a "recombinant DNA millenium" is not around the corner.[73] Among the most promising projects are anticancer agents like the interferons (e.g., alpha, beta, gamma) and lymphokines (e.g., interleukin-2), fibrinolytic agents (e.g., alteplase, human urokinase), blood-related products (e.g., erythropoietin, factor VIII, human serum albumin), and products such as human growth hormone, human insulin, and calcitonin.

Although different from traditional pharmacologic agents, products based on biotechnology should be evaluated in the pharmaceutical context rather than upon the production techniques that are employed (i.e., recombinant DNA). The products of biotechnology are essentially a new class of human therapeutic agents, and as such, will have to go through the conventional regulatory approval process and marketing channels. However, because of the unique production techniques used and their different mode of action, it is likely that new pharmacoepidemiologic methodologies will need to be developed. Biotechnology agents constitute a new arena of study for pharmacoepidemiology.

Summary

Drugs present problems to researchers that are uncommon in epidemiologic studies of other types of exposures, such as environmental pollutants, occupational toxins, or food additives. Close attention needs to be paid to the complex mechanisms of reasoning and decision making that usually involve the use of drugs, in which both physicians and patients play important roles. All factors leading to prescription drug use, self-medication, and compliance must be considered in the study design.

Assumptions that hold in other epidemiologic and clinical studies are rarely valid when studying drugs. For example, independence of exposure classification and disease classification cannot be realized if a physician, pharmacist, or nurse intervenes in the data collection process. Knowledge that a particular drug has been taken guides the search for specific effects, the assessment of these effects, and their labeling. A particular diagnosis (e.g., Stevens-Johnson syndrome) is more likely to be determined if it is known that the patient took a particular drug (e.g., a sulfonamide). Sackett has called diagnostic suspicion bias the distortion that occurs when knowledge of the subject's prior exposure to a putative use influences both the intensity and the outcome of the diagnostic process.[24] As Inman points out, UDEs, with few exceptions, are clinically and pathologically indistinguishable from events that can occur spontaneously in untreated patients.[74] For example, thrombosis in a woman taking oral contraceptives cannot be distinguished from thrombosis in a nonuser. The diagnosis could be verified by a professional blinded to the patient's drug history. However, referral to the clinic may have been influenced by the patient's drug history. Thus, a hospital-based study would still suffer from selection bias.[75] Pharmacoepidemiology is a rather peculiar branch of epidemiology due to the many and subtle factors that affect drug exposure and the assessment of drug effects.

Although it formerly may not have been recognized as a distinct discipline, the practice of pharmacoepidemiology is not new: epidemiologic, clinical, and laboratory studies of drugs and vaccines have captured epidemiologists' interest at least since the beginning of this century.[1,76] What is different today is the technologic, scientific, societal, and regulatory context within which drugs are developed and used. Proper scientific evaluation of the actual contributions and accomplishments of pharmacoepidemiology has been undertaken only partially;[3,13,47-51,77-80] however, in recent years drug epidemiology has experienced many developments in substantive, methodologic, and operational issues. Important questions are addressed, meaningful answers to these questions are generated and, increasingly, policy makers implement a reasonable proportion of recommendations.[80] Clinical pharmacologists and other health professionals often use epidemiologic methods and pharmacoepidemiologic findings in their research, practice, and teaching.

One can contend that pharmacoepidemiology constitutes classic quantitative epidemiology techniques applied to a specific content area, namely drugs. The specificity of the techniques employed in drug studies and the unique problems that drugs present to practitioners and researchers define the discipline of pharmacoepidemiology. Conversely, drugs can help to study the frequency and origins of human illness, as well as the functioning of the healthcare system. Development of new therapeutic agents based on biotechnology will stimulate the design of innovative, feasible, and valid pharmacoepidemiologic techniques to foster the optimal use of these agents.

The authors thank Linda Wastella, Ferran Sanz, Magi Farre, and the students of "Methods and Issues of Pharmacoepidemiology" for their helpful comments to previous versions of this manuscript. This work was partially made possible by a grant of The Wellcome Fund to the University of North Carolina School of Public Health (Dr. Porta).

References

1. Porta MS, Ruiz X, Hartzema AG. Pharmacoepidemiology: the name is new; what else is new? *Drug News Perspect* 1988;1:243-5.

2. Porta MS, Carné X. Pharmacoepidemiology. In: Olsen J, Trichopoulos D, eds. Teaching of epidemiology. Oxford: Oxford University Press, 1990.

3. Strom BL, ed. Pharmacoepidemiology: the science of postmarketing drug surveillance. New York: Churchill Livingstone, 1989.

4. Strom BL, Miettinen OS, Melmon KL. Postmarketing studies of drug efficacy: why? *Am J Med* 1985;78:475-80.

5. Slone D, Shapiro S, Miettinen OS, Finkle WD, Stolley PD. Drug evaluation after marketing. *Ann Intern Med* 1979;90:257-61.

6. Lasagna LL. A plea for the "naturalistic" study of medicines. *Eur J Clin Pharmacol* 1974; 7:153-4.

7. Miettinen OS. Efficacy of therapeutic practice: will epidemiology provide the answers? In: Melmon KL, ed. Drug therapeutics. New York: Churchill Livingstone, 1980:201-8.

8. Jick H, Miettinen OS, Shapiro S, Lewis GP, Siskind V, Slone D. Comprehensive drug surveillance. *JAMA* 1970;213:1455-60.

9. Wardell WM, Tsianco MC, Anavekar SN, Davis HT. Postmarketing surveillance of new drugs: I. Review of objectives and methodology. *J Clin Pharmacol* 1979;19:85-94; and II. Case studies. *J Clin Pharmacol* 1979;19:169-84.

10. Strom BL, Melmon KL. Can postmarketing surveillance help to effect optimal drug therapy? *JAMA* 1979;242:2420-3.

11. Castle WM, Nicholls JT, Downie CC. Problems of postmarketing surveillance. *Br J Clin Pharmacol* 1983;16:581-5.

12. Bell RL, O'Brian Smith E. Clinical trials in post-marketing surveillance of drugs. *Controlled Clin Trials* 1982;3:61-8.

13. Rossi AC, Knapp DE, Anello C, et al. Discovery of adverse drug reactions: a comparison of selected phase IV studies with spontaneous reporting methods. *JAMA* 1983;249:2226-8.

14. Borden EK, Gardner JS, Westland MM, Gardner SD. Postmarketing drug surveillance (letter). *JAMA* 1984;251:729.

15. Sackett DL, Haynes RB, Gent M, Taylor DW. Compliance. In: Inman WHW, ed. Monitoring for drug safety. 2nd ed. Lancaster, England: MTP Press, 1986:471-83.

16. Rogers AS, Tilson HH. Postmarketing surveillance: the sponsor's viewpoint. Proceedings of the Drug Information Association 20th annual meeting. San Diego, CA, 1984.

17. Schwartz D, Flamant L, Lelloch J. L'essai therapeutique chez l'homme (2nd ed.). Paris: Flammarion, 1981. (The English translation of the first edition is: Clinical Trials. London: Academic Press, 1980.)

18. Porta M. The relevance of the explanatory/pragmatic distinction for experimental and observational studies (abstract). *Clin Res* 1986;34:831A.

19. Charlson ME, Horwitz RI. Applying results of randomized trials to clinical practice: impact of losses before randomization. *Br Med J* 1984;259:1281-4.

20. Last JM, ed. A dictionary of epidemiology. 2nd ed. New York: Oxford University Press, 1988:110.

21. Office of Technology Assessment. The impact of randomized clinical trials on health policy and medical practice: background paper. Washington, DC: U.S. Congress Printing Office, OTA-BP-H/22, 1983.

22. Meinert CL. Clinical trials: design, conduct, and analysis. New York: Oxford University Press, 1986:49-62.

23. Feinstein AR. Clinical epidemiology. The architecture of clinical research. Philadelphia: WB Saunders, 1985:44-5, 285-7, 303-5, 461-7.

24. Sackett DL. Bias in analytic research. *J Chronic Dis* 1979;32:51-63.

25. Miettinen OS. The need for randomization in the study of intended effects. *Stat Med* 1983;2:267-71.

26. Strom BL, Miettinen OS, Melmon KL. Postmarketing studies of drug efficacy: when must they be randomized? *J Clin Pharmacol* 1983;34:1-7.

27. Strom BL, Miettinen OS, Melmon KL. Postmarketing studies of drug efficacy: how? *Am J Med* 1984;77:703-8.

28. Shuster J, van Eys J. Interaction between prognostic factors and treatment. *Controlled Clin Trials* 1983;4:209-14.

29. Horwitz RI, McFarlane MJ, Brennan TA, Feinstein AR. The role of susceptibility bias in epidemiologic research. *Arch Intern Med* 1985;145:909-12.

30. Crooks J. Drug epidemiology and clinical pharmacology: their contributions to patient care. *Br J Clin Pharmacol* 1983;16:351-7.

31. Colin-Jones DG, Langman MJS, Lawson DH, Vessey MP. Postmarketing surveillance of the safety of cimetidine: twelve-month morbidity report. *Q J Med* 1985;54:253-68.

32. Colin-Jones DG, Langman MJS, Lawson DH, Vessey MP. Postmarketing surveillance of the safety of cimetidine: mortality during second, third, and fourth years of follow-up. *Br Med J* 1985;*291*:1084-8.

33. Stolley PD. The use of vital and morbidity statistics for the detection of adverse drug reactions and for monitoring of drug safety. *J Clin Pharmacol* 1982;*22*:499-504.

34. Stolley PD. Asthma mortality: why the United States was spared an epidemic of deaths due to asthma. *Am Rev Respir Dis* 1972;*105*:883-90.

35. Edlavitch SA, Feinleib M, Anello C. A potential use of the National Death Index for postmarketing drug surveillance. *JAMA* 1985;*253*:1292-5.

36. Jick H, Vessey MP. Case control studies in the evaluation of drug induced illness. *Am J Epidemiol* 1978;*107*:1-7.

37. Ibrahim MA, ed. The case-control study: consensus and controversy. New York: Pergamon Press, 1979.

38. Royal College of General Practitioners. Oral contraceptives and health. London: Pitman, 1974.

39. Vessey M, Doll R, Peto R, Johnson B, Wiggins P. Long-term follow-up study of women using different methods of contraception—an interim report. *J Biosoc Sci* 1976;*8*:373-427.

40. WHO Collaborating Centre for Drug Statistics Methodology. Drug Utilization bibliography. Copenhagen: World Health Organization. Regional Office for Europe, 1989.

41. Sjoqvist F, Agenas I, eds. Drug utilization studies: implications for medical care. Proceedings from ANIS Symposium, Sanga-Saby, Sweden, June 8-9, 1982. *Acta Med Scand* 1984; *683*(suppl):127-34.

42. Laporte JR, Porta M, Capella D. Drug utilization studies: a tool for determining the effectiveness of drug use. *Br J Clin Pharmacol* 1983;*16*:301-4.

43. Colombo F, Shapiro S, Slone D, Tognoni G, eds. Epidemiological evaluation of drugs. Amsterdam: Elsevier North-Holland, 1977.

44. Tognoni G, Bellantuono C, Lader M, eds. Epidemiological impact of psychotropic drugs. Amsterdam: Elsevier North-Holland, 1981.

45. Inman WHW, ed. Monitoring for drug safety. Lancaster, England: MTP Press, 1980.

46. Walker SR, Goldberg A, eds. Monitoring for adverse drug reactions. Lancaster, England: MTP Press, 1984.

47. Venning GR. Identification of adverse reactions to new drugs. I. What have been the important adverse reactions since thalidomide? *Br Med J* 1983;*286*:199-202.

48. Venning GR. Identification of adverse reactions to new drugs. II. How were 18 important adverse reactions discovered and with what delays? *Br Med J* 1983; *286*:289-92.

49. Venning GR. Identification of adverse reactions to new drugs. II. (continued) How were 18 important adverse reactions discovered and with what delays? *Br Med J* 1983;*286*:365-8.

50. Venning GR. Identification of adverse reactions to new drugs. III. Alerting processes and early warning systems. *Br Med J* 1983;*286*:458-60.

51. Venning GR. Identification of adverse reactions to new drugs. IV. Verification of suspected adverse reactions. *Br Med J* 1983;*286*:544-7.

52. Matoren GM, ed. The clinical research process in the pharmaceutical industry. New York: Marcel Dekker, 1983.

53. Jones JK, Van de Carr SW, Rosa F, Morse L, LeRoy A. Medicaid drug-event data: an

emerging tool for evaluation of drug risk. *Acta Med Scand* 1984;*683*(suppl):127-34.

54. Jick H, Madsen S, Nudelman PM, Perera DR, Stergachis A. Postmarketing follow-up at Group Health Cooperative of Puget Sound. *Pharmacotherapy* 1984;4:99-100.

55. Tilson HH. Getting down to bases—record linkage in Saskatchewan (editorial). *Can J Public Health* 1985;76:222-3.

56. Roos LL, Roos NP, Cageorge SM, Nicol JP. How good are the data? Reliability of one health care data bank. *Med Care* 1982;20:266-76.

57. Roos LL, Nicol JP. Building individual histories with registries. A case study. *Med Care* 1983;21:955-69.

58. Feinleib M. Data bases, data banks and data dredging: the agony and the ecstasy. *J Chronic Dis* 1984;37:783-90.

59. Strand LM. Drug epidemiology resources and studies: the Saskatchewan data base. *Drug Inf J* 1985;19:253-6.

60. Strom BL, Carson JL, Morse L, LeRoy AA. The computerized on-line Medicaid pharmaceutical analysis and surveillance system: a new resource for postmarketing drug surveillance. *Clin Pharmacol Ther* 1985;38:359-64.

61. Shapiro S. The role of automated record linkage in the postmarketing surveillance of drug safety: a critique. *Clin Pharmacol Ther* 1989;46:371-86.

62. Byar DP. Why data bases should not replace randomized clinical trials. *Biometrics* 1980; 36:337-42.

63. Green SB, Byar DP. Using observational data from registries to compare treatments: the fallacy of onmimetrics. *Stat Med* 1984;3:361-73.

64. Hulka BS. Epidemiological applications to health services research. *J Commun Health* 1978;4:140-9.

65. Hulka BS, Wheat J. Utilization patterns. *Med Care* 1985;23:438-60.

66. Tognoni G, Liberati A, Pello L, Sasanelli F, Spagnoli A. Drug utilization studies and epidemiology. *Rev Epidemiol et Sante Publ* 1983;31:59-71.

67. Tognoni G. Drug use and monitoring. In: Holland WW, ed. Evaluation of health care. Oxford: Oxford University Press, 1983:207-25.

68. Kunin CM, ed. Conference on pharmacoepidemiology. INCLEN program. Tarrytown, NY: The Rockefeller Foundation, 1988.

69. Aquilonius SM, Granat M, Hartvig P. Utilization of antiparkinson drugs in Norway, Sweden, Denmark and Finland in 1975-1979. *Acta Neurol Scand* 1981;64:47-53.

70. Parish PA. Sociology of prescribing. *Br Med Bull* 1974;30:214.

71. Haynes RB, Taylor DW, Sackett DL. Compliance in health care. Baltimore: Johns Hopkins University Press, 1981.

72. Baksaas I, Lunde PKM. Drug utilization: pharmacokinetics in the community. *Trends Pharmacol Sci* 1981 (February):V-VII.

73. Script yearbook 1986. Richmond, England: PJB Publications, 1985:7.

74. Inman WHW. Prescription-event monitoring. *Acta Med Scand* 1984;683(suppl):119-26.

75. Miettinen O, Slone D, Shapiro D. Current problems in drug-related epidemiologic research. In: Colombo F, Shapiro S, Slone D, Tognoni G, eds. Epidemiological evaluation of drugs. Littleton, MA: PSG Publishing, 1977:295-303.

76. Porta MS, Ruiz X. Pharmacoepidemiological studies in the *American Journal of Epi-*

demiology (1925-1985). In: Edlavitch SA, ed. Proceedings of the 4th International Conference on Pharmacoepidemiology. Chicago: Lewis Publishers, 1990.

77. Susser M. Epidemiology in the United States after World War II: the evolution of technique. *Epidemiol Rev* 1985;7:147-77.

78. Rossi AC, Knapp DE. Discovery of adverse drug reactions: a review of the Food and Drug Administration's spontaneous reporting system. *JAMA* 1984;252:1030-3.

79. Weinshilboum RM. The therapeutic revolution. *Clin Pharmacol Ther* 1987; 42:481-4.

80. Edlavitch SA. The 3rd International Conference on Pharmacoepidemiology—Contributions of pharmacoepidemiology to public health: industry, government, academic, and clinical practice perspectives. The convener's overview. *J Clin Res Drug Dev* 1987;1:237-62.

2

Pharmacogenetics and Biologic Markers of Unintended Drug Effects

Stephen P. Spielberg
Denis M. Grant

Abstract

This chapter reviews some basic principles of so-called idiosyncratic unintended drug effects (UDEs), which are not based on the pharmacologic mechanism of the drug administered and typically are unrelated to the dose. Fundamentals of human pharmacogenetics are covered next. Examples of pharmacogenetic variants with potential as biologic markers in the diagnosis and prediction of drug toxicity are provided. Such examples include: thiopurine methyltransferase and UDEs from azathioprine and mercaptopurine, debrisoquin oxidation polymorphism, and acetylation polymorphism. The availability of safe in vivo probes of drug metabolism pathways exhibiting genetic polymorphisms, of cellular models for assaying enzymes and studying drug toxicity in cell types, and rapid advances in molecular and cell biology, hold great promise for pharmacogenetics. Biologic markers of susceptibility to UDEs based on pharmacogenetic considerations will increasingly be used in early drug development to define outliers in the population and consequences of polymorphic drug metabolism for new compounds. The integration of epidemiologic and pharmacogenetic studies has the potential for more accurate diagnosis of true UDEs amidst events occurring during therapy, prediction of individual as well as population risk, and ultimately, UDE prevention.

Outline

The introduction of the sulfonamides into therapy in the 1930s heralded the beginning of rational therapeutics.[1] In the short span of 60 years, myriad compounds have been developed possessing remarkable efficacy against specific diseases and producing minimal toxicity in patients. Nonetheless, unintended effects of drug therapy remain a major problem, contributing to perhaps 3 percent of hospital admissions and occurring in up to 20 percent of inpatients. It was also adverse reactions such as the tragedies associated with elixir of sulfanilamide and thalidomide[2-4] that led to our present regulatory milieu with the Pure Food and Drug Act of 1938 and the Kefauver-Harris Amendments in 1963.

The current drug development process does an excellent job screening out compounds with excessively high toxicity risk for the population at large. Preclinical animal toxicology studies provide data on most mechanism- and dose-related toxicities. Unexpected outcomes, such as nonmechanism-based organ toxicity (e.g., hepatotoxicity), or an increased incidence of tumors or birth defects, may or may not have any relevance to human risk. Compounds may be lost to further development because of such toxicities, even if they are indeed false positive with respect to humans. If development continues, animal toxicology results can form the basis for epidemiologic hypothesis generation and follow-up studies.

In Phase I–III clinical studies, a small number of relatively homogeneous subjects are exposed to a new drug. Since perhaps only 3000–5000 patients are studied in premarketing trials, it is not surprising that even life-threatening unintended drug effects (UDEs) with an incidence of 1/10 000 are unlikely to be seen prior to large population exposure to the drug in the postmarketing period. Similarly, if an unexpected event such as aplastic anemia is reported during the clinical trials, it is difficult to assess if the event is a UDE and, if it is, what the true incidence will be. In the face of uncertainty in diagnosis and incidence, such events can have severe consequences for the licensing and subsequent labeling of a new drug.

Table 1 provides a comparison of traditional animal toxicology studies with the real world of human patients, and the characteristics of patients in preclinical trials and those taking the drugs postmarketing. It is becoming increasingly apparent that the basis for many of the serious UDEs that cause significant patient morbidity and withdrawal or failure of licensing of otherwise useful medications is variability in response to foreign compounds in the heterogeneous human population. The sources of variability include age, sex, disease state, diet, habits (e.g., alcohol, tobacco), drug interactions, and an increasingly recognized role of inherited differences in drug handling and response (pharmacogenetics). Epidemiologic studies, including postmarketing surveillance, can help detect unexpected UDEs, define their incidence, and determine risk factors such as age and drug interactions. Basic investigation of the mechanisms of drug toxicity and of pharmacogenetic factors predisposing to risk have the potential for the development of "biologic markers" that can be used to confirm the diagnosis of complex UDEs, predict who in the population is at risk, and help guide epidemiologic studies. Most progress made in understanding the pathogenesis and decreasing the incidence of UDEs is likely to arise from the collaboration between pharmacoepidemiologists and pharmacogeneticists.

In this chapter, we review some basic principles of so-called idiosyncratic UDEs, fundamentals of human pharmacogenetics, and provide some examples of pharmacogenetic variants with potential as biologic markers useful in the diagnosis and prediction of drug toxicity risk.

Idiosyncratic Drug Reactions

Idiosyncratic UDEs are not based on the pharmacologic mechanism of the drug in question and typically are unrelated to the dose administered. As alluded to above, preclinical toxicology studies performed on inbred animals rarely detect or predict human idiosyncratic reactions. Similarly, since the reactions are not related directly to dose or serum concentration, monitoring of drug serum concentrations will not prevent UDEs. Indeed, one of the main problems with such UDEs is that the usual clinical setting is a patient correctly diagnosed, given the correct drug for the indication, and given the correct dose, and yet a potentially severe UDE unexpectedly develops.

Many of the reactions, including "hypersensitivity reactions," present major diagnostic quandaries. In the absence of confirmatory diagnostic laboratory data, events occurring during therapy such as fever, skin rash, liver function abnormalities, and bone marrow abnormalities could be attributed to a wide spectrum of infectious and autoimmune processes, and, with frequent multidrug therapy, to any of the medications. Various approaches to evaluating clinical data (e.g., Bayesian methods) may help in the diagnosis, and large epidemiologic studies may suggest a statistically significant association between use of a drug and a given event; however, there remains a major need to develop diagnostic tests both to confirm epidemiologic data as well as the diagnosis. Even with possible drug-induced birth defects, epidemiologic studies can ascertain the relative risk in exposed and unexposed populations, yet individual risk remains undefined. Here too, the challenge is to understand the pathogenesis of the undesired effect of the drug, and to turn understanding of the mechanism into a valid biologic marker of drug effect and susceptibility to toxicity.

In perspective, many idiosyncratic reactions that currently elude our predictive capacity occur with incidences of less than 1/1000, often less than 1/10000. This has several consequences when considering possible biologic approaches to help in diagnosis and prediction. Recommendations are given for routine monitoring of liver function tests (serum enzymes and bilirubin) or blood counts for many drugs associated with liver or bone marrow toxicity. When applied to large populations, however, most of the currently available tests exhibit considerable day-to-day variability with a significant percentage of the population having abnormal values at any given time. In a population of patients taking a specific medication, then, several percent of the patients might reach the criteria for abnormal liver

Preclinical Toxicology and Human Risk		
	Animals	Humans
Genetics	inbred	heterogeneous
Environment	defined	heterogeneous
Diet	defined	heterogeneous
Disease	well	sick
Other drugs	none	many
Habits	none	many
Clinical Trials and Postmarketing Risk		
	Trials	Postmarketing
Age	limited	unrestricted
Sex	mostly male	unrestricted
Race	limited	unrestricted
Indication	defined	unrestricted
Other drugs	defined	unrestricted
Habits	defined	unrestricted

Table 1
Preclinical Toxicology, Clinical Trials, and UDE Risk

function tests, while only about 1/10 000 would be true drug-induced events. In other words, the vast majority of abnormal screening values represent false positives, and the positive predictive value of such tests is very poor. The consequences of relying on these types of tests to prevent rare UDEs include: diagnostic confusion; pursuit of medically irrelevant laboratory variation; unnecessary discontinuation of medication, with potential exposure of patients to other medications with undefined UDE risk; and substantial costs in laboratory screening and other tests if a value comes back abnormal. In addition, patients may have entirely normal laboratory values, only several days or weeks later to present with a true UDE. Routine laboratory tests are very far removed biologically from the mechanism of toxicity of any drug and are rather nonspecific markers of organ function; therefore, it is not surprising that under most circumstances such tests are of limited value. The closer a biologic marker is to the approximate mechanisms of toxicity of a compound, the more likely it is to have both diagnostic and predictive utility (see below).

The second issue with respect to relatively infrequent events is that it is intuitively unlikely that risk is distributed evenly throughout the population, just as it is medically unsatisfying to tell a patient that they have a 1/10 000 chance of having a specific UDE. We are increasingly recognizing the role of individual differences in the metabolism of and response to drugs based on inherited differences in enzymes and receptors as a basis for many idiosyncratic drug reactions. It is likely that most of the population has essentially no risk of specific UDEs from a specific drug, while a subpopulation is at very high risk. Markers of susceptibility based on pharmacogenetic mechanisms hold the promise of providing individual estimates of risk and predicting such risk, thus decreasing UDEs both for individuals and the population as a whole.

Pharmacogenetics

Pharmacogenetic variants represent a subclass of inborn errors of metabolism. Perhaps their main distinguishing feature is that they usually are "silent" in the absence of exposure to a drug or other foreign chemical. The presence of a variant gene usually is manifest upon exposure to specific chemical structures and can result in: (1) functional overdose in patients unable to eliminate an active drug, (2) lack of therapeutic effect in patients unable to convert a prodrug into its active form, and (3) idiosyncratic reactions that often result from overproduction or failure to detoxify a potentially toxic metabolite. Pharmacogenetic traits are divided arbitrarily between rare defects and polymorphisms where a variant gene product results in a phenotype with a frequency of at least one percent in the population. Similar to other genetic abnormalities, allelic variation is common. It also is common for there to be several variant alleles at a given locus. Finally, it would be expected that gene frequencies for variant alleles will differ among different human populations, and that UDE frequencies thus will vary among different human ethnic and racial groups. The latter considerations have obvious consequences for epidemiologic studies and international drug development.

Pharmacogenetic variants often come to light in the context of investigating variation in drug response in the population. Most well-defined disorders are abnormalities in enzymes responsible for drug metabolism. Unexpected variability in serum concentrations, pharmacologic effect, or unanticipated UDEs may provide the impetus for investigation of the basis for the variability, with family studies used to confirm inheritance. Techniques for study have traditionally included examination of metabolic profiles and clearance of drugs, population and family studies of a specific drug or in vivo test compound, and investigation of drug handling in monozygotic and dizygotic twins. Increasingly, in vitro approaches using human cells to measure specific enzymes and the toxicologic potential of drugs, and direct molecular genetic analysis of gene polymorphisms are being used. The explosive advances of molecular biology in human genetic disease are being applied to pharmacogenetic variants at an ever-increasing rate.

Examples of Pharmacogenetic Variants as Possible Markers of UDEs and UDE Susceptibility

Several good reviews of the area of pharmacogenetics are available.[5-10] A few examples are discussed from the vantage point of the possible development of biologic markers of drug toxicity or susceptibility.

THIOPURINE METHYLTRANSFERASE AND UDEs FROM AZATHIOPRINE AND MERCAPTOPURINE

Many drugs undergo metabolism by several different pathways mediated by different drug metabolism enzymes. Figure 1 presents the pathways of metabolism

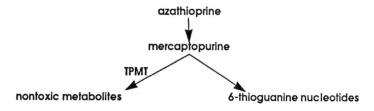

Figure 1
Pathways of
Metabolism of
Azathioprine and
Mercaptopurine.
TPMT = thiopurine
methyltransferase

of azathioprine and mercaptopurine, drugs used in immunologic disorders and cancer chemotherapy. One of the major adverse effects of the drugs is bone marrow suppression. It has been demonstrated that the enzyme thiopurine methyltransferase (TPMT) is polymorphic in the human population; approximately 0.3 percent of the population has essentially no TPMT activity and 11 percent has intermediate activity.[11-14] Low enzyme activity is inherited as a simple autosomal recessive trait. These studies employed peripheral blood erythrocytes for measurement of enzyme activity after proving that enzyme activity in these easily obtained cells correlated with activity in other organs, such as the liver. Furthermore, it has been suggested that low TPMT activity might shunt intracellular metabolism toward 6-thioguanine nucleotides, which might mediate the bone marrow toxicity.[15] Using erythrocyte TPMT activity as a marker, it was found that patients receiving azathioprine who developed severe bone marrow suppression at conventional doses were in the 0.3 percent of people with absent enzyme activity.[16] Furthermore, the level of 6-thioguanine nucleotides in their erythrocytes was far higher than among patients who tolerated the drug without excessive myelosuppression.

Several issues are raised by these studies. First, given that the incidence of absent enzyme activity is relatively rare in the population, absent enzyme activity in 5 patients with marrow suppression compared with only 16 controls is highly statistically significant. If a rare pharmacogenetic defect is postulated to play a critical role in a given UDE, epidemiologic and clinical ascertainment of only a relatively small number of patients with UDEs is necessary to prove or disprove the hypothesis. Second, for azathioprine or mercaptopurine therapy, it would appear that absent TPMT activity may preclude use of the drug. Prescreening patients who might be exposed to the drugs may lead to selection of alternative therapy, or, if the drugs are used, to dose adjustments with careful monitoring of intracellular 6-thioguanine nucleotide concentrations. Here, then, is a potential example of a biologic marker of susceptibilty to a UDE that could be employed in selected patients prior to therapy, coupled with a monitoring technique closely linked to the biologic basis of the UDE to monitor patients during treatment. Third, to be useful, markers must be reasonably simple tests (peripheral blood cells in this example), and correlation must be demonstrated with other potential target tissues in vivo. Finally, drug action and UDE mechanisms are rarely simple. 6-Thioguanine nucleotides also may be involved in the mechanism of desired action of these drugs as immunosuppressants and cancer chemotherapy agents. Further data are needed to ascertain the importance of the relative balances of the production of different metabolites in determining the overall outcome of therapy. It will also be of significant interest to fit the gene frequency of TPMT deficiency together with the incidence of marrow suppression from epidemiologic studies to determine if this abnormality is both necessary and sufficient for a UDE to occur. This may be one of the most interesting aspects of the interaction between drug epidemiology and basic investigation, as each approach generates hypotheses useful by the other discipline.

DEBRISOQUIN OXIDATION POLYMORPHISM

This example illustrates the successful progression, within little more than a decade, from an initial set of clinical observations of variable drug response to an advanced level of understanding concerning its underlying molecular mechanisms. Such knowledge presently is being used to devise tests that will predict UDE risk for compounds metabolized by a specific cytochrome P-450 enzyme.

Considering that the majority of lipid-soluble drugs are metabolized at least to some extent through oxidation by members of the liver microsomal monooxygenase (cytochrome P-450) enzyme system, it is somewhat surprising that, until the mid-1970s, only a few isolated reports of inherited defects of drug oxidation had been published. This may be due largely to the known multiplicity and overlapping substrate specificity of this enzyme superfamily,[17] implying that for many drugs multiple biotransformation pathways exist. Thus, compensatory metabolism by alternate pathways could prevent the clinical manifestations associated with a defect in a particular metabolic reaction.

The first clear demonstration of polymorphic drug oxidation involving cytochrome P-450 was provided during independent studies of the antihypertensive drug debrisoquin[18] and the oxytocic agent sparteine.[19] Maghoub et al. published population evidence that previously observed wide interpatient variations in the required dose of debrisoquin for achieving a hypotensive response were due primarily to genetic differences in the extent to which debrisoquin is hydroxylated to 4-hydroxydebrisoquin.[18] By using a metabolic ratio of the parent drug to its hydroxylated metabolite excreted in urine following a single oral dose, it was possible to construct a population frequency histogram that was distinctly bimodal, dividing subjects into extensive and poor metabolizers. Further population and family pedigree analyses established that the hydroxylation of debrisoquin was genetically controlled by what appeared to be two alleles at a single autosomal gene locus, with poor metabolizer phenotype frequencies ranging from six to ten percent in various Caucasian populations.

At about the same time, studies of variations in the response to sparteine showed that a similar percentage of German subjects were almost entirely unable to metabolize the compound to its two major metabolites, 2- and 5-dehydrospar-teine.[19] Correlation studies subsequently established that defective metabolism of debrisoquin and sparteine are under identical genetic control. Moreover, since these initial observations the polymorphism has been shown to control, either fully or partially, the rate of oxidation of a number of other drugs as well (Table 2). One of these, dextromethorphan, shows promise as a particularly safe in vivo marker for determining the debrisoquin oxidation phenotype. Simple determination of the urinary excretion of dextromethorphan and its metabolites allows phenotyping of subjects for this polymorphic enzyme.

The clinical consequences of the debrisoquin-type drug oxidation defect have been investigated thoroughly for a number of the affected drugs in Table 2.[20] In this regard it is important to recognize that, although the biotransformation of each of these compounds is affected by the polymorphism, not all result in UDEs. For example, genetically poor metabolizers experience a greater incidence of excessive beta-blockade and loss of cardioselectivity due to elevated plasma drug concentrations after administration of the beta-adrenergic antagonist metoprolol, but not after closely related propranolol, even though both are linked to the oxidation defect. The reason for this is that propranolol undergoes several additional metabolic pathways which, along with renal elimination, can compensate for defective biotransformation by debrisoquin oxidase.[20] On the other hand, the genetically variable pathway of encainide oxidation gives rise to an active metabolite that is responsible for most of the pharmacologic activity of the drug, so that poor metabolizers respond poorly to the antiarrhythmic effects of this compound.[21] Finally, certain drugs (e.g., quinidine, many neuroleptics) are potent competitive inhibitors of the polymorphic enzyme without necessarily being significantly metabolized by it.[22] Coadministration of these with any of the drugs in Table 2 could lead to potentially significant drug–drug interactions, or even misclassification of normal individuals as having genetically poor drug metabolism.[23]

Much progress has been made in determining the biochemical and molecular mechanisms leading to the occurrence of the poor metabolizer phenotype in human populations. Earlier in vitro studies conclusively established that defective metabolism of debrisoquin and other drugs was related to alterations in the catalytic activity of a specific isozyme of cytochrome P-450,[24,25] but two general questions remained to be answered: (1) at the protein level, were the decreases in cat-

			Table 2
Alprenolol	Dextromethorphan	Phenacetin	Some Drugs Affected by the Debrisoquin-Type Oxidation Polymorphism
Amiflamine	Encainide	Phenformin	
Amphetamine	Guanoxan	Propaphenone	
Bufuralol	Methoxyphenamine	Propranolol	
Captopril	Metiamide	Sparteine	
Codeine	Metoprolol	Timolol	
Debrisoquin	Nortriptyline		
Desipramine	Perhexiline		

alytic activity in affected individuals due to alterations in the quantity of a specific P-450 isozyme present, or to changes in substrate specificity of a structurally altered variant protein? and (2) at the gene level, what mutations were underlying these enzyme expression characteristics?

Using biochemical, immunological, and recombinant DNA methods, and with access to liver tissues from individuals whose metabolizer phenotypes often could be determined, the following conclusions have been reached. With respect to the enzyme protein itself, it is now clear that in livers from phenotypically poor metabolizers of debrisoquin, there is a marked decrease in the quantity of a specific isozyme of cytochrome P-450 (most recently designated P-450IID6), determined by immunoblotting methods using specific antibodies raised against the purified human enzyme or its rat homologue.[26] At the gene level, the above-mentioned antibodies also were used as a tool in molecular cloning procedures to isolate a full-length cDNA probe corresponding to the gene transcript that encodes cytochrome P-450IID6. With this cDNA probe, experiments were designed to investigate the nature of the defect(s) in poor metabolizers with respect to transcript prevalence and gene structure.[27,28] There appear to be at least three different mutant alleles at the P-450IID6 locus that contribute to the poor metabolizer phenotype in humans. Recent advances in gene amplification techniques coupled with specific oligonucleotide hybridization methods hold the promise of simple, direct gene assays that could be applied to widespread determination of the P-450IID6 genotype.

As indicated above, the consequences of abnormal metabolism by this polymorphic P-450 depend on the compound in question. The outcomes can vary from trivial effects on kinetics, which would be overwhelmed by other sources of variability, to major kinetic perturbation, and idiosyncratic reactions by shunting metabolism. For compounds whose metabolism may involve P-450IID6, it should now be possible to include poor metabolizers in early studies to establish how important the polymorphism is for that compound even prior to reported UDEs. When unusual events are noted, it becomes possible to rapidly assess the role of the enzymopathy in causing a specific UDE. If the UDE occurs with high frequency in subjects deficient in the enzyme, prescreening patients for risk potential becomes possible.

ACETYLATION POLYMORPHISM

The story of the acetylator polymorphism lends historical perspective to the field of pharmacogenetics.[29,30] Indeed, it was more than 30 years ago, before the term pharmacogenetics was even formulated, that high interindividual variations were observed in the urinary excretion of the tuberculostatic drug isoniazid.[31] This observation was followed by the finding that frequency histograms of plasma isoniazid concentrations after a single oral dose in a normal population were distinctly bimodal, allowing for classification of subjects as "rapid" or "slow" eliminators of the drug.[32] Genetic involvement initially was suggested by (1) a greater concor-

4-Aminobiphenyl	Clonazepam	Nitrazepam	**Table 3**
2-Aminofluorene	Dapsone	Phenelzine	Some Drugs and
Aminoglutethimide	Dipyrone	Procainamide	Chemicals Affected
Amrinone	Hydralazine	Sulfamerazine	by the Acetylation
Benzidine	Isoniazid	Sulfamethazine	Polymorphism
Caffeine	β-Naphthylamine	Sulfapyridine	

dance among monozygotic than dizygotic twins in isoniazid urinary excretion rates;[33] and (2) an observed ethnic difference in the proportions of the two classes of isoniazid eliminators, with Oriental populations displaying a markedly lower frequency of the slow eliminator phenotype than that seen in Caucasian groups.[34] Family pedigrees verified this hypothesis and showed that the ability to eliminate isoniazid was controlled by the action of two major alleles at a single autosomal gene locus, with rapid elimination as the apparently dominant trait.[35] Numerous subsequent investigations confirmed these findings, and demonstrated that the disposition of a wide variety of drugs and xenobiotics containing a primary arylamine or hydrazine group is under identical genetic control (Table 3).

It soon was established that the basis of the observed population variations was related to differences in the rate of arylamine and hydrazine N-acetylation taking place to a large extent in the liver.[36] The enzymatic reaction is now known to be catalyzed by cytosolic arylamine N-acetyltransferase, which uses the essential cofactor acetyl coenzyme A as acetyl group donor to conjugate primary amino and hydrazino groups with acetate, producing an amide.

The clinical and toxicological consequences of the acetylation polymorphism have been studied in considerable detail.[30] For instance, slow acetylators are more prone to develop a drug-induced systemic lupus erythematosus-like syndrome during prolonged therapy with procainamide or hydralazine, hematological UDEs from dapsone, or polyneuropathy after isoniazid treatment. The slow acetylator phenotype also appears to be one of the predisposing factors in the etiology of sulfonamide-induced idiosyncratic UDEs.[37] In addition, numerous studies indicate that there is an increased incidence of bladder cancer in slow acetylators exposed to carcinogenic arylamines, which presumably are substrates for arylamine N-acetyltransferase. On the other hand, rapid acetylators encounter therapeutic failure more often when receiving isoniazid dosage regimens once weekly. They require higher doses of hydralazine to control hypertension or of dapsone for dermatitis herpetiformis. However, reported associations of acetylator phenotype with some apparently unrelated disorders such as Gilbert's syndrome, diabetes, and leprosy require further validation and explanation.

Because of the potential clinical and toxicological importance of the acetylation polymorphism in determining the response to arylamine drugs and toxins, numerous in vivo methods for determining the acetylator phenotype have been developed. These make use of "probe" drugs which are polymorphically acetylated.

Isoniazid was the first drug used for this purpose, and has been followed by tests using sulfamethazine, procainamide, and dapsone.[30] However, recent observations that the urinary excretion of a caffeine metabolite, 5-acetylamino-6-formylamino-3-methyluracil, is also governed by the acetylation polymorphism, have led to the development of a caffeine test for acetylator phenotype.[38] This test has gained widespread popularity for its safety, simplicity, and sensitivity in the phenotyping of a variety of normal and patient populations. For example, accurate phenotype determination may be achieved in a single spot urine sample from small children after administration of caffeinated cola beverages.[37] Moreover, the test is sensitive enough to discriminate the three genotypes of acetylation capacity in human populations,[38,39] a considerably valuable feature for assessing the differential susceptibility of heterozygous and homozygous individuals to toxicity from specific chemicals. Finally, recent in vivo/in vitro correlation studies have verified that the caffeine test specifically and precisely measures only the activity of the genetically polymorphic liver acetylating enzyme.[40]

The underlying mechanism of the acetylation polymorphism has recently been investigated using similar biochemical and molecular approaches to those outlined above for the debrisoquin oxidase studies. Although studies are still in progress, the following observations have been made. To date, two independent human N-acetyltransferase genes, designated NAT1 and NAT2, at separate loci on chromosome 8, have been isolated and characterized.[41,42] The expressed product of the NAT2 gene shows protein immunoreactivity and kinetic properties identical to those of a human liver N-acetyltransferase whose content varies with acetylator phenotype. We therefore presume that the NAT2 locus is the site of the human acetylation polymorphism. The possibility of a defect in a promoter region is currently being explored. Thus, similar to the debrisoquin polymorphism, a safe in vivo probe (caffeine) and the molecular probes being developed can be applied to determining acetylator phenotype in patients.

The frequency of slow acetylation varies among different populations: roughly 50 percent in white and black populations in North America, and 10 percent or less among Oriental populations. This would predict possible interethnic differences in UDE rates where the acetylator polymorphism plays a major role.

Since neither of the two acetylator phenotypes is rare, and many of the UDEs that correlate with phenotype are considerably less frequent than 50 or even 10 percent, acetylation cannot be the only risk factor. However, the fact that N-acetylation is relatively protective against toxicity in certain circumstances can focus basic studies on UDE mechanisms. For example, slow acetylation appears to be a major risk factor for hypersensitivity reactions to sulfonamides.[37] This suggests that alternate pathways of metabolism of the arylamine may play a role in the UDE. In fact, oxidation of the amine to reactive hydroxylamine and nitroso metabolites, with subsequent inherited inability to detoxify the latter, may be involved in the pathogenesis.[37,43,44] In this case, acetylation alone would not be an adequate marker of risk since 50 percent of the patients would be excluded from using the drugs.

However, a marker tapping the detoxification defect for the reactive metabolites of the drugs might well serve such a purpose. The use of cellular models as markers for diagnosis and prediction is discussed in the context of the aromatic anticonvulsants.

ANTICONVULSANT HYPERSENSITIVITY SYNDROME AND BIRTH DEFECTS

Hypersensitivity reactions to phenytoin and related anticonvulsants can be life-threatening, and association with both major and minor birth defects is a major concern in managing pregnancies in epileptic patients. However, it remains striking that the drugs do not cause such toxicities in the majority of patients who are exposed. The precise incidence of hypersensitivity reactions is uncertain—somewhere between 1/1000 and 1/10 000 patients.[45] Similarly, there appears to be approximately a two- to threefold increased risk of major birth defects in pregnancies in epileptic patients taking phenytoin (5–10 percent of exposed fetuses), and up to a 30-percent risk of minor abnormalities often classified as the fetal hydantoin syndrome.[46] The challenge, then, is to define the pathogenesis of both the hypersensitivity reactions and fetal effects, and to ascertain if genetic differences in the handling of or response to the drug determine susceptibility to toxicity.

The hypersensitivity reactions typically are delayed in onset after institution of therapy (often several weeks), and are characterized by fever, skin rash, lymphadenopathy, and variable involvement of other organs including liver, kidney, bone marrow, lung, and heart.[45] The pathogenesis appears to involve both direct toxicity to cells as well as an immunologic response. The reactions might be mediated by cytochrome P-450-generated metabolites of the parent drug, possibly arene oxides.[47-50] Current understanding of susceptibility to toxicity is that there is an inherited abnormality in detoxification of such unstable, potentially toxic metabolites. When peripheral blood lymphocytes from patients who have had phenytoin UDEs are exposed to reactive metabolites of phenytoin, the cells exhibit far more toxicity than do normal cells.[48-50] An intermediate pattern of the toxicity of metabolites has been demonstrated in cells from the parents of patients, and cells from the siblings are distributed among normal, abnormal, and intermediate responses. The molecular and biochemical bases of the defects are currently under investigation. Prime candidates for the abnormality are mutations in epoxide hydrolase, altering the substrate specificity of the enzyme for reactive metabolites of phenytoin, thereby leading to accumulation of the reactive intermediate, increased covalent binding to cell macromolecules, and resultant cell death and immunologic response to neoantigens (Figure 2).

The decision to use peripheral blood lymphocytes for performing in vitro toxicology experiments depends on the assumption that enzyme activities are expressed in this tissue similarly to that in the major organs of xenobiotic biotransformation, such as the liver. However, once this has been established, the method opens up possibilities for aiding in the diagnosis of complex diseases in the face of drug therapy, and also of prospectively screening patients for possible toxicity. Understanding the molecular defects involved will help in the selection of other anticonvulsant therapy for patients who have had phenytoin UDEs. Studies suggest that the defect in metabolite detoxification is shared in most pedigrees among phenytoin, phenobarbital, and carbamazepine.[50] In other families, the abnormality is somewhat more restricted. Heterogeneity of defects is likely to be the case among most pharmacogenetic variants. Knowing the specific defects, the structures of alternative anticonvulsants, and their pathways of metabolism may help in selecting compounds with the least toxicity risk for specific patients, and in designing newer, safer anticonvulsants in the future.

The role of anticonvulsants in the etiology of birth defects among mothers with epilepsy is controversial. Phenytoin use has been associated with a two- to threefold increased risk of major defects, and a variable risk of minor abnormalities. Regardless of the precise epidemiologic risk, most fetuses exposed to the drug in utero do not have birth defects. In studies in the rat, there was a correlation between birth defects (e.g., cardiac anomalies, cleft palate) and the amount of covalently bound phenytoin metabolites in the fetuses.[51] Inhibition of epoxide hydrolase increased metabolite binding and the yield of malformations. The detoxification ability of peripheral blood lymphocytes was examined in patients exposed to phenytoin in utero who did and did not have birth defects, and from their parents.[52] There was a strong correlation between abnormal detoxification (in all cases characterized by an intermediate pattern of detoxification defect) and major birth defects. No correlation was found with minor stigmata of the fetal hydantoin syndrome. For each patient with an abnormality in detoxification, cells from one of the parents were also abnormal. Mothers with intermediate detoxification defects tolerated phenytoin without hypersensitivity reactions.

The results suggest that an inherited abnormality in detoxification of phenytoin metabolites may play a role in the development of birth defects upon exposure to the compound. If the intermediate response truly represents a heterozygous state, a single abnormal gene may be sufficient to place a developing fetus at risk for toxicity. Homozygosity is required for hypersensitivity reactions in children or adults. This emphasizes the complex nature of the interaction between devel-

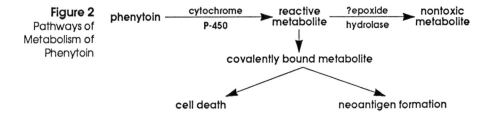

Figure 2
Pathways of
Metabolism of
Phenytoin

phenytoin → (cytochrome P-450) → reactive metabolite → (?epoxide hydrolase) → nontoxic metabolite

reactive metabolite → covalently bound metabolite

covalently bound metabolite → cell death / neoantigen formation

opmental processes regulating drug metabolic pathways and inborn errors of metabolism of those pathways. Balances of rates down several potential pathways of metabolism may determine the ultimate outcomes.

In addition, not all effects of a drug such as phenytoin will be mediated by the same metabolites or processes. In our study, we found no correlation between detoxification defects and minor birth defects. In adults, facial coarsening, hirsutism, and gingival hyperplasia are very common events compared with hypersensitivity reactions. Similarly, some of the minor abnormalities associated with phenytoin occur with much higher frequency than major structural birth defects. Once molecular probes are available for pathways critical in phenytoin toxicity, it will become possible to sift through various clinical presentations and determine what abnormalities are and are not related to pharmacogenetic disorders. Ultimately, it may be possible to assign individual maternal-fetal pairs with individual estimates of risk of an abnormal outcome of pregnancy and be able to ensure a successful outcome for the vast majority of patients.

Summary

Pharmacogenetics is having an increasing impact on our concepts of the pathogenesis of human UDEs. The availability of safe in vivo probes of drug metabolism pathways exhibiting genetic polymorphisms, of cellular models for assaying enzymes and studying drug toxicity in readily available cell types, and the rapid advances in molecular biology hold great promise for future progress in this area. Biologic markers of susceptibility to UDEs based on pharmacogenetic considerations will be used in early drug development to define outliers in the population and the consequences of polymorphic drug metabolism for new compounds under development. Similarly, the integration of epidemiologic studies and basic pharmacogenetic investigation has the potential for more accurate determination of true UDEs amidst events occurring during therapy (improved diagnosis), prediction of individual as well as population risk, and ultimate UDE prevention.

References

1. Weinshilboum RM. The therapeutic revolution. *Clin Pharmacol Ther* 1987; 42:481-4.

2. Geiling EMK, Cannon PR. Pathologic effects of elixir of sulfanilamide (diethylene glycol) poisoning. *JAMA* 1938;*111*:919-26.

3. McBride WG. Thalidomide and congenital abnormalities. *Lancet* 1961; 2:1358.

4. Lenz W. Thalidomide and congenital abnormalities. *Lancet* 1962;*1*:45.

5. Kalow W. Pharmacogenetics. Heredity and the response to drugs. Philadelphia: WB Saunders, 1962.

6. Evans DAP. Pharmacogenetics. *Am J Med* 1963;34:639-62.

7. Propping P. Pharmacogenetics. *Rev Physiol Biochem Pharmacol* 1978;83:123-73.

8. Vesell ES. Pharmacogenetics. In: Yaffe SJ, ed. Pediatric pharmacology: therapeutic principles in practice. New York: Grune & Stratton, 1980.

9. Roots I, Heinemeyer G, Drakoulis N, Kampf D. The role of pharmacogenetics in drug epidemiology. In: Kewitz H, Roots I, Voigt K, eds. Epidemiological concepts in clinical pharmacology. Berlin: Springer-Verlag, 1987.

10. Ayesh R, Smith RL. Genetic polymorphism in human toxicology. In: Turner P, Volans GN, eds. Recent advances in clinical pharmacology and toxicology, number 4. Edinburgh: Churchill Livingstone, 1989.

11. Weinshilboum RM, Sladek L. Mercaptopurine pharmacogenetics: monogenic inheritance of erythrocyte thiopurine methyltransferase activity. *Am J Hum Genet* 1980;32:651-62.

12. Van Loon J, Weinshilboum RM. Thiopurine methyltransferase biochemical genetics: human lymphocyte activity. *Biochem Genet* 1982;20:637-58.

13. Woodson LC, Dunnette JH, Weinshilboum RM. Pharmacogenetics of human thiopurine methyltransferase: kidney-erythrocyte correlation. *J Pharmacol Exp Ther* 1982;222:174-81.

14. Szymlanski CL, Scott MC, Weinshilboum RM. Thiopurine methyltransferase pharmacogenetics: human liver enzyme activity. *Clin Pharmacol Ther* 1988; 43:134-40.

15. Lennard L, Van Loon JA, Lilleyman JS, Weinshilboum RM. Thiopurine pharmacogenetics in leukemia: correlation of erythrocyte thiopurine methyltransferase activity and 6-thioguanine nucleotide concentrations. *Clin Pharmacol Ther* 1989;46:18-25.

16. Lennard L, Van Loon JA, Weinshilboum RM. Pharmacogenetics of acute azathioprine toxicity: relationship to thiopurine methyltransferase genetic polymorphism. *Clin Pharmacol Ther* 1989;46:149-54.

17. Gonzalez FJ. The molecular biology of cytochrome P450s. *Pharmacol Rev* 1989;40:243-88.

18. Mahgoub A, Dring LG, Idle JR, Lancaster R, Smith RL. Polymorphic hydroxylation of debrisoquine in man. *Lancet* 1977;2:584-6.

19. Eichelbaum M, Spannbrucker N, Dengler HJ. N-oxidation of sparteine in man and its interindividual differences. *Naunyn Schmiedebergs Arch Pharmacol* 1975;287 (suppl):R94.

20. Evans DAP. Therapy. In: Kalow W, Goedde HW, Agarwal DP, eds. Ethnic differences in reactions to drugs and xenobiotics. New York: Alan R. Liss, 1986.

21. Wang T, Roden DM, Wolfenden HT, Woosley RL, Wood AJJ, Wilkinson GR. Influence of genetic polymorphism on the metabolism and disposition of encainide in man. *J Pharmacol Exp Ther* 1984;228:605-11.

22. Fonne-Pfister R, Meyer UA. Xenobiotic and endobiotic inhibitors of cytochrome P450db1 function, the target of the debrisoquine/sparteine type polymorphism. *Biochem Pharmacol* 1988;37:3829-35.

23. Leeman T, Dayer P, Meyer UA. Single-dose quinidine treatment inhibits metoprolol oxidation in extensive metabolizers. *Eur J Clin Pharmacol* 1986;29:739-41.

24. Davies DS, Khan GC, Murray S, Brodie MG, Boobis AR. Evidence for an enzymatic defect in the 4-hydroxylation of debrisoquine by human liver. *Br J Clin Pharmacol* 1981;11:89-91.

25. Meier PJ, Mueller HK, Dick B, Meyer UA. Hepatic monooxygenase activities in subjects with a genetic defect in drug oxidation. *Gastroenterology* 1983; 85:682-92.

26. Zanger UM, Vilbois F, Hardwick JP, Meyer UA. Absence of hepatic cytochrome

P450buff causes genetically deficient debrisoquine oxidation in man. *Biochemistry* 1988;27: 5447-54.

27. Gonzalez FJ, Skoda RC, Kimura S, et al. Characterization of the common genetic defect in humans deficient in debrisoquine metabolism. *Nature* 1988; *331*:442-6.

28. Skoda RC, Gonzalez FJ, Demierre A, Meyer UA. Two mutant alleles of the human cytochrome P-450db1 gene (P450C2D1) associated with genetically deficient metabolism of debrisoquine and other drugs. *Proc Natl Acad Sci USA* 1988; *85*:5240-3.

29. Weber WW. The acetylator genes and drug response. Oxford: Oxford University Press, 1987.

30. Evans DAP. *N*-acetyltransferase. *Pharmacol Ther* 1989;*42*:157-234.

31. Bönicke R, Reif W. Enzymatic inactivation of isonicotinic acid hydrazide in humans and animals. *Arch Exp Pathol Pharmak* 1953;*220*:321-33.

32. Mitchell RS, Bell JC. Clinical implications of isoniazid, PAS and streptomycin blood levels in pulmonary tuberculosis. *Trans Am Clin Chem Assoc* 1957; *69*:98-105.

33. Bönicke R, Lisboa BP. On the inherited basis of intraindividual constancy of isoniazid elimination in man (studies of monozygotic and dizygotic twins). *Naturwissenschaften* 1957;*44*:314.

34. Mitchell RS, Riemensnider DK, Harsch JR, Bell JC. New information on the clinical implications of individual variations in the metabolic handling of antituberculous drugs, particularly isoniazid. Transactions of the 17th Conference on Chemotherapy of Tuberculosis. Washington, DC: Veterans Administration, 1958.

35. Evans DAP, Manley KA, McKusick VA. Genetic control of isoniazid metabolism in man. *Br Med J* 1960;2:485-91.

36. Evans DAP, White TA. Human acetylation polymorphism. *J Lab Clin Med* 1964;*63*:394-403.

37. Shear NH, Spielberg SP, Grant DM, Tang BK, Kalow W. Differences in metabolism of sulfonamides predisposing to idiosyncratic toxicity. *Ann Intern Med* 1986;*105*:179-84.

38. Grant DM, Tang BK, Kalow W. A simple test for acetylator phenotype using caffeine. *Br J Clin Pharmacol* 1984;*17*:459-64.

39. Gascon M-P, Leeman T, Dayer P. Evaluation d'un test à la caféine pour déterminer le phénotype de la *N*-acétyltransférase (NAT). *Schweiz Med Wochenschr* 1987;*117*:1974-6.

40. Grant DM, Mörike K, Eichelbaum M, Meyer UA. Acetylation pharmacogenetics: the slow acetylator phenotype is caused by decreased or absent arylamine *N*-acetyltransferase in human liver. *J Clin Invest* 1990;*85*:968-72.

41. Grant DM, Blum M, Demierre A, Meyer UA. Nucleotide sequence of an intronless gene for a human arylamine *N*-acetyltransferase related to polymorphic drug acetylation. *Nucl Acids Res* 1989;*17*:3978.

42. Blum M, Grant DM, McBride OW, Heim M, Meyer UA. Human arylamine *N*-acetyltransferase genes: isolation, chromosomal localization and functional expression. *DNA* 1990; 9:193-203.

43. Rieder MJ, Uetrecht J, Shear NH, Cannon M, Miller M, Spielberg SP. Diagnosis of sulfonamide hypersensitivity reactions by in vitro rechallenge with hydroxylamine metabolites. *Ann Intern Med* 1989;*110*:286-9.

44. Cribb AE, Spielberg SP. Hepatic microsomal metabolism of sulfamethoxazole to the hydroxylamine. *Drug Metab Dispos* 1990; in press.

45. Thomsick RS. The phenytoin syndrome. *Cutis* 1983;32:535-41.

46. Kelly TE. Teratogenicity of anticonvulsant drugs: review of the literature. *Am J Med Genet* 1984;19:413-34.

47. Spielberg SP, Gordon GB, Blake DA, Mellits ED, Bross DS. Anticonvulsant toxicity in vitro: possible role of arene oxides. *J Pharmacol Exp Ther* 1981;217:386-9.

48. Spielberg SP, Gordon GB, Blake DA, Goldstein DA, Herlong HF. Predisposition to phenytoin hepatotoxicity assessed in vitro. *N Engl J Med* 1981;305:722-7.

49. Gerson WT, Fine DG, Spielberg SP, Sensenbrenner LL. Anticonvulsant induced aplastic anemia: increased susceptibility to toxic drug metabolites in vitro. *Blood* 1983;61:889-93.

50. Shear NH, Spielberg SP. Anticonvulsant hypersensitivity syndrome: in vitro assessment of risk. *J Clin Invest* 1988;82:1826-32.

51. Martz F, Failinger C, Blake DA. Phenytoin teratogenesis: correlation between embryopathic effect and covalent binding of putative arene oxide metabolite in gestational tissue. *J Pharmacol Exp Ther* 1977;203:231-9.

52. Strickler SM, Dansky LV, Miller MA, Seni M-H, Andermann E, Spielberg SP. Genetic predisposition to phenytoin-induced birth defects. *Lancet* 1985;2:746-9.

3

Safety Profiles of New Drugs at the Time of Initial Marketing

Bert Spilker

Abstract

This chapter addresses how a company may identify the amount of safety data required when a new drug is marketed. The perspective is primarily that of a pharmaceutical company developing a drug, but perspectives of a regulatory agency and a practicing physician also are mentioned. Limitations of safety data usually present at the time a drug is initially marketed are presented. The greater the benefit-to-risk ratio of a new drug over existing treatments, the smaller the safety package may be at the time of the drug's initial approval. The two most important groups that influence the size of the safety package usually are the sponsor and the regulatory agency. A third major element is the nature of the disease being treated. Acceptable safety packages are discussed for the following types of drugs: breakthrough drugs, "me-too" drugs, average new drugs with substantial medical value, lifesaving drugs, and orphan drugs that are not lifesaving. Delaying some safety studies from Phase III to Phase IV affects major breakthrough drugs and does not represent a trend that will affect the development of most new drugs.

Outline

R esearch- and development-based pharmaceutical companies frequently address the question of how much clinical safety data, efficacy data, and other types of data (e.g., pharmacokinetic, quality of life) should be included in the initial regulatory submission (i.e., product license application [PLA] or new drug application [NDA]) for each new drug under development. This chapter discusses how a company may identify the amount of safety data required when a new drug is marketed. Both general and specific factors that influence this decision are discussed. The perspective used is primarily that of a pharmaceutical company developing a drug, but perspectives of a regulatory agency and a practicing physician also are mentioned.

Limitations of Safety Data at the Time of Initial Marketing

Before describing the factors that influence the decision of how much data to collect, it is important to understand the limitations of safety data that usually are present when a drug is initially marketed. The reasons for those limitations should also be understood. It would be ideal if the full profile of the unintended drug effects (UDEs), as well as the incidence of each of these, were known at the time of marketing. This is impossible for several reasons.

First, only several hundred to a few thousand patients usually are evaluated at the time a new drug is marketed. This number is insufficient to identify the nature and clinical importance of rare UDEs, although most common and unusual ones will be known. It was estimated that zomepirac sodium was administered to 15 million patients before it was withdrawn as a result of a rare, severe anaphylactic reaction. An incidence of 0.007 percent resulted in five deaths (0.00003 percent of all users).[1] The number of patients that must be studied to be reasonably sure of having observed any specific adverse reaction usually is three times the UDE incidence. Thus, to identify a UDE with an incidence of 1 in 5000 patients, 15 000 patients must be studied. Algorithms, global introspection, and other techniques are used to identify whether any specific adverse event is drug related. See Chapters 6 and 10 for a more detailed discussion of these issues.

The problem of having safety data on too few patients to understand which uncommon adverse reactions are drug related at the time of initial marketing is even more severe when a drug is developed to treat a rare disease. Data on fewer than 100 patients may be all that can be included in a regulatory application; therefore, relatively little safety data will be available at the time of marketing. In the 1980s pimozide was approved for Tourette's syndrome, using data from approximately 60 patients, although it did not have an orphan drug designation (personal communication, Abbey Meyers, National Organization for Rare Disorders, September 1989). Since the Orphan Drug Act in 1983, several drugs have been approved for marketing with data on fewer than 100 patients (e.g., hemin, L-carnitine, sodium benzoate, sodium phenylacetate; personal communication from Aleta Sindelar, R.N., Office of Orphan Products Development, FDA, October 1989). Risk-to-benefit considerations often suggest that orphan drugs should be made available rapidly to patients, despite what may be obvious shortcomings in their safety profile.

The second reason why limited safety information usually is available when a new drug is first marketed is that some severe UDEs may not be recognized until many years after the drug is marketed. Diethylstilbestrol (DES) is an example of this situation.[2] The potential for precancerous and cancerous genital lesions that sometimes occur with this agent many years after maternal exposure is difficult, if not impossible, to recognize in the early years of a drug's development and marketing. Major improvements in toxicologic methods and standards used to evaluate drugs since DES was first marketed should minimize and perhaps prevent future occurrences of this type of problem. These changes include the necessity of conducting teratology studies and more elaborate reproduction studies in animals to evaluate fertility, reproductive function, and perinatal and postnatal aspects.

Third, it is impossible to study fully or even to predict all areas where safety problems may arise. There is an almost infinite combination of concurrent diseases, potential drug interactions, patient ages, genetic predispositions, and other factors that may affect the safety of a new drug. Few of these possible factors can or should be specifically studied during Phase III, unless there are particular reasons to do so.

Fourth, drugs often are used for nonapproved indications in patients who differ significantly from those entered in clinical trials. These patients may have quite different UDE profiles.

Fifth, there are increasing pressures in society to make important new efficacious drugs (i.e., breakthrough drugs) available for medical treatment at an earlier time than ever before. This means that some of the human safety studies traditionally conducted during Phases II and III are now delayed until Phase IV. This is appropriate when the benefit-to-risk ratio favors the new treatment over existing therapy. Examples of types of drugs targeted for abbreviated Phase III development and for rapid regulatory review include important anti-AIDS and anticancer drugs.

Sixth, certain patient populations are either excluded from all clinical trials or so few patients are studied that their UDE profile is virtually unknown. This includes both children and pregnant women.

Seventh, the optimal method of treating patient overdose often is not established when the drug is marketed initially. The profile of clinical effects observed after an accidental or purposeful overdosage may be incomplete or even unknown, because few cases of overdose may have occurred. As a result, determining the method to treat those patients would be mere speculation.

Total Safety Package Required for New Drugs

There is no simple formula to define an acceptable size of a safety package for new drugs. The algebraic sum of interactions, pressures, and opinions of groups shown in Figure 1 will determine the appropriate size. Not all groups shown in Figure 1 are always involved, and additional groups may express opinions on this issue, particularly for controversial drugs. *Although a single, precise formula cannot be established, an important principle is that the greater the benefit-to-risk ratio of a new drug over existing treatments, the smaller the safety package may be at the time of the drug's initial approval.* In situations where the benefit-to-risk ratio of a new drug represents a clinically significant improvement over current therapy, there should be a shifting of some (or all) of the Phase III trials to Phase IV. This last point has not been generally accepted by the regulatory agencies, except for a number of clinically important breakthrough drugs.

The two most important groups that influence the size of the safety package are usually the sponsor and the regulatory agency. Other groups generally play little, if any, role. For novel and newsworthy drugs such as anistreplase (tissue plasminogen activator), most of the groups shown in Figure 1 became heavily involved in attempting to influence the size and nature of the efficacy package required.

Three types of safety studies are conducted on new drugs. These are: (1) the basic package of safety studies, which is generally similar in nature, and often size, for most new drugs; (2) specialized safety studies that depend on the particular

Figure 1
Groups That
Influence the
Relative Size of a
New Drug's Safety
Package

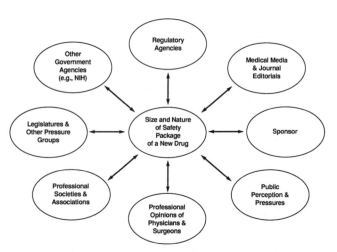

The arrows are double-headed to illustrate that there may be influences moving back and forth between each group and those people responsible for establishing the size and nature of the safety package of a new drug.

drug (e.g., ophthalmological, gonadal, electroencephalogram, or sleep studies); and (3) additional safety studies that explore abnormalities observed or possible safety issues raised during clinical trials.

BASIC PACKAGE OF SAFETY STUDIES

The basic package of safety studies required on all new drugs includes evaluations of laboratory parameters (e.g., electrolytes, basic chemistry analytes, basic hematology analytes), complete physical examinations with vital signs and body weights, electrocardiograms, ophthalmological examinations, and assessment of any UDEs observed. The number of patients who should have a complete battery of assessments generally is at least 100 for almost any new drug. Virtually all patients exposed to a drug during the investigational period should have at least a minimal safety profile obtained. This number usually varies from 1000 to 3000 patients, but numerous exceptions occur that may make the safety package required for marketing either greater or lesser than this range. There must be some balance in the number of patients studied in each of the separate tests of the basic safety package. This means that it makes little sense to have data on only 25 patients with complete hematological profiles to demonstrate a lack of drug effect, and totally negative data on 500 patients with multiple 12-lead electrocardiograms on a new drug to treat a noncardiac disease. Any abnormal safety findings or unexpected signals of potential safety issues require a sufficient number of additional studies to convince the sponsor, regulatory agencies, and physicians that there is either no problem or that the problem has been adequately explored and described.

NUMBER OF PATIENTS EXPOSED TO A DRUG

Clinical safety evaluations must be determined at therapeutic dose concentrations of a drug. If a drug studied for several years at a dose of 50 mg/d is found to be ineffective, and 250 mg/d is necessary to provide clinical benefits, then the basic safety package must be reassembled for the higher dose.

The number of patients required to be evaluated with a new drug does not refer to the total number of patients entered in a study, but to those exposed to therapeutic concentrations. The total number of patients treated with a therapeutic dose for the full treatment period usually is far fewer than the number who receive the drug under various other conditions. Numerous reports state, for example, that the safety profile of drug X is based on data from 3000 patients. However, closer examination of the data often reveals that this number includes patients given placebo, subtherapeutic doses, therapeutic doses for inadequate treatment periods, doses for patients with other indications in pilot studies, or patients receiving active drugs who were used as controls.

SPECIALIZED PACKAGE OF SAFETY STUDIES

A number of specialized safety studies are almost always conducted prior to a drug's approval, based on data from the basic package of safety and efficacy studies, as well as knowledge of the chemical class of a drug. These studies may focus on a particular target organ (e.g., eyes, heart, liver, lungs) or a particular physiological function (e.g., digestion, metabolism, absorption), or certain interactions (e.g., with other drugs, with food). The exact nature of these specialized studies varies from drug to drug, but the most important principle in determining how much data are required is: Enough data must be gathered so that a physician prescribing the drug can understand the relative risks of the drug from the package insert, and can assess the benefit-to-risk ratio for the particular patient being treated.

The specialized package of safety studies overlaps the third category of safety studies, which explore any abnormal results observed. The principles for guiding both types of studies are similar, so a separate discussion of this type of study is not presented.

Three major factors affect the decision of how much clinical safety data to include in the initial submission of a new drug for marketing approval: the regulatory strategy adopted, type of drug being developed, and nature of the disease being treated. Each of these is discussed below.

Regulatory Strategies

Regulatory agencies vary widely in the type and amount of clinical safety data they require before they are willing to approve a new drug for marketing.[3] A company that first attempts to attain regulatory approval in a less-demanding country may take either of two views. It may decide to seek more rapid approval by submitting a minimal safety data package, or it may wait until a relatively complete safety package of data has been assembled. The strategy of submitting a minimal amount of safety data may easily backfire if the regulatory agency requests more data, and this delays the drug's approval. If a company desires to minimize the total amount of work required for rewriting reports, assembling and reassembling documents, and submitting regulatory applications, it makes sense to obtain a relatively complete amount of data before submitting the initial application.

The actual quantity of safety data included in regulatory applications on a single drug submitted to different national agencies often varies widely. This depends on the year of submission, rather than on an attempt to withhold data. Figure 2 illustrates two models of how clinical safety packages are assembled for multiple regulatory submissions. Model A minimizes the difference in time between regulatory submissions compared with potential differences that arise if a company follows Model B. In Model B, it is possible that safety reports in regulatory applications sent to agencies A, D, and H not only contain different quantities of safety

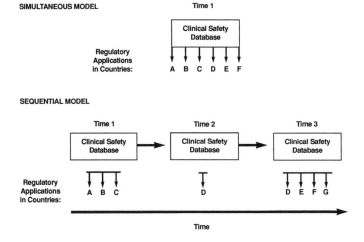

SIMULTANEOUS MODEL

Time 1

Regulatory
Applications
in Countries:

Clinical Safety
Database

A B C D E F

SEQUENTIAL MODEL

Time 1   Time 2   Time 3

Clinical Safety
Database

Clinical Safety
Database

Clinical Safety
Database

Regulatory
Applications
in Countries:

A B C   D   D E F G

Time

Figure 2
Models of Clinical
Safety Package
Assembly for
Multiple Regulatory
Submissions

data, but also may contain conflicting information, interpretations, and conclusions. This could readily lead to multiple regulatory problems for a company if different safety results or interpretations were present, although the company would not be guilty of any wrongdoing. In fact, pending PLA and NDA regulatory submissions in multiple countries may (and in some sense should) be updated periodically to minimize any substantial differences between them. The practice of frequent updating, however, is frowned upon by regulatory agencies, although they generally are interested in a final updating of safety data shortly before the drug's approval.

Companies may be unable to utilize Model A for a variety of practical reasons. In situations where the sequential Model B is used, the duration of time between submissions to major agencies should be kept to a minimum. The longer this time becomes, the greater the chance that conflicting information, interpretations, or conclusions will arise. In addition, the longer the time that elapses between submissions, the greater the number of new personnel at both the company and the regulatory agencies. The new people will have to familiarize themselves with the data and are more likely to challenge the conclusions reached than are the individuals who previously worked with the data.

The contents of regulatory applications in Model A vary in the amount of data presented, but the database from which the information is drawn does not. Expert reports are critical evaluations of up to 25 pages that summarize one type of study (e.g., clinical, preclinical safety). These reports are required for PLA regulatory submissions in many countries and usually are prepared by experts either in academia or within the pharmaceutical company. It becomes more problematic to prepare multiple versions of these reports when they are based on a changing database. The question that must be addressed concerns the types of changes in the database that require a new expert report to be written.

A company may initially submit an application to a less-demanding regulatory agency, but intend to follow up rapidly with applications to more demanding authorities. Model A still makes the most sense to use in that situation. One of the difficulties in using Model A is that it requires more time and effort to acquire necessary data than if a company desired to market their drug as rapidly as possible. The counterargument is that aquiring postmarketing data in one or more countries often helps speed regulatory approval elsewhere. A corollary of this view is that a drug should be marketed first in a major area where postmarketing data may be obtained and not in a minor market with little scientific or commercial significance.

The preceding discussion demonstrates that the regulatory strategy established for a particular drug depends on more than just the nature of the drug and its therapeutic usefulness. Other critical factors that influence regulatory strategies are the nature and traditions of the company, its leaders' personalities, and the degree of risk they are comfortable taking.

The clinical development plan indicates which studies will be conducted for a regulatory submission. At some stage during a drug's development, each of the studies that will be conducted is identified. The number of studies and number of patients targeted for enrollment in each study for any specific drug varies with different companies. At one extreme, these clinical development plans are designed to be lean or skimpy; the company decides to accumulate the least amount of safety and efficacy data possible to achieve marketing authorization. At the other extreme, the company adopts a "fat" plan and accumulates much more data than necessary for market approval. Of course, it is possible to propose a development plan where a fat plan is chosen for efficacy data and a lean plan for safety data (or vice versa).

Type of Drug Being Developed

A company that uses Model A for regulatory submissions must determine the standards to be used in acquiring clinical data. These standards depend to a large degree on the type of drug being developed. An acceptable safety package is discussed for the following types of drugs. This classification is a convenient one proposed for this discussion.

- Breakthrough drugs
- "Me-too" drugs
- Average new drugs with substantial medical value
- Lifesaving drugs
- Orphan drugs that are not lifesaving

A single drug may fit two of these categories. In describing these categories the primary question to discuss is what safety questions should be addressed, if not answered, at the time of initial marketing. A related question is: What safety information may be reasonably delayed to Phase IV?

BREAKTHROUGH DRUGS

The amount of safety data necessary at the time of initial marketing for a breakthrough drug traditionally has been viewed as approximately the same as an average new drug with substantial medical value. One of the arguments for requiring a smaller safety package for marketing this category of drugs would be the desire of companies, physicians, and the public to reach the market more rapidly with an acknowledged medically superior drug. Whether regulatory agencies agree with this premise and would approve a drug for earlier marketing under these circumstances is uncertain. However, they do not always agree whether a drug represents a breakthrough.

Most regulatory agencies accept the logic of deferring some safety assurances for breakthrough drugs to the postmarketing period. Nonetheless, two successive drugs of this type could be treated entirely differently by a single regulatory agency. Discussions with regulatory authorities to achieve an agreement and commitment to defer some safety studies to Phase IV would be an ideal solution to reach at the end of Phase II. The FDA welcomes these discussions. Unfortunately, those types of discussions and commitments are the exception worldwide rather than the rule, and companies must use their own judgment about whether or not to submit a PLA without Phase III data. Propranolol and cimetidine are examples of breakthrough drugs that were not lifesaving treatments of previously untreatable diseases. The sponsors of these drugs had to conduct substantial Phase III trials prior to their approval for marketing in the U.S. and other countries.

ME-TOO DRUGS

Me-too drugs represent agents that are relatively equivalent to one or more drugs already on the market. The exact number is arbitrary and depends on the type of drug, the differences between them, and the views of the person referring to them as me-too. These drugs often are developed because some or many patients are not receiving adequate treatment with their current therapy or have developed tolerance or UDEs. The rationale for developing and marketing me-too drugs is that some of the patients who are being inadequately treated might be helped with a related, but different drug. This occurred with nonsteroidal antiinflammatory drugs (NSAIDs). Another reason for the development of the NSAIDs is that some of these drugs were major breakthroughs at the time of their discovery and early development, but were beaten to the market by a number of competitors. Yesterday's breakthrough drugs may become today's me-too drugs.

A commercial reason for developing me-too drugs is that attaining even a small share of a very large market often justifies the development effort. Market research may suggest that there is a chance the total market will expand, the drug will become widely used, or that other drugs will lose market share and development should continue.

Two points of view are often expressed about safety packages for me-too drugs. The first is that since there are several (or many) similar drugs on the market (e.g., beta-blockers, thiazide diuretics, calcium-channel blockers), their safety has been firmly established and potential problems are well understood. The proponents of this view state that companies and regulatory agencies should not require as substantial a total safety package as for a new drug that is chemically and medically unique.

The opposite perspective states that because there are other similar drugs available, it is mandatory to acquire as much, if not more, safety data on a me-too drug to get its application approved. Companies that develop me-too drugs with the philosophy of acquiring a limited safety package prior to regulatory submission risk the chance that their drug will not be expeditiously approved in a major market. They also risk the possibility that regulatory agencies will raise safety questions that brand the drug with a negative stigma. Most stigmas usually are difficult to erase. The company also may be branded with a negative stigma within the regulatory agency.

Little, if any, pressure is ever placed on a regulatory agency to approve me-too drugs, and in numerous cases, these applications sit for many years on regulators' desks. If these applications eventually were picked up and reviewed, the safety data may be found lacking by new, higher standards used at that time. The regulators then can easily justify their denial of marketing approval for the drug, or they may request additional safety data. The latter response places companies in a difficult position because of the possibility that this cycle will continue. Similar problems also may occur for efficacy data.

This negative approach to me-too drugs usually is found in practice at important regulatory agencies, and must be considered if a decision is made to develop a me-too drug. Nonetheless, there often are sound medical and commercial reasons (described above) for developing me-too drugs, and no company should eschew this practice. Additional points about me-too drugs are presented in reference 4.

AVERAGE NEW DRUGS WITH SUBSTANTIAL MEDICAL VALUE

This category represents drugs that do not have special labels such as breakthrough, lifesaving, orphan, or me-too. The safety package of drugs in this group is judged on an individual basis as described in other sections.

LIFESAVING DRUGS

There is universal agreement that the safety package of a new lifesaving drug may be smaller than that for most other new drugs. Despite this agreement, there is no consensus on the definition of lifesaving drugs and exactly how much smaller the safety package may be.

The difficulty of defining lifesaving drugs arises because most clinical situations and diseases cannot be described easily. Some of the issues that complicate this definition are:

- If alternative therapies currently used to treat the disease are adequate or almost adequate, should the new drug be considered as lifesaving?
- Must a new drug be more effective than existing therapy to be considered lifesaving?
- If a drug is agreed to be lifesaving, but the quality of a patient's life is severely compromised, should the size of the safety package be smaller than for other drugs at the time of initial approval?
- What percentage of patients with a disease must find the drug to be lifesaving before that label is appropriate?

After these and other issues are determined, the issue of how much smaller the safety package may be for the new drug remains to be determined. This should be addressed in the same manner as for breakthrough drugs.

ORPHAN DRUGS THAT ARE NOT LIFESAVING

The safety package for orphan drugs that are not lifesaving must be determined case by case. Each of the factors influencing the safety package must be considered. Various myths abound about orphan drugs and rare diseases. Regardless of which general definition of orphan drugs is accepted, there are many types or categories of orphan drugs, representing a heterogeneous group of investigational and marketed drugs. The vast majority do not represent breakthrough or lifesaving treatments. In fact, many are developed for diseases that already have treatments, albeit inadequate ones. A well-known example is Wilson's disease, which is treated with penicillamine, dimaval (2,3, dimercaptopropane 1-sulfonate), trientine, or zinc sulfate. The need for new therapies varies widely among orphan diseases, and the appropriate safety package for a new orphan drug depends on the need for the drug in terms of its medical value and safety.

Nature of the Disease Being Treated

The third major element in the equation for determining the amount of safety data to obtain on a new drug relates to the disease being treated. If the disease is one with high morbidity or mortality and is not adequately treated (e.g., primary pulmonary hypertension, adult respiratory distress syndrome), then a smaller safety package may be acceptable at the time of initial marketing. The less the morbidity and mortality of a disease (e.g., allergic rhinitis, nausea, hiatal hernia), the greater must be the safety package of a drug used to treat it. The exact size of the safety package required depends, however, on an overall assessment by various regulatory agencies of the medical importance of the drug being developed, as well as other factors described in this chapter. Drugs given on a chronic basis to prevent a disease (e.g., by decreasing a risk factor such as hypertension) must have a relatively complete safety package at the time of marketing.

Summary

There has been a change in recent years to delay some safety studies on new drugs from Phase III to Phase IV, but this primarily affects major breakthrough drugs that are also lifesaving and does not represent a trend that will affect the development of most new drugs. The optimal relationship between Phase III and Phase IV requirements for safety is a relative one, depending on the perspective of the person or group addressing the question, the medical importance of the drug, its relative safety as demonstrated in investigational trials, and the time when this relationship is being defined.

References

1. Reines SA, Fong D. Clinical evaluation of drug candidates. In: Williams M, Malick JB, eds. Drug discovery and development. Clifton, NJ: Humana Press, 1987: 327-52.

2. Chalmers TC. The impact of controlled trials on the practice of medicine. *Mt Sinai J Med* 1974;41:753-9.

3. Walker SR, Griffin JP. International medicines regulations: a forward look to 1992. Dordrecht, The Netherlands: Kluwer Academic Publisher, 1989.

4. Spilker B, Cuatrecasas P. Inside the drug industry. Barcelona: Prous Scientific Publisher, 1990.

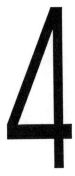

The Drug Approval Process and the Information It Provides

Ann Myers
Steven R. Moore

Abstract

This chapter presents an overview of the drug approval process in the U.S. By law, the commissioner of the FDA is responsible for determining whether a new drug is safe and efficacious before it is approved for marketing in the U.S. and for monitoring its use after approval. A brief description is provided of the approval process, in terms of responsibilities of the sponsor in submitting an application for review to the FDA, and the FDA's responsibilities and organizational procedures for reviewing and approving those applications. A brief history of the legislation regarding the FDA's responsibility in the drug approval area is discussed along with recent regulations, legislation, and FDA initiatives aimed at improving the drug approval process. Specific information that can be released to the public upon request is also presented. The discussion is limited to the regulation of drugs; somewhat different regulations govern the review and regulation of biological products and abbreviated new drug applications.

Outline

Food and Drug Administration (FDA) authority over drug review and approval began with the Food and Drug Act of 1906. This act (often referred to as the Wiley Act or Heyburn Act) made it unlawful to manufacture adulterated or misbranded foods or drugs within any territory of the U.S. and the District of Columbia and banned adulterated or misbranded foods or drugs from interstate commerce. However, the law was limited in that the burden of proof was on the FDA to show that the labeling was false or fraudulent before the product could be taken off the market.

The limitations of the 1906 act prompted further legislation, and in 1938 Congress passed the Federal Food, Drug, and Cosmetic (FD&C) Act, which prohibited marketing new drugs unless they had been tested adequately to show they were safe for use under the conditions prescribed on their labels. This legislation was passed the year following the elixir of sulfanilamide tragedy in which more than 100 people died as a result of ingesting an untested, poisonous new drug formulation. This act put the burden on manufacturers to prove the product was safe.

In 1962 Congress passed the Kefauver-Harris Amendments to the FD&C Act, stating that drug manufacturers had to provide scientific proof that new products were efficacious, as well as safe, before marketing them. This requirement was applied retroactively to 1938, when the FD&C Act was passed. Pre-1938 drugs were "grandfathered" provided no evidence of problems with safety or efficacy developed. The amendment also stated that the FDA must be notified when drugs are being tested on humans.

Recent Changes in the New Drug Evaluation Process

The past several years have been a period of enormous change due to Congressional actions, regulatory changes, and FDA initiatives to improve the drug approval process. In the legislative area, Congress enacted the Orphan Drug Act in 1983 which allows manufacturers developing drugs and other products for rare diseases the benefits of tax deductions for much of the cost of clinical development. Firms also are granted exclusive marketing rights for seven years when their orphan products are approved.

The Drug Price Competition and Patent Term Restoration Act of 1984 (the Waxman-Hutch amendments) encourages drug price competition by simplifying the approval process for drugs shown to be safe and effective that are identical to previously approved drug products. Among other provisions, the act codified and expanded the acceptance by the agency of abbreviated new drug applications (ANDAs). Patent term restoration refers to the addition of as many as 5 years to the original 17 years of legal protection given a firm for each drug patent. This is meant to offset the amount of time used while the drug goes through the approval process.

In the regulatory area, the revised new drug regulations (also known as the NDA Rewrite) were published in the *Federal Register* on February 22, 1985, and were made effective May 23, 1985. The major objective of the NDA Rewrite was to establish an efficient, but thorough, drug approval process in order to (1) facilitate the approval of drugs shown to be safe and effective, and (2) ensure the disapproval of drugs not shown to be safe and effective.[1] The Rewrite also established an improved flow of communications between the applicant and the agency and improves the FDA's surveillance of marketed drugs.[2-4]

In July 1985, the revised regulations for investigational new drugs (the IND Rewrite) were signed. The final IND regulations were published in the *Federal Register* March 19, 1987, and were made effective June 17, 1987. These regulations are intended to facilitate the development of new drug therapies while ensuring FDA's ability to monitor the safety of patients participating in clinical investigations.[5]

Regulations on treatment INDs were published May 22, 1987, and made effective June 22, 1987. These regulations allow new drugs to be available to patients with serious or life-threatening diseases for which no comparable or satisfactory alternative drug or other therapy exists.[6]

Interim regulations (21 CFR 312 Subpart E), published in the *Federal Register* on October 21, 1988, speed the availability of promising new experimental drugs in early phases of development. Procedures are designed to facilitate the development, evaluation, and marketing of new therapies intended to treat life-threatening and severely debilitating illnesses, especially when no satisfactory alternative exists.

The Center for Drug Evaluation and Research and the Review Process

The Center for Drug Evaluation and Research (CDER) is the FDA component responsible for regulating the review and approval of new drug products intended for human use. The director and staff in CDER provide the highest level of policy making and program management in the center. Within the center, the two main offices directly responsible for drug review are the Offices of Drug Evaluation (ODE) I and II. Five review divisions report to the Office Director in ODE I. ODE II has three review divisions. Recently, a new reviewing component, the Pilot Drug Evaluation Staff, was added which reports directly to the center director.

When an investigational new drug (IND) application or a new drug application (NDA) is submitted to the agency, it is assigned an application number and checked for completeness. Specific data are entered into the management information system for tracking purposes and the application is assigned and distributed to one of nine drug review divisions. The drug review divisions are responsible for specific classes of drugs and are organizationally similar in composition (Figure 1). Each has a division director and some, but not all, have a deputy director who usually handles administrative responsibilities. Group leaders who are medical officers serve primarily as leaders of the review team, which is loosely structured around a clinical reviewer, chemist, pharmacologist, and consumer safety officer.

There also are consulting reviewers in biopharmaceutics and statistics located organizationally outside of the immediate reviewing division. In addition, outside consultants and other support personnel (i.e., advisory committee members) are used to complement the FDA review staff. Each member of the team performs his own review based on regulatory guidelines and precedents and the review eventually becomes part of the basis for approval or nonapproval of the application. Periodically, the reviewers meet to discuss issues, progress, and problems, and frequently meetings are arranged with the applicant to discuss certain issues or summarize the status of the application.

Once all reviews have been completed (including any necessary statistical and biopharmaceutical review), a package consisting of a draft action letter, the reviews, and possibly a summary basis of approval is prepared by the consumer safety officer. The package is circulated to the review staff, including supervisors and the division director, for concurrence and signatures. New molecular entities, new combinations, significant new indications, and novel routes of administration are then forwarded to the appropriate ODE director's office for final clearance.

IND Submission

The filing of an IND application and subsequently an NDA marks the inception of a sequence of events that may lead to the approval and eventual marketing of a new drug. The FD&C Act provides exemptions for interstate shipment of investigational new drugs from the requirement of having an approved NDA. Regulations permit the interstate shipment of new drugs if they are intended solely for investigational use by experts whose scientific training and experience qualify them to investigate the safety and effectiveness of a drug.

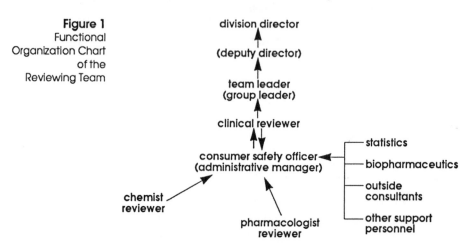

Figure 1
Functional
Organization Chart
of the
Reviewing Team

Figure 2a

DEPARTMENT OF HEALTH AND HUMAN SERVICES PUBLIC HEALTH SERVICE FOOD AND DRUG ADMINISTRATION **INVESTIGATIONAL NEW DRUG APPLICATION (IND)** *(TITLE 21, CODE OF FEDERAL REGULATIONS (CFR) Part 312)*	Form Approved: OMB No. 0910-0014. Expiration Date: June 30, 1991. See OMB Statement on Reverse. NOTE: No drug may be shipped or clinical investigation begun until an IND for that investigation is in effect (21 CFR 312.40).

1. NAME OF SPONSOR	2. DATE OF SUBMISSION

3. ADDRESS *(Number, Street, City, State and Zip Code)*	4. TELEPHONE NUMBER *(Include Area Code)*

5. NAME(S) OF DRUG *(Include all available names: Trade, Generic, Chemical, Code)*	6. IND NUMBER *(If previously assigned)*

7. INDICATION(S) *(Covered by this submission)*

8. PHASE (S) OF CLINICAL INVESTIGATION TO BE CONDUCTED: ☐ PHASE 1   ☐ PHASE 2   ☐ PHASE 3   ☐ OTHER _____
(Specify)

9. LIST NUMBERS OF ALL INVESTIGATIONAL NEW DRUG APPLICATIONS *(21 CFR Part 312)*, NEW DRUG OR ANTIBIOTIC APPLICATIONS *(21 CFR Part 314)*, DRUG MASTER FILES *(21 CFR 314.420)*, AND PRODUCT LICENSE APPLICATIONS *(21 CFR Part 601)* REFERRED TO IN THIS APPLICATION.

10. IND submissions should be consecutively numbered. The initial IND should be numbered "Serial Number: 000." The next submission (e.g., amendment, report, or correspondence) should be numbered "Serial Number: 001." Subsequent submissions should be numbered consecutively in the order in which they are submitted.	SERIAL NUMBER: _ _ _

11. THIS SUBMISSION CONTAINS THE FOLLOWING: *(Check all that apply)*
    ☐ INITIAL INVESTIGATIONAL NEW DRUG APPLICATION (IND)   ☐ RESPONSE TO CLINICAL HOLD

PROTOCOL AMENDMENT(S):	INFORMATION AMENDMENT(S):	IND SAFETY REPORT(S):
☐ NEW PROTOCOL	☐ CHEMISTRY/MICROBIOLOGY	☐ INITIAL WRITTEN REPORT
☐ CHANGE IN PROTOCOL	☐ PHARMACOLOGY/TOXICOLOGY	☐ FOLLOW-UP TO A WRITTEN REPORT
☐ NEW INVESTIGATOR	☐ CLINICAL	

☐ RESPONSE TO FDA REQUEST FOR INFORMATION   ☐ ANNUAL REPORT   ☐ GENERAL CORRESPONDENCE

☐ REQUEST FOR REINSTATEMENT OF IND THAT IS WITHDRAWN,   ☐ OTHER _____
    INACTIVATED, TERMINATED OR DISCONTINUED   *(Specify)*

CHECK ONLY IF APPLICABLE

JUSTIFICATION STATEMENT MUST BE SUBMITTED WITH APPLICATION FOR ANY CHECKED BELOW. REFER TO THE CITED CFR SECTION FOR FURTHER INFORMATION.

    ☐ TREATMENT IND 21 CFR 312.35(b)   ☐ TREATMENT PROTOCOL 21 CFR 312.35(a)   ☐ CHARGE REQUEST/NOTIFICATION 21 CFR 312.7(d)

FOR FDA USE ONLY

CDR/DBIND/DGD RECEIPT STAMP	DDR RECEIPT STAMP	IND NUMBER ASSIGNED:
		DIVISION ASSIGNMENT:

FORM FDA 1571 (12/90)   PREVIOUS EDITION IS OBSOLETE.

The investigator must submit the IND in triplicate with signed forms 1571 and 1572 (Figures 2a, b and 3a, b). The following information needs to be submitted: descriptive name of the drug and the route of administration, complete list of components, quantitative composition, source of the new drug, chemical and manufacturing information, preclinical test results (any clinical studies or experience), clinical protocol, scientific training and experience of investigators, statements to the effect that the sponsor will notify the FDA when and why studies have been discontinued, and notice that an institutional review board will be responsible for continuing review of the proposed study. The sponsor also must submit results of all animal studies that were conducted prior to submitting the IND in order to document that the drug may be safe in humans and will not impose an unreasonable risk.

The sponsor must wait 30 days after submitting the IND before beginning any tests in humans. This provides a reasonable amount of time for the FDA to determine whether there are any safety problems involving the use of the drug. If there are concerns, the FDA places the application on clinical hold and the investigator may not begin testing in humans until changes are made to eliminate the safety problems. In the absence of a clinical hold the investigator may begin testing in humans.

Figure 2b

12.   CONTENTS OF APPLICATION

This application contains the following items: *(check all that apply)*

☐ 1. Form FDA 1571 *[21 CFR 312.23 (a) (1)]*

☐ 2. Table of contents *[21 CFR 312.23 (a) (2)]*

☐ 3. Introductory statement *[21 CFR 312.23 (a) (3)]*

☐ 4. General investigational plan *[21 CFR 312.23 (a) (3)]*

☐ 5. Investigator's brochure *[21 CFR 312.23 (a) (5)]*

6. Protocol(s) *[21 CFR 312.23 (a) (6)]*

   ☐ a. Study protocol(s) *[21 CFR 312.23 (a) (6)]*

   ☐ b. Investigator data *[21 CFR 312.23 (a) (6)(iii)(b)] or completed Form(s) FDA 1572*

   ☐ c. Facilities data *[21 CFR 312.23 (a) (6)(iii)(b)] or completed Form(s) FDA 1572*

   ☐ d. Institutional Review Board data *[21 CFR 312.23 (a) (6)(iii)(b)] or completed Form(s) FDA 1572*

☐ 7. Chemistry, manufacturing, and control data *[21 CFR 312.23 (a) (7)]*

   ☐ Environmental assessment or claim for exclusion *[21 CFR 312.23 (a) (7)(iv)(e)]*

☐ 8. Pharmacology and toxicology data *[21 CFR 312.23 (a) (8)]*

☐ 9. Previous human experience *[21 CFR 312.23 (a) (9)]*

☐ 10. Additional information *[21 CFR 312.23 (a) (10)]*

13. IS ANY PART OF THE CLINICAL STUDY TO BE CONDUCTED BY A CONTRACT RESEARCH ORGANIZATION? ☐ YES   ☐ NO

IF YES, WILL ANY SPONSOR OBLIGATIONS BE TRANSFERRED TO THE CONTRACT RESEARCH ORGANIZATION? ☐ YES   ☐ NO

IF YES, ATTACH A STATEMENT CONTAINING THE NAME AND ADDRESS OF THE CONTRACT RESEARCH ORGANIZATION, IDENTIFICATION OF THE CLINICAL STUDY, AND A LISTING OF THE OBLIGATIONS TRANSFERRED.

14. NAME AND TITLE OF THE PERSON RESPONSIBLE FOR MONITORING THE CONDUCT AND PROGRESS OF THE CLINICAL INVESTIGATIONS

15. NAME(S) AND TITLE(S) OF THE PERSON(S) RESPONSIBLE FOR REVIEW AND EVALUATION OF INFORMATION RELEVANT TO THE SAFETY OF THE DRUG

I agree not to begin clinical investigations until 30 days after FDA's receipt of the IND unless I receive earlier notification by FDA that the studies may begin. I also agree not to begin or continue clinical investigations covered by the IND if those studies are placed on clinical hold. I agree that an Institutional Review Board (IRB) that complies with the requirements set forth in 21 CFR Part 56 will be responsible for the initial and continuing review and approval of each of the studies in the proposed clinical investigation.   I agree to conduct the investigation in accordance with all other applicable regulatory requirements.

16. NAME OF SPONSOR OR SPONSOR'S AUTHORIZED REPRESENTATIVE	17. SIGNATURE OF SPONSOR OR SPONSOR'S AUTHORIZED REPRESENTATIVE	
18. ADDRESS *(Number, Street, City, State and Zip Code)*	19. TELEPHONE NUMBER *(Include Area Code)*	20. DATE

(WARNING: A willfully false statement is a criminal offense. U.S.C. Title 18, Sec. 1001.)

Public reporting burden for this collection of information is estimated to average 30 minutes per response, including the time for reviewing instructions, searching existing data sources, gathering and maintaining the data needed, and completing and reviewing the collection of information. Send comments regarding this burden estimate or any other aspect of this collection of information, including suggestions for reducing this burden to:

Reports Clearance Officer, PHS   and to: Office of Management and Budget
Hubert H. Humphrey Building, Room 721-B   Paperwork Reduction Project (0910-0014)
200 Independence Avenue, S.W.   Washington, DC 20503
Washington, DC 20201
Attn: PRA   Please DO NOT RETURN this application to either of these addresses.

Figure 3a

DEPARTMENT OF HEALTH AND HUMAN SERVICES PUBLIC HEALTH SERVICE FOOD AND DRUG ADMINISTRATION **STATEMENT OF INVESTIGATOR** *(TITLE 21, CODE OF FEDERAL REGULATIONS (CFR) Part 312)* (See instructions on reverse side.)	Form Approved: OMB No. 0910-0014 Expiration Date: November 30, 1990 *See OMB Statement on Reverse.* NOTE: No investigator may participate in an investigation until he/she provides the sponsor with a completed, signed Statement of Investigator, Form FDA 1572 (21 CFR 312.53(c)).

1. NAME AND ADDRESS OF INVESTIGATOR.

2. EDUCATION, TRAINING, AND EXPERIENCE THAT QUALIFIES THE INVESTIGATOR AS AN EXPERT IN THE CLINICAL INVESTIGATION OF THE DRUG FOR THE USE UNDER INVESTIGATION. ONE OF THE FOLLOWING IS ATTACHED:

    ☐ CURRICULUM VITAE   ☐ OTHER STATEMENT OF QUALIFICATIONS

3. NAME AND ADDRESS OF ANY MEDICAL SCHOOL, HOSPITAL, OR OTHER RESEARCH FACILITY WHERE THE CLINICAL INVESTIGATION(S) WILL BE CONDUCTED.

4. NAME AND ADDRESS OF ANY CLINICAL LABORATORY FACILITIES TO BE USED IN THE STUDY.

5. NAME AND ADDRESS OF THE INSTITUTIONAL REVIEW BOARD (IRB) THAT IS RESPONSIBLE FOR REVIEW AND APPROVAL OF THE STUDY(IES).

6. NAMES OF THE SUBINVESTIGATORS *(e.g., research fellows, residents, associates)* WHO WILL BE ASSISTING THE INVESTIGATOR IN THE CONDUCT OF THE INVESTIGATION(S).

7. NAME AND CODE NUMBER, IF ANY, OF THE PROTOCOL(S) IN THE IND FOR THE STUDY(IES) TO BE CONDUCTED BY THE INVESTIGATOR.

FORM FDA 1572 (7/90)   PREVIOUS EDITION IS OBSOLETE.

Testing is conducted in three regulatory phases:

Phase I: The first phase of human testing is directed at determining safety of the drug, the ways it is absorbed into the body, and possible levels of toxicity. These tests usually are conducted on 20–80 normal, healthy volunteers. About 70 percent of drugs successfully complete this phase and go on to Phase II.

Phase II: The second phase of human testing is performed on closely monitored patients to learn more about the drug's safety and effectiveness. The number of patients monitored in this phase depends on the nature of the drug, but seldom is more than 200. Most Phase II testing is directed at treatment of prevention of a specific disease. Additional animal testing usually is undertaken to gain further safety information. If the tests show the drug may be useful in treating a disease and the long-term animal testing indicates no unwarranted harm, the sponsor then proceeds to Phase III. Approximately 33 percent of drugs successfully complete this phase and go on to Phase III.

Phase III: This phase involves the most extensive testing. Phase III studies are intended to assess the safety, effectiveness, and most desirable dosage of the drug in treating a specific disease in a large group of patients (usually several hundred to several thousand, depending on the drug). During Phase III, the drug is used

Figure 3b

8. ATTACH THE FOLLOWING CLINICAL PROTOCOL INFORMATION:

☐ FOR PHASE 1 INVESTIGATIONS, A GENERAL OUTLINE OF THE PLANNED INVESTIGATION INCLUDING THE ESTIMATED DURATION OF THE STUDY AND THE MAXIMUM NUMBER OF SUBJECTS THAT WILL BE INVOLVED.

☐ FOR PHASE 2 OR 3 INVESTIGATIONS, AN OUTLINE OF THE STUDY PROTOCOL INCLUDING AN APPROXIMATION OF THE NUMBER OF SUBJECTS TO BE TREATED WITH THE DRUG AND THE NUMBER TO BE EMPLOYED AS CONTROLS, IF ANY; THE CLINICAL USES TO BE INVESTIGATED; CHARACTERISTICS OF SUBJECTS BY AGE, SEX, AND CONDITION; THE KIND OF CLINICAL OBSERVATIONS AND LABORATORY TESTS TO BE CONDUCTED; THE ESTIMATED DURATION OF THE STUDY; AND COPIES OR A DESCRIPTION OF CASE REPORT FORMS TO BE USED.

9. COMMITMENTS:

I agree to conduct the study(ies) in accordance with the relevant, current protocol(s) and will only make changes in a protocol after notifying the sponsor, except when necessary to protect the safety, rights, or welfare of subjects.

I agree to personally conduct or supervise the described investigation(s).

I agree to inform any patients, or any persons used as controls, that the drugs are being used for investigational purposes and I will ensure that the requirements relating to obtaining informed consent in 21 CFR Part 50 and institutional review board (IRB) review and approval in 21 CFR Part 56 are met.

I agree to report to the sponsor adverse experiences that occur in the course of the investigation(s) in accordance with 21 CFR 312.64.

I have read and understand the information in the investigator's brochure, including the potential risks and side effects of the drug.

I agree to ensure that all associates, colleagues, and employees assisting in the conduct of the study(ies) are informed about their obligations in meeting the above commitments.

I agree to maintain adequate and accurate records in accordance with 21 CFR 312.62 and to make those records available for inspection in accordance with 21 CFR 312.68.

I will ensure that an IRB that complies with the requirements of 21 CFR Part 56 will be responsible for the initial and continuing review and approval of the clinical investigation. I also agree to promptly report to the IRB all changes in the research activity and all unanticipated problems involving risks to human subjects or others. Additionally, I will not make any changes in the research without IRB approval, except where necessary to eliminate apparent immediate hazards to human subjects.

I agree to comply with all other requirements regarding the obligations of clinical investigators and all other pertinent requirements in 21 CFR Part 312.

INSTRUCTIONS FOR COMPLETING FORM FDA 1572
STATEMENT OF INVESTIGATOR:

1. Complete all sections. Attach a separate page if additional space is needed.

2. Attach curriculum vitae or other statement of qualifications as described in Section 2.

3. Attach protocol outline as described in Section 8.

4. Sign and date below.

5. FORWARD THE COMPLETED FORM AND ATTACHMENTS TO THE SPONSOR. The sponsor will incorporate this information along with other technical data into an Investigational New Drug Application (IND). INVESTIGATORS SHOULD NOT SEND THIS FORM DIRECTLY TO THE FOOD AND DRUG ADMINISTRATION.

10. SIGNATURE OF INVESTIGATOR   11. DATE

Public reporting burden for this collection of information is estimated to average 1 hour per response, including the time for reviewing instructions, searching existing data sources, gathering and maintaining the data needed, and completing reviewing the collection of information. Send comments regarding this burden estimate or any other aspect of this collection of information, including suggestions for reducing this burden to:

Reports Clearance Officer, PHS   and to: Office of Management and Budget
Hubert H. Humphrey Building, Room 721-B   Paperwork Reduction Project (0910-0014)
200 Independence Avenue, S.W.   Washington, DC 20503
Washington, DC 20201
Attn: PRA

☆U.S. Government Printing Office: 1990-261-200/13866

Figure 4a

DEPARTMENT OF HEALTH AND HUMAN SERVICES
PUBLIC HEALTH SERVICE
FOOD AND DRUG ADMINISTRATION
**APPLICATION TO MARKET A NEW DRUG FOR HUMAN USE
OR AN ANTIBIOTIC DRUG FOR HUMAN USE**
(Title 21, Code of Federal Regulations, 314)

Form Approved: OMB No. 0910-0001
Expiration Date; March 31, 1990.
See OMB Statement on Page 3.

FOR FDA USE ONLY

DATE RECEIVED	DATE FILED
DIVISION ASSIGNED	NDA/ANDA NO. ASS.

NOTE: No application may be filed unless a completed application form has been received (21 CFR Part 314).

NAME OF APPLICANT

DATE OF SUBMISSION

TELEPHONE NO. (Include Area Code)

ADDRESS (Number, Street, City, State and Zip Code)

NEW DRUG OR ANTIBIOTIC APPLICATION NUMBER (If previously issued)

DRUG PRODUCT

ESTABLISHED NAME (e.g., USP/USAN)   PROPRIETARY NAME (If any)

CODE NAME (If any)   CHEMICAL NAME

DOSAGE FORM   ROUTE OF ADMINISTRATION   STRENGTH(S)

PROPOSED INDICATIONS FOR USE

LIST NUMBERS OF ALL INVESTIGATIONAL NEW DRUG APPLICATIONS (21 CFR Part 312), NEW DRUG OR ANTIBIOTIC APPLICATIONS (21 CFR Part 314), AND DRUG MASTER FILES (21 CFR 314.420) REFERRED TO IN THIS APPLICATION:

INFORMATION ON APPLICATION
TYPE OF APPLICATION (Check one)

☐ THIS SUBMISSION IS A FULL APPLICATION (21 CFR 314.50) ☐ THIS SUBMISSION IS AN ABBREVIATED APPLICATION (ANDA) (21 CFR 314.55)

IF AN ANDA, IDENTIFY THE APPROVED DRUG PRODUCT THAT IS THE BASIS FOR THE SUBMISSION

NAME OF DRUG   HOLDER OF APPROVED APPLICATION

STATUS OF APPLICATION (Check one)

☐ PRESUBMISSION ☐ AN AMENDMENT TO A PENDING APPLICATION ☐ SUPPLEMENTAL APPLICATION
☐ ORIGINAL APPLICATION ☐ RESUBMISSION

PROPOSED MARKETING STATUS (Check one)

☐ APPLICATION FOR A PRESCRIPTION DRUG PRODUCT (Rx)   ☐ APPLICATION FOR AN OVER - THE - COUNTER PRODUCT (OTC)

FORM FDA 356h (10/89)   Page 1

the way it would be administered when marketed. Additional testing intended to define more specifically any drug-related adverse effects is also done in Phase III. Approximately 25–30 percent will clear Phase III.

As the investigational studies progress, the IND must be amended to include new protocols, progress reports, and stability data. Once Phase III is completed and the sponsor believes the drug is safe and effective under specific conditions, the sponsor can apply to the FDA for approval to market the drug. Several new initiatives (subpart E and "parallel track") are efforts aimed at speeding the availability of certain drugs in early stages of development to patients with life-threatening diseases.

NDA Submission

By the time an NDA is submitted, a drug usually has been studied in several hundred to several thousand patients. The applicant must submit a signed 356H (Figures 4a, b) and two copies of the NDA, and an archival and review copy. The archival copy is a complete copy of the application that serves as a reference source for agency reviewers and as a repository for the case report forms and tabulations on the clinical studies.

Figure 4b

CONTENTS OF APPLICATION
This application contains the following items: *(Check all that apply)*
1. Index
2. Summary (21 CFR 314.50 (c))
3. Chemistry, manufacturing, and control section (21 CFR 314.50 (d) (1))
4. a. Samples (21 CFR 314.50 (e) (1)) (Submit only upon FDA's request)
b. Methods Validation Package (21 CFR 314.50 (e) (2) (i))
c. Labeling (21 CFR 314.50 (e) (2) (ii))
i. draft labeling *(4 copies)*
ii. final printed labeling (12 copies)
5. Nonclinical pharmacology and toxicology section (21 CFR 314.50 (d) (2))
6. Human pharmacokinetics and bioavailability section (21 CFR 314.50 (d) (3))
7. Microbiology section (21 CFR 314.50 (d) (4))
8. Clinical data section (21 CFR 314.50 (d) (5))
9. Safety update report (21 CFR 314.50 (d) (5) (vi) (b))
10. Statistical section (21 CFR 314.50 (d) (6))
11. Case report tabulations (21 CFR 314.50 (f) (1))
12. Case reports forms (21 CFR 314.50 (f) (1))
13. Patent information on any patent which claims the drug (21 U.S.C. 355 (b) or (c))
14. A patent certification with respect to any patent which claims the drug (21 U.S.C. 355 (b) (2) or (j) (2) (A))
15. OTHER *(Specify)*

I agree to update this application with new safety information about the drug that may reasonably affect the statement of contraindications, warnings, precautions, or adverse reactions in the draft labeling. I agree to submit these safety update reports as follows: (1) 4 months after the initial submission, (2) following receipt of an approvable letter and (3) at other times as requested by FDA. If this application is approved, I agree to comply with all laws and regulations that apply to approved applications, including the following:
    1. Good manufacturing practice regulations in 21 CFR 210 and 211.
    2. Labeling regulations in 21 CFR 201.
    3. In the case of a prescription drug product, prescription drug advertising regulations in 21 CFR 202.
    4. Regulations on making changes in application in 21 CFR 314.70, 314.71, and 314.72.
    5. Regulations on reports in 21 CFR 314.80 and 314.81.
    6. Local, state and Federal environmental impact laws.
If this application applies to a drug product that FDA has proposed for scheduling under the controlled substances Act I agree not to market the product until the Drug Enforcement Administration makes a final scheduling decision.

NAME OF RESPONSIBLE OFFICIAL OR AGENT	SIGNATURE OF RESPONSIBLE OFFICIAL OR AGENT	DATE
ADDRESS *(Street, City, State, Zip Code)*	TELEPHONE NO. *(Include Area Code)*	

(WARNING: A willfully false statement is a criminal offense. U.S.C. Title 18, Sec.1001.)

FORM FDA 356h (10/89)   Page 2

Table 1. Contents of Application

Elements of NDA		Sections of the Review Copy					
	Archival Blue	Chemistry Red	Pharmacology Yellow	Pharmacokinetics Orange	Microbiology White	Clinical Light-Brown	Statistics Green
Application form (Form 356h)	X	X	X	X	X	X	X
cover letter	X	X	X	X	X	X	X
patent information	X	X	X	X	X	X	X
letter of authorization (if applicable)	X	X	X	X	X	X	X
1. Index to application index to section[a]	X	X	X	X	X	X	X
2. Summary	X	X	X	X	X	X	X
3. Chemistry manufacturing controls	X	X					
4. Samples[b]	X						
Methods validation[c]	X	X					
Labeling:[d]							
draft labeling (4 copies) or	X	X	X			X	
FPL (12 copies)	X						
5. Nonclinical pharmacology toxicology	X		X				
6. Human pharmacokinetics bioavailability	X			X			
7. Microbiology (if required)	X				X		
8. Clinical data	X					X	X

a Review sections should contain a copy of the index to the entire application, in addition to the index for the specific section.
b Samples should be submitted upon request.
c One copy of methods validation should be submitted in the archival copy; three copies should be submitted in the chemistry section of the review copy.
d The applicant should submit 4 copies of draft labeling or 12 copies of FPL (if available). The archival copy should contain one copy of all proposed labeling for the product (draft labeling or FPL and carton labeling, if available).
FPL = final printed labeling.

The review copy of an application is divided into five sections (or six, if a microbiology section is required) containing the scientific information needed by FDA reviewers. Submission of the review copy in sections permits concurrent review by experts in the FDA review disciplines: clinical, pharmacology, chemistry, statistics, biopharmaceutics, and microbiology (when required). A breakdown of the information that should be submitted in each copy of the application appears in Table 1.

The FDA reviews the entire NDA to determine whether the benefits of the drug, when used properly, outweigh the risks. The FDA is required by law to review the application within 180 days. This time period, called the regulatory review period, starts the day the application is received at the agency and lasts until a final decision is made. During the review process (Figure 5), the FDA may request additional information from the applicant. When significant changes are submitted to the application undergoing review, the time in the review period may be extended, but not more than 180 days. After the application is approved, the applicant is required to report to the FDA on a scheduled basis (with annual or periodic reports) and when significant changes are made. The FDA is responsible for monitoring the use of the drug after its approval to ensure that changes and reports of unintended drug effects (UDEs) are reflected accurately in the labeling and that the drug continues to be safe for public use.

Early in the review process, all NDAs and commercially sponsored INDs are classified by chemical type and therapeutic potential. Classification of a particular drug product is determined by comparing the active ingredient(s) with other products previously approved or marketed (Appendixes I and II). This system provides a convenient way of describing drug applications upon initial receipt and throughout the drug approval process, and also is used as a basis for reporting the types of approved new drug products. Although the classification of any new drug may

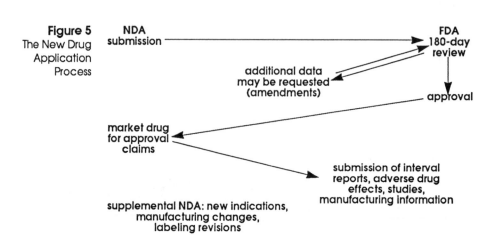

Figure 5
The New Drug Application Process

Year	NDA Approved	NME Approved
1979	94	14
1980	114	12
1981	96	27
1982	116	28
1983	94	14
1984	142	22
1985	100	30
1986	98	20
1987	69	21
1988	67	20
1989	87	23

Table 2
Number of NDA and
NME Approved
1979–1989

NDA = new drug application; NME = new molecular entity.

Year	Total	Original IND Commercial	Noncommercial	Original NDA	Supplements
1979	940	249	691	182	2641
1980	1087	269	818	162	2907
1981	1184	247	937	129	2934
1982	1467	297	1170	202	2677
1983	1798	402	1396	269	2062
1984	2112	391	1721	217	2429
1985	1904	326	1578	148	2220
1986	1596	330	1266	120	2077
1987	1346	302	1044	142	1889
1988	1337	363	974	126	1857
1989	1345	308	1037	118	1867

Table 3
Number of IND, NDA,
and Supplements
Received 1979–1989

IND = investigational new drug; NDA = new drug application.

change during the IND phase or during NDA review, once the NDA is approved, its chemical and therapeutic classification will remain the same.

Statistics on the Drug Review Process

A great deal of interest surrounds the data resulting from the drug review process. Given the monetary interest of sponsors and the potential health impact of the approval of new drug entities, this interest can be reasonably explained.

The number of NDAs approved between 1979 and 1989 is shown in Table 2.[6] Of this number, those that were new molecular entities (NMEs) (i.e., drug entering the market for the first time) are shown in column 2.

Some of the accomplishments made in the drug review area from 1987 to 1989 include approving a total of 41 NMEs in the three-year period. Some of the more significant of the NME approvals are:

- Zidovudine (Retrovir), the first AIDS drug, approved in 3.5 months;
- Lovastatin (Mevacor), the first drug in a class of cholesterol-lowering agents, approved in only 9.5 months;
- Apraclonidine hydrochloride (Iopidine), an adrenergic agonist used for post-surgical intraocular pressure reduction, approved in just 3 months;
- Misoprostol (Cytotec), indicated for the reduction of stomach ulcers in high-risk users of nonsteroidal antiinflammatory drugs, approved 9 months after receipt of the submission supporting the approved indication;
- Clozapine (Clozaril), indicated for the management of severely ill schizophrenic patients who fail to respond to standard antipsychotic drug treatment;
- Clomipramine (Anafranil), approved in 6.4 months for the treatment of obsessive-compulsive disorders.

Access to Review Information

A large amount of scientific and statistical data is generated by the IND and NDA processes. Even after the application is approved, reports must be submitted by the applicant to update the original application. Unfortunately, due to the trade secret nature of the material, the FDA is under legislative mandate not to release much of the information, such as that pertaining to formulas, manufacturing processes, or patient identification. However, specially prepared information from which the confidential and trade secret information has been deleted is available for public disclosure through the Freedom of Information Act, although there may be a cost involved to obtain the information.

For newly approved drugs, outside sources can obtain a copy of the scientific reviews as well as the summary basis for the approval, which is the document prepared by the agency to explain the scientific basis for the approval. After the drug is approved and the applicant submits data to update the application, edited copies of the submission data from the FDA's reports also can be obtained by writing to the Freedom of Information Office (HFI-35), Food and Drug Administration, 5600 Fisher's Lane, Rockville, MD 20857.

Other documents available to the public include the FDA Drug Device Product Approvals (DDPA), the Offices of Drug Evaluation Statistical Report, and the Approved Drug Products List (ADP). The DDPA is a monthly report identifying certain review actions completed during the previous month. It includes approval actions for all NDAs and ANDAs, approvable actions for NDAs, and registration and licensing actions for veterinary, biological, and medical device products. The Statistical Report is a compilation of summaries and statistics representing the results of the review process, showing trends in the numbers of various documents received and reviewed (Table 3). Both publications are available to the public through the National Technical Information Service, 5285 Port Royal Road, Springfield, VA 22161.

The ADP List, also referred to as the Therapeutic Equivalence List, identifies all products by virtue of NDA and ANDA approvals. This publication is available through the Government Printing Office, Washington, DC 20402.

Summary

The process by which an NDA is submitted to the FDA, reviewed, and eventually approved for marketing is long, laborious, and very costly, both to the FDA and the applicant.

Type 1. New molecular entity: A drug for which the active moiety (either as the unmodified base [parent] compound or an ester, salt, clathrate, or other noncovalent derivative of the base [parent] compound) has not been previously marketed in the U.S. for use in a drug product, either as a single ingredient or as part of a combination product, or as part of a mixture of stereoisomers.

Type 2. New ester, new salt, or other noncovalent derivative: A drug for which the active moiety has been previously marketed in the U.S., but for which the particular ester, salt, clathrate, or other noncovalent derivative or the unmodified base (parent) compound is not yet marketed in the U.S., either as a single ingredient or as part of a combination product.

A drug product previously marketed only as a part of a combination or mixture of stereoisomers will also be considered a Type 2 drug.

Type 3. New formulation: The compound is marketed in the U.S. by the same or another manufacturer, but the particular dosage form or formulation is not.

Type 4. New combination: The product contains two or more compounds that have not previously been marketed together in a drug product in the U.S. by any manufacturer.

Type 5. Already-marketed drug product: The product duplicates a drug product (same active moiety, same salt, same formulation, or same combination) already marketed in the U.S. by another firm.

Type 6. New indication: The product adds a new indication for a drug product already marketed in the U.S. by the same firm.

Appendix I
Classification System
for Chemical Types*

---

*These chemical types are not mutually exclusive: a new formulation (Type 3) or a new combination (Type 4) may also contain a new molecular entity (Type 1) or a new salt (Type 2). In such cases, both numbers should be included in the overall classification number for the drug. For example, a new molecular entity would be classified 1; if the entity also were in a new combination it would be classified 1, 4.

Appendix II
Classification System
for Therapeutic
Potential*

Type A. Important therapeutic gain: The drug may provide effective therapy or diagnosis for a disease not adequately treated or diagnosed by any marketed drug, or provide improved treatment of disease through improved effectiveness or safety (including decreased abuse potential).

Type B. Modest therapeutic gain: The drug has a modest, but real, potential advantage over other available marketed drugs, for example, greater patient convenience, elimination of an annoying but not dangerous adverse reaction, potential for large cost reduction, less frequent dosage schedule, or usefulness in specific subpopulation or those with disease (e.g., those allergic to other available drugs).

Type C. Little or no therapeutic gain: The drug essentially duplicates in medical importance and therapeutic usage one or more already marketed drugs.

*A, B, and C therapeutic potentials are mutually exclusive. Only one of these letters may be included in the overall classification.

References

1. 21 CFR 314.

2. Romansky MA. Protest for reform of the IND/NDA processes: part II. *J Clin Psychopharmacol* 1982;2:424-6.

3. Romansky MA. NDA rewrite: here at last. *J Clin Psychopharmacol* 1983;3:110-2.

4. Faich G. Reporting adverse drug experiences under the NDA rewrite. Presented before the Food and Drug Law Institute, New York, May 13, 1985.

5. 21 CFR 312.

6. Offices of Drug Evaluation Statistical Report. Springfield, VA: National Technical Information Services, 1987-1988: PB89-233530/AS.

Methodologic
Considerations

5

Unintended Drug Effects: Identification and Attribution

Audrey Smith Rogers

Abstract

The central thesis developed here is that the definition of an unintended drug effect (UDE) should be tailored to one's purpose in examining the incident. Although the more specific of these definitions is required for scientific evaluation of the link between drug and effect, other less stringent definitions usually are adequate for clinical purposes. As Chapter 3 indicated, knowledge about the safety profile of a drug in humans is limited at the time of marketing. The mechanisms for supplementing safety data during the postmarketing phase include: (1) the Spontaneous Reporting System maintained by the Food and Drug Administration, (2) formal projects to assemble safety data on larger or more complex populations, and (3) formal projects designed to answer specific research questions. Judgments about attribution can be no better than the data that support them. The criteria applied by the clinician to the individual UDE to determine association differ from those required to establish causation based on epidemiologic evidence. In most situations, regulatory action on drug recall should be based on epidemiologic evidence. This chapter discusses the choice of a definition for UDE, examines the extent and nature of the safety data assembled on a drug at the time it is marketed, proposes the best methods for collecting additional information after marketing, and designates factors to be considered in judging a drug to be causally related to a UDE.

Outline

The development of a precise and generally accepted definition of an unintended drug effect (UDE) has been complicated by the number of factors that can be considered. Simple definitions ("…any undesirable effect produced by a drug"[1]) include experiences such as overdose, drug abuse, and expected adverse effects. Although appropriate for such a purpose as cost-benefit analysis of societal impact, this approach complicates the estimate or determination of risk associated with therapeutic drug use. It is critical to tailor the definition of UDEs to one's purpose in examining a drug's undesirable effects.

For the physician managing the patient the broadest definition of a UDE might apply. During drug therapy, any event unacceptable to either the patient or physician can be viewed as an adverse experience. Examples include a patient's proclivity to abuse a particular agent, intolerance of fully expected adverse effects, and even therapeutic failure.

Research efforts to determine a drug's safety profile, however, require a more precise definition of outcome. One simple classification, proposed by Rawlins, categorizes events as type A or type B reactions.[2] Type A reactions are those consistent with the agent's pharmacology, are commonly occurring, usually dose-dependent, and fairly predictable. Type B reactions represent allergic and idiosyncratic reactions to the drug and are independent of its pharmacologic action. These occurrences are rare, not dose-related, and cannot be predicted. Other classifications are available.[3-5] The choice of one to employ in any research protocol will be determined by the study design and the availability of data.

There can never be an absolute guarantee of drug safety but it is important to determine how much safety information is necessary, when it should be required in the process of drug development, and how much this knowledge will cost. The probable timing of UDE detection is discussed in the following sections (Table 1).

Premarketing Clinical Research

Premarketing clinical research (Phases I–III) should define all common unfavorable dose-related drug effects, whether or not they are predictable on the basis of the drug's pharmacology. These effects are likely to be exhibited with varying intensity in most patients. Allergic or idiosyncratic reactions, because they occur so infrequently, have little likelihood of detection during the premarketing phase, as discussed in Chapter 1. Other UDEs unlikely to emerge prior to marketing include those (1) that occur rarely (1 in 10 000–1 in 100 000), (2) require a long induction period, or (3) result from a specific interaction with personal characteristics, concurrent disease, or concomitant drug therapies. This lack of detection is a consequence of the five "too's" of premarketing drug evaluation: too few, too simple, too median-aged, too narrow, and too brief.

Too Few: The number of people exposed to a drug prior to its approval in the U.S. is usually less than 2000. However, to have a 95 percent probability of detecting an adverse medical event that an investigational drug is suspected of producing once in every 10 000 exposed persons, the drug experience of 30 000 individuals would have to be studied. To accept a reduced probability of 80 percent still requires the evaluation of 16 000 drug exposures (see Chapter 1). In fact, with the 2000 or so exposed persons commonly studied, the risk of the UDE associated with the drug exposure would have to be substantial for it to be detected prior to marketing (e.g., the investigational drug would have to increase about 13 times the risk of a medical event that would normally occur in the population once per 1000 individuals to be detected with 95 percent probability). Thus, to establish drug safety to this extent prior to marketing would entail prohibitive expense and usually is not feasible.

Too Simple: Because an ineffective drug, however safe, is useless, the primary objective of premarketing studies is the determination of efficacy. Patients with complicated medical conditions or receiving concurrent drug therapies usually are excluded from premarketing studies to simplify the evaluation of drug efficacy.

Too Median-Aged: The very young and the very old are rarely represented in clinical trials. Once marketed, the agent will be prescribed to both groups if there is a perceived need.

Too Narrow: The indications for which an investigational drug is employed are specified and well defined in all study protocols. Once a drug is marketed, however, it may be used for other related conditions for which the risk-benefit ratio can be radically different.

Too Brief: UDEs that occur after years of chronic therapy with an agent or that require an extended induction period after a single exposure (e.g., vaginal carcinoma after intrauterine exposure to diethylstilbestrol) cannot be known when a drug is approved for marketing.

In summary, then, the only safety information that is definitively available at the time a drug is approved for marketing consists of a frequency description of expected side effects, dose-related toxicity information from dosing studies (Phase I), and the toxicologic, teratogenic, and carcinogenic evaluations in animals. (The extent, duration, and number of animal studies performed depends on the expected length of therapy with the drug, its proposed indication, and characteristics of the target population. Positive findings in animal studies can indict the drug, but negative studies can never fully guarantee the drug's safety.) If serious UDEs exist, the ones with any reasonable probability of detection by this stage of limited drug use are those that occur commonly. For a drug frequently exhibiting serious UDEs to reach this stage of approval, a special case must exist. Such situations include treatment of uniformly fatal diseases for which there are no therapeutic alternatives or serious diseases in which the new drug represents a demonstrated improvement in safety.

There are two cases in which these data limitations should be addressed before the drug is brought to market: when the drug is indicated for use in a highly prevalent disease and large subsets of people with unusual genetic and physical characteristics may be treated, and when the drug is indicated for use in medically complicated populations. It is essential that the occurrence of occasional serious

Table 1
Probable Timing of Unintended Drug Effect Detection

If a UDE exists:
Increasing probability of detection ————————————————————→

——————Premarketing evaluation——————			Approval marketing	——————Postmarketing evaluation——————		
Phase I 3 years normal volunteers	**Phase II** 3 years selected patients	**Phase III** 4 years multicenter patients		**Phase IV-A** 2 years preliminary experience in limited populations	**Phase IV-B** 8 years routine use in general population	**Phase IV-C** > 10 years chronic effects and dose accumulation

expected adverse effects

limited dose-related toxicity from dose-finding studies

toxicity/overdose experience*

excessive pharmacologic effects in some patients*

unexpected, unintended effects in some patients*

allergic or hypersensitivity events in a few patients*
idiosyncratic events in a few patients

cancer, other chronic diseases

*Detection will always be a function of the size of the population exposed and the true rate of the UDE of interest.

events (1 in 100–1 in 500) be clinically proven unlikely to occur in the target populations or, if demonstrated, be worth the risk given the expected benefit. Therefore, if either of these cases hold, Phase III trials should widen the detection net by increasing the numbers and/or medical complexity of enrollees.

It is unlikely that other, more infrequent UDEs, if they exist, will be observed at this stage of limited exposure. The detection of these events will occur after the drug is marketed and used for extended periods of time in larger numbers of patients of all ages with more complicated disease states.

Postmarketing Surveillance of Drug Safety

THE SPONTANEOUS REPORTING SYSTEM

After drug marketing, safety data are collected from spontaneous reporting and formal research projects. The Spontaneous Reporting System (SRS) in the U.S. is maintained by the Food and Drug Administration (FDA). Case reports of UDEs are received directly from health professionals or indirectly through pharmaceutical manufacturers. The SRS may serve as an early warning system for serious UDEs but depends on voluntary professional reporting. In 1982, the rate of UDE reports in the U.S. was 57.6 per 1000 physicians; this is one-third to one-half the report rate in Canada, New Zealand, the United Kingdom, Sweden, and Denmark.[6] For the system to be an effective sentinel, practicing clinicians must be aware of it, have the means of reporting (this includes ease of access and convenience), and be willing to participate. The degree of underreporting in the U.S. attests that these conditions are not being met.

Rossi and Knapp examined the sources of spontaneous reports received in 1970 and their influence on subsequent labeling changes for the drug.[7] Of the nearly 18 000 reports received by the FDA during 1970 from all sources (including manufacturers, physicians and other professionals, and hospitals), 17 of these were ultimately incorporated into the labeling information for the drug in the 1980 *Physicians' Desk Reference* (PDR). They found that manufacturers submitted nearly 10 000 of the reports in 1970 and, of these, 7 resulted in labeling changes in the 1980 *PDR*. Due most assuredly to the efforts of pharmacists, hospitals submitted 7500 reports in 1970 and these resulted in 35 percent of all subsequent labeling changes by 1980. Although it represented about 1 percent of all spontaneous reports received in 1970, direct reporting by physicians and other health professionals accounted for 24 percent of all labeling changes in the 1980 *PDR*. On the basis of this study, it appears that reporting by this last group may represent the most efficient and productive approach to early detection of serious events. The FDA is sponsoring pilot studies of physician behavior, knowledge, and attitudes about the SRS in an effort to devise innovative methods that encourage physician reporting. Milstien et al. have demonstrated that pharmacists play an important role in encouraging direct physician reporting to the FDA.[8]

For the SRS to function effectively, it must be selective in data collection. It should focus on serious UDEs that cause new hospitalizations, prolong current hospitalizations, are associated with a congenital anomaly, cause cancer, or lead to death. Events that are serious clinical conditions (e.g., drug-induced liver disease or renal impairment) not meriting hospitalization under new regulations should also be reported. Of all these events, the two that should be the most difficult for the individual physician to detect would be congenital anomalies and cancers, because considerable time must elapse between drug exposure and clinical outcome. Further, it is not important for the physician to be convinced that the suspected drug was implicated in the untoward event (although certain circumstances to be reviewed later must hold). If the system is operating effectively, it is the frequency and the pattern of these kinds of events that signal the need for closer examination. Thus, every serious UDE should be reported, whether it is documented in the literature or not, because no one physician would be in a position to detect trends in the frequency or nature of rare events.

If reports are received in a timely manner, appropriate action can occur more quickly. Should a specific drug be implicated in producing serious reactions, other individuals can be spared a similar fate. It remains crucial, however, that the anecdotal reports generated by this system never assume more importance than they merit, because many require verification and some may be no more than false positive reports. Venning assessed the validity of all suspected UDEs reported in four major medical journals in 1963 to determine what proportion was ultimately verified 18 years later.[9] Ten percent of the 52 UDE articles were planned scientific studies; the remaining 90 percent consisted of anecdotal reports. Three of the four anecdotal reports ultimately proved correct in their assertion of a drug-event association (28 of 35 demonstrating satisfactory evidence at the time of publication). Seven of the remaining 19 have since been satisfactorily verified, leaving 12 with unclear status. Eight of these 12 were rare clinical events (7 hematologic) which may represent conditions with such extremely low incidences that similar cases have not yet occurred or been reported. The other four involve the association between frequently used drugs and common clinical syndromes and would require epidemiologic evaluation not yet performed. With varying probabilities corresponding to the evidence in each case, there also exists the possibility that all 12 may represent false positive reports. No reason exists to assume that the nature of reports in the FDA system is any different from that of these published reports. Indeed, without the editorial filter that journals provide and adequate government staffing to pursue missing data, the quality of the reports is probably worse. Yet, despite its limitations, the SRS may be the only affordable system for detecting rare and serious UDEs and attempts to improve its functioning are necessary. The contribution of the pharmacist in monitoring, collecting, and reporting the UDE of drug therapy is a vitally important component of the SRS.

FORMAL POSTMARKETING PROJECTS

Event Monitoring. Formal postmarketing research projects can differ in nature according to the time period in which they are initiated. The purpose of projects that begin within the first three years is generally to collect information on the nature, severity, and incidence of UDEs in the general population and, in effect, to compensate for the premarketing study deficiencies discussed above. Although these studies have defined populations and specified exposures, the outcomes of interest are not limited to any one medical condition; rather they employ the "event-monitoring" approach of Inman. An outcome is defined as "any new diagnosis, unexpected deterioration, or improvement in a preexisting condition (whether or not related to the condition for which the drug has been prescribed), and any accident or any complaint of symptoms that were not present before the treatment was started."[10] Postmarketing surveillance projects employing this outcome definition were conducted in the evaluation of cimetidine in Great Britain[11,12] and in the U.S.[13] Obviously, a project that follows many patients and records all events over a long period is expensive, and the technical and statistical problems encountered in analysis of such data are formidable.

Every drug brought to market merits a systematic, thorough, and scientific review of unanswered safety questions. However, a large-scale evaluation of every marketed drug would be neither cost effective nor possible. Public health and clinical considerations may necessitate supplemental epidemiologic information on drug safety.[14,15]

The decision to perform an event-monitoring postmarketing study should result from a careful examination of these factors: (1) known safety information for the drug including animal data, premarketing clinical data, and evidence from population use in countries where the drug may already have been marketed; (2) prevalence and severity of the disease for which the drug is indicated and the probability of exposure; and (3) currently available treatment.

Specific Research Hypotheses. The other type of formal research project occurring after the drug is marketed and has been in general use for four or more years is designed to answer a specific research hypothesis. These drug safety questions are usually generated from case reports of UDEs associated with drug use and require validation by accepted epidemiologic methods. Such projects have a defined population, stated exposure criteria, and specific medical conditions of interest. Data from these studies produce incidence and risk estimates of specific UDEs with a given drug exposure. Safety information gathered is limited to the research questions posed but, if the study design and analysis are valid and the study has adequate statistical power, that information can be considered definitive as it relates to the specific question studied.

In summary, probable timing of the detection of any event depends on the size of the susceptible, exposed population and the rate of exposure as well as the true rate of the UDE itself. A drug's safety profile is dynamic rather than static; it may be modified as the drug is used to treat different conditions, or is used in combination with new or unusual therapies. The natural history of its original indication may change and thereby alter the risk-benefit ratio for the drug's use.

Attribution

Judgments about attribution can be no better than the data supporting them. A comprehensive UDE report should contain information specific to the event, the drug, and the patient (Table 2). Information on demographics, concurrent disease, and concomitant drug therapy permits the examination of risk in particular subsets. Information on dose, duration, and route gives an indication of any dose-response relationship. An examination of the event itself may elucidate the pharmacologic mechanism of action for the adverse experience and demonstrate any necessary induction time.

For those planning to submit the UDE for publication as a case report, Soffer lists the following additional necessary information: the individual's prior adverse experiences with drugs of similar class, ancillary information from pharmaceutical manufacturers and regulatory agencies, and data on any previous publications relating to the same or similar events.[16]

Determining the exact role a drug plays in a UDE can become a difficult process of sorting out the effects of the disease being treated, other therapies, and the influence of lifestyle (e.g., smoking, obesity, alcoholism). Numerous algorithms have been devised to aid in this determination, and they propose that certain common criteria be applied to clinical situations to assess causation.[4,5,17]

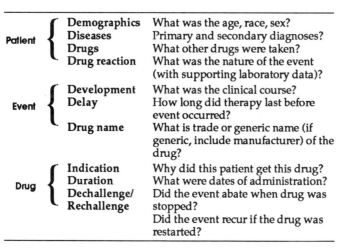

Patient	Demographics	What was the age, race, sex?
	Diseases	Primary and secondary diagnoses?
	Drugs	What other drugs were taken?
	Drug reaction	What was the nature of the event (with supporting laboratory data)?
Event	Development	What was the clinical course?
	Delay	How long did therapy last before event occurred?
	Drug name	What is trade or generic name (if generic, include manufacturer) of the drug?
Drug	Indication	Why did this patient get this drug?
	Duration	What were dates of administration?
	Dechallenge/ Rechallenge	Did the event abate when drug was stopped? Did the event recur if the drug was restarted?

Table 2
Information Required in a Comprehensive Unintended Drug Effect Report

In routine clinical practice, causality can be assumed when these criteria are met:

1. Timing: The event occurred after an appropriate interval and was consistent with pharmacologic and pharmacokinetic parameters of the drug.
2. Dose: The intensity of the event was related to the dose or serum concentration of the drug. Serum concentrations were higher than predicted based on dose.
3. Nature: The character of the UDE is consistent or predictable based on the pharmacology of the drug; i.e., it is a known or predictable response to the drug.
4. Experience: Events of this nature have previously been reported in the literature.
5. Dechallenge/Rechallenge: The event abated when the drug was withdrawn. It recurred if the drug was restarted.
6. Alternative etiologies: The effects of the disease being treated, other therapies being employed, or the influence of lifestyle could be responsible for the event.

Although these criteria appear clear and direct, their application in the clinical situation is not always manageable. Data on the influence of such other factors as interactions with other drugs or lifestyle characteristics are often unavailable. Therefore, most algorithms weigh the evidence supporting various factors and score the event as possible, probable, or definite, based on the examining clinician's assessment.

Causation judgments based on epidemiologic evidence accumulated in well-designed case control or cohort studies rely on these accepted criteria:[18]

1. Strength of the association: What value is the relative risk estimate derived from the study and what values are bounded by the associated confidence intervals?
2. Specificity of the association: Does this medical event occur frequently and has it been linked to other, perhaps multiple, causes? Alternatively, the association is more likely to be real when the outcome event is a specific form of medical condition; e.g., a site- and histological-specific cancer is a more credible candidate than a drug association with cancer in general.
3. Consistency of the association: Does the association between drug and event remain the same when different subgroups of the study population are examined? It may be true that a particular subset is at greater risk or the only group at risk, but this is a conclusion that can only be reached if it can be determined that the increased risk in that particular subset is not due to an extraneous factor operating only in that subset.
4. Dose response: When controlled for all other factors, if the dose is increased does the intensity and/or frequency of the UDE increase in the population?

5. Biologic plausibility: Are there experimental or animal data that support the cause and effect link?

6. Concordance among investigators: Do all epidemiologic investigations concur on the presence, direction, and strength of the drug-event relationship?

Often, the event does not emerge from a controlled observational study, but rather is reported as a single occurrence demanding a regulatory response. In this situation, it is imperative to obtain as detailed and comprehensive a report as possible on the individual case and evaluate the type of evidence provided. In the absence of valid epidemiologic data from controlled studies, Venning proposes using the following criteria to develop operating guidelines for regulatory agencies deciding on the drug-event link: (1) rechallenge data, (2) experimental data demonstrating mechanisms of pathogenesis, (3) immediate and acute UDEs, (4) local reactions at the site of administration, (5) a first report of reaction with a new route previously recognized with another method of administration, and (6) repeated occurrence of rare events.[9] Given these types of evidence, regulators must weigh the nature of the event: Is it reversible and at what cost? Does it result in permanent disability or death? They must estimate the incidence of the event and the proportion of the population who may be exposed: How many individuals could experience this event? They must evaluate the contribution this agent makes to the overall treatment of the disorder for which it is indicated: Is this the only drug available or one of many? All these factors must be carefully considered in deciding on regulatory action.

Summary

Attempts to strengthen the Spontaneous Reporting System and new methods for examining drug safety after marketing may be useful in preventing unnecessary delay in the public availability of new and efficacious agents while fulfilling safety requirements. At the same time, examination of past drug safety issues has clarified the type of evidence required to link event with drug. Certainly no one believes a drug could and therefore should be certified as safe before human use. Given the new appreciation of the limits of our knowledge about a drug's safety at any point of its temporal evolution, the current task is to make wise decisions about drug safety evaluation that safeguard the public health, provide physicians with therapeutic options, and secure industry investment in necessary research.

References

1. Karch FE, Lasagna L. Adverse drug reactions: a critical review. *JAMA* 1975;234:1236-41.

2. Rawlins MD. Clinical pharmacology: adverse reactions to drugs. *Br Med J* 1981;282:974-6.

3. Koch-Weser J. Panel I: definition and classification of adverse drug reactions. *Drug Inf Bull* 1968:72-8.

4. Karch FE, Lasagna L. Toward the operational identification of adverse drug reactions. *Clin Pharmacol Ther* 1977;21:247-54.

5. Kramer MS, Leventhal JM, Hutchinson TA, Feinstein AR. An algorithm for the operational assessment of adverse drug reactions. I. Background, description, and instructions for use. *JAMA* 1979;242:623-32.

6. Griffin JP, Weber JCP. Voluntary systems of adverse reaction reporting—part II. *Adverse Drug React Acute Poisoning Rev* 1986;1:23-55.

7. Rossi AC, Knapp DE. Discovery of new adverse drug reactions: a review of the Food and Drug Administration's spontaneous reporting system. *JAMA* 1984;252:1030-3.

8. Milstien JB, Faich GA, Hsu JP, Knapp DE, Baum C, Dreis MW. Factors affecting physician reporting of adverse drug reactions. *Drug Inf J* 1986;20:157-64.

9. Venning GR. Validity of anecdotal reports of suspected adverse drug reactions: the problem of false alarms. *Br Med J* 1982;284:249-52.

10. Inman WHW. Postmarketing surveillance of adverse drug reactions in general practice. II: Prescription-event monitoring at the University of Southampton. *Br Med J* 1981;282:1216-7.

11. Colin-Jones DG, Langman MJS, Lawson DH, Vessey MP. Postmarketing surveillance of the safety of cimetidine: 12 month mortality report. *Br Med J* 1983;286:1713-6.

12. Colin-Jones DG, Langman MJS, Lawson DH, Vessey MP. Postmarketing surveillance of the safety of cimetidine: mortality during second, third, and fourth years of follow up. *Br Med J* 1985;291:1084-8.

13. Gifford LM, Aeugle ME, Myerson RM, Tannenbaum PJ. Cimetidine postmarket outpatient surveillance program: interim report on phase I. *JAMA* 1980;243:1532-5.

14. Rogers AS, Tilson H. Postmarketing surveillance: the sponsor's viewpoint. Proceedings of the annual meeting of the Drug Information Association, San Diego, CA: June 17-21, 1984:101-5.

15. Rogers AS, Porta MS, Tilson H. Postmarketing surveillance of drugs: decision-making based on expert consensus (abstract no. 1573). Third World Conference on Clinical Pharmacology and Therapeutics, Stockholm, Sweden: July 26-August 1, 1986.

16. Soffer A. The practitioner's role in detection of adverse drug reactions (editorial). *Arch Intern Med* 1985;145:232-3.

17. Naranjo CA, Busto U, Sellers EM, et al. A method for estimating the probability of adverse drug reactions. *Clin Pharmacol Ther* 1981;30:239-45.

18. Lilienfeld AM, Lilienfeld DE. Foundations of epidemiology. Oxford: Oxford University Press, 1980:289-321.

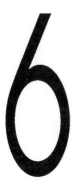

Causality Assessment for Unintended Drug Effects

David A. Lane

Abstract

This chapter presents the elements of a quantitative approach to causality assessment, based on the use of subjective probability. Causality assessment problems are typically complex and fraught with uncertainty. Qualitative causality assessment methods (e.g., global introspection) and standardized assessment methods (which range from simple flowcharts to lengthy questionnaires) are reviewed. The role of subjective probability and the use of Bayes' theorem are justified, and a strategy based on the following steps is proposed: (1) decompose the causality assessment problem into subproblems, each of which is accessible to the knowledge and experience of the assessor; (2) express the assessor's uncertainty about the solutions to the subproblems in quantitative form, as subjective probabilities; (3) use the rules of probability theory to merge the solutions to these subproblems into a coherent solution to the overall causality assessment problem. Steps to implement the strategy are shown. Finally, technical issues, such as handling multiple drugs, missing information, conditioning and decomposition, and estimating prior odds, are presented.

Outline

A patient takes a drug and subsequently experiences an unintended drug effect (UDE). Did the drug cause the event to happen? Answering this question is the goal of causality assessment. Causality assessment plays a role in clinical decision making, in the discovery of previously unsuspected UDEs, in pharmacoepidemiology, and in liability litigation. General discussions of causality assessment and its applications can be found in Venulet et al.,[1] Herman,[2] Jones and Herman,[3] Stephens,[4] and Lane.[5]

This chapter presents the elements of a quantitative approach to causality assessment, based on the use of subjective probability. This approach is introduced, discussed, and illustrated in Auriche,[6] Lane et al.,[7,8] Jones and Herman,[3] and Lane.[5]

To appreciate the advantages of the probabilistic approach to causality assessment, it is important first to consider what makes causality assessment problems difficult and then to see that alternative existing methods of causality assessment fail to address these difficulties.

Why is Causality Assessment Difficult?

There are two features of causality assessment problems that contribute substantially to their difficulty: they are typically complex and they are fraught with uncertainty. Consider the following example, paraphrased from a report submitted to the manufacturer of one of the drugs.[9]

EXAMPLE 1

A 42-year-old woman was found dead in her home in the evening following a 1 p.m. appointment with her dentist for a wisdom tooth extraction. The woman had been taking propranolol for high blood pressure, but was reportedly otherwise in good health. The dentist related that she had given a history of heart murmur on her previous visit and that he had instructed her to take two penicillin V tablets one hour before her appointment; she gave no history of drug allergy. Prior to the oral surgery, she had an injection of xylocaine. The extraction procedure lasted 40 minutes. She was instructed to go home and rest and was given a prescription for five zomepirac tablets 100 mg q4–6h prn for pain. She was also instructed to continue the penicillin for one day. Filled prescriptions for zomepirac, penicillin V, and propranolol were found in her home. Autopsy revealed pulmonary congestion and some hyperinflation, along with evidence of laryngeal edema and swelling of the extremities. An analysis of the stomach contents revealed no drugs associated with abuse, such as narcotics, amphetamines, or barbiturates. The coroner estimated the time of death as 4:00 pm ± 2 hours.

COMPLEXITY

Was the woman's death caused by a drug? If so, which one? Several factors have evidentiary significance for the causality assessment problem. First, there are several possible causes of the woman's death to consider, including the fact that three of the drugs mentioned in the report can cause sudden death from anaphylaxis (xylocaine, penicillin, and zomepirac). Second, there are details of the patient's history (her high blood pressure and history of heart murmur) that may have placed her at special risk for possible nondrug causes of death. The fact that she was taking propranolol may have increased the chance that she suffered an immunologic reaction to the other drugs. The relation between the time at which she took the various drugs and when she died also may provide evidence about what killed her, as may the autopsy findings.

To interpret the evidence provided by each of these factors, the assessor can access relevant information obtained from many different sources: observations and findings for the particular case at hand, his or her own previous clinical experience, other case reports and epidemiologic studies, and facts and theories derived from pharmacology and other basic sciences. The quality of the data derived from these different sources can vary enormously, from "relatively hard" to "very soft."

UNCERTAINTY

The assessor cannot know all the relevant information with certainty. In particular, this report leaves out some of the most important facts of the case: Did the woman actually take the zomepirac (nobody seems to have counted how many pills were left)? If so, when? Exactly when did she die? In addition, the assessor may be uncertain about background information that affects how the facts of the case are interpreted. For example, what is the incidence of anaphylaxis due to penicillin? To zomepirac? To xylocaine? Is there any mechanism other than anaphylaxis whereby any of the drugs could cause sudden death? What other causes of sudden death are consistent with the findings in this case?

In summary, to solve causality assessment problems, it is necessary to weigh information about a variety of factors coming from a variety of sources, and in the presence of a large amount of residual uncertainty, to arrive at an overall measure of how plausible it is that a particular drug caused the UDE in question.

Qualitative Causality Assessment Methods

GLOBAL INTROSPECTION

The usual approach to a causality assessment problem is to refer it to an expert, who solves it by an act of global introspection. That is, the expert collects all the facts that are relevant to the problem, mixes them together, and then decides what the answer is. In the causality assessment context, this answer usually is expressed in terms of a qualitative probability scale: for example, "definite," "probable," "possible," "doubtful," or "unrelated."

Unfortunately, global introspection does not work well. Cognitive psychologists have shown that the ability of the human brain to make unaided assessments of uncertainty in complicated situations is poor, especially when assessing the probability of a cause given an effect, precisely the task of causality assessment.[10] In fact, several groups of clinical pharmacologists have demonstrated how unreliable global introspection is as a causality assessment method, by comparing their individual evaluations of a series of suspected UDEs and documenting the extent of their disagreement.[11-13] Another problem with global introspection is that it is uncalibrated: one assessor's "possible" might mean the same thing as another assessor's "probable." Other shortcomings of global introspection as a causality assessment method are discussed in Lane[14] and Kramer.[15]

STANDARDIZED ASSESSMENT METHODS

Because of the difficulties with global introspection, during the past decade much effort has been devoted to developing decision aids for causality assessment. Physicians from industry, regulatory agencies, and academia now have published more than a dozen standardized assessment methods (SAMs).[1,2,4,16]

These methods range from simple flowcharts posing 10 or fewer questions to lengthy questionnaires containing up to 84 items. However, they share a common basic structure. They divide the considerations that bear on causality assessment into a number of factors or axes: for example, the timing of the UDE in relation to administration of the drug; alternative etiologic candidates; previous recognition of the event as a possible adverse reaction to the drug; the response when the drug is discontinued (dechallenge) and when the drug is subsequently readministered (rechallenge). Information relevant to each factor is elicited by a series of questions, the answers to which are restricted to yes/no/(and for some methods) do not know. The answers to these questions then are converted to a score for each factor, the factor scores are summed, and this overall score is converted into a value on a qualitative probability scale.

Although SAMs have advantages compared with global introspection,[14] they are not free from criticism. Some experts in UDEs complain that SAMs, with their preset series of questions and limited range of possible answers, are too inflexible to deal with all the kinds of evidence that may differentiate between drug and non-drug causation.[17] In particular, SAMs cannot handle uncertainty about the facts of a case, such as whether or not the woman in Example 1 actually took zomepirac. Moreover, even adherents of SAMs agree that their procedures for converting answers into probability ratings are arbitrary.

The following hypothetical example points out a more serious difficulty with SAMs: in situations in which quantitative probability calculations are appropriate, the methods give answers that contradict the results of these calculations.

EXAMPLE 2

An analgesic (D) commonly is taken to relieve pain associated with influenza (M). Data from a large epidemiologic study indicate that about one in eight patients who take D subsequently experience nausea (E); one in ten patients who do not take D experience nausea due to their influenza. The mechanism of D-induced nausea is well understood, and it implies that such nausea always occurs within one hour of drug administration. On the other hand, M-caused nausea may occur any time within two days following the onset of M.

Problem: A patient takes D as soon as the symptoms of M begin and becomes nauseated within 45 minutes. What is the chance that the nausea is D-induced?

Solution: Bayes' theorem can be applied to solve this problem. Let B represent the background incidences reported above, and Ti the fact that the nausea occurred in the first hour after administration of D. Then:

$$\frac{P(\text{D caused E} \mid \text{B, Ti})}{P(\text{M caused E} \mid \text{B, Ti})} = \frac{P(\text{D caused E} \mid \text{B})}{P(\text{M caused E} \mid \text{B})} \cdot \frac{P(\text{Ti} \mid \text{D caused E, B})}{P(\text{Ti} \mid \text{M caused E, B})}$$

$$= \frac{1/5}{4/5} \cdot \frac{1}{1/48} \qquad \text{Eq. 1}$$

$$= 12$$

That is, using the odds to probability transformation (Appendix I):

$$P(\text{D caused E} \mid \text{B, Ti}) = \frac{12}{13} = 0.92 \qquad \text{Eq. 2}$$

The evaluations of $P(\text{D caused E} \mid \text{B})$ and $P(\text{M caused E} \mid \text{B})$ follow from the epidemiologic data. That is, assuming that the incidence of M-caused nausea is the same among those patients who take D and those who do not, $1/8 - 1/10 = 1/40$ of the influenza patients taking D suffer from D-induced nausea, and $1/10$ suffer from M-caused nausea. Thus, $1/5$ of the nausea suffered by influenza patients taking D is caused by D. The evaluations of $P(\text{Ti} \mid \text{M caused E, B})$ and $P(\text{Ti} \mid \text{M caused E, B})$ follow from the given timing information. All D-induced nausea begins in the first hour after administration, so $P(\text{Ti} \mid \text{D caused E, B}) = 1$. Assuming a uniform distribution for onset of M-caused nausea over the assumed two-day vulnerable period, only $1/48$ of the M-caused nausea begins in the first hour, therefore $P(\text{Ti} \mid \text{M caused E, B}) = 1/48$.

INCONSISTENCY BETWEEN SAMs AND BAYES' THEOREM

When SAMs are applied to this case, they yield answers ranging from "doubtful" to "possible," much too conservative to characterize a quantitative probability of 0.92. There are several reasons for this inconsistency. First, SAMs do not allow sharp information about a single factor (in this case, timing) to override neutral or weakly negative data relating to other factors (e.g., the absence of dechallenge and rechallenge information, or the existence of an alternative etiologic candidate, M). Second, SAMs do not directly compare how consistent the observed data are with each alternative etiology, while Bayes' theorem measures the evidence in each piece of data by its relative plausibility, given each competing etiological hypothesis. Finally, SAMs do not process quantitative evidence directly, so that the strength of the evidence about timing and about background incidences in the example cannot be adequately assessed. Hutchinson and Lane provided further discussion of the weaknesses of SAMs.[18]

The Role of Subjective Probability

PROBABILITY, FREQUENCIES, AND COHERENCE

The key to the solution of Example 2 is the use of Bayes' theorem, which isolates the separate effects of the two sources of evidence, B and Ti, and determines how the given information from each of these sources is converted into the appropriate measure of evidence for (or against) D-causation. What justifies this use of Bayes' theorem? The axioms of probability theory and, hence, Bayes' theorem hold for relative frequencies in finite populations. At first glance, the calculation seems to be about such frequencies: the calculation determines only what fraction of patients suffer D-induced nausea among all patients with influenza who take D and become nauseated within one hour.

However, a closer look makes it clear that more than information about frequencies is involved in assessing and interpreting the probabilities that appear in Equation 1. First, the probabilities for Ti are calculated conditionally on unobserved causes, so they could not be based directly on observed frequencies; in fact, the probability given D-causation derives from a model for the mechanism whereby D causes nausea. Second, the probabilities appearing on the left side of Equation 1 refer only to the patient being discussed. The relevance of the given frequency information (used in evaluating the first ratio on the right of Equation 1) follows from a judgment by the assessor that this patient is fungible with those on whom the frequency information is available. If, for example, the assessor learns that this patient had had nausea within two hours of his five previous influenza attacks when he did not take D, the questions posed by the probabilities on the left of Equation 1 still have meaning, but the frequencies given by the background incidence figures are no longer directly relevant. In fact, all the probabilities that appear in Equation 1 refer to the case at hand, and they can be interpreted reasonably only as measures of the assessor's degree of belief, even though frequencies may be used to help assess some of them.

If Equation 1 is interpreted as a statement of subjective probability, the ratio on the left side represents the assessor's odds in favor of D-causation for the case at hand, which is what the assessor must evaluate to solve the causality assessment problem.[19,20] The first ratio on the right side of Equation 1 represents the assessors' odds in favor of D-causation, not taking into account just when the nausea occurred. The second represents the ratio between her probability that D-induced nausea would happen in the first hour and her evaluation of the same probability for M-induced nausea. The probabilities in the latter two ratios now are easy for her to evaluate, using the given information (and her judgment of fungibility between this patient and the patients to whom the frequency information refers). The laws of probability presented in Appendix I tell the assessor that there is only one possible relationship between the opinions expressed in the two ratios that are easy to evaluate and the ratio she wants, her odds in favor of D-causation taking into account when the nausea occurred. That relationship follows from Bayes' theorem and is given by Equation 1. Thus, the assessor should use Equation 1 to determine her solution to the causality assessment problem. If she evaluates it differently, she is, in effect, expressing an opinion that contradicts her own, better-founded beliefs.

It is a psychological fact that not all uncertainty is easy to measure in probability terms. On the other hand, as the solution to Example 2 indicates, some probabilities are easy to assess. The advantage of a probabilistic approach to problems like causality assessment is that the rules of probability theory can be used to relate the probabilities you want to assess to probabilities that available information makes it possible (even easy) for you to assess.

COHERENCE AND CAUSALITY ASSESSMENT

These considerations suggest the following strategy for a solution to the causality assessment problem based on subjective probability:

1. Decompose the causality assessment problem into subproblems, each of which is accessible to the knowledge and experience of the assessor.
2. Express the assessor's uncertainty about the solutions to the subproblems in quantitative form, as subjective probabilities.
3. Use the rules of probability theory to merge the solutions to these subproblems into a coherent solution to the overall causality assessment problem.

The first step in implementing this strategy is to define the goal of causality assessment in probabilistic terms. This is accomplished by the following expression, called the posterior odds in favor of D-causation:

$$\frac{P(D \to E \mid B, C)}{P(D \nrightarrow E \mid B, C)} \qquad \text{Eq. 3}$$

where E is a UDE suffered by a particular patient, and D is a drug expected to cause E. The proposition $D \to E$ (D caused E) means that E would not have happened as and when it did had D not been administered (i.e., D is a necessary, but not necessarily sufficient, cause of E). $D \nrightarrow E$ denies that $D \to E$. B represents background information, including everything the assessor knows about the connection between the drug D and events similar to E (from his own clinical experience, published case series and epidemiologic studies, facts and theories from pharmacology, and other basic sciences). The only case-specific information in B is the proposition that a patient with a specified clinical condition M who has been administered D in a specified way subsequently develops a UDE of type E_t. (M and E_t, discussed in the next section, are generic characterizations describing essential elements of the patient's condition and the event E, respectively.) C represents case information: details about the particular patient and his UDE E.

Just as in the solution to Example 2, Bayes' theorem can be applied to the posterior odds to yield the following equation:

$$\underbrace{\frac{P(D \to E \mid B, C)}{P(D \not\to E \mid B, C)}}_{\text{posterior odds}} = \underbrace{\frac{P(D \to E_t \mid B)}{P(D \not\to E_t \mid B)}}_{\text{prior odds}} \cdot \underbrace{\frac{P(C \mid D \to E, B)}{P(C \mid D \not\to E, B)}}_{\text{likelihood ratio}} \qquad \text{Eq. 4}$$

Both the posterior and prior odds are calculated conditionally on B and so refer to a patient with clinical condition M who has been given D and experienced an event of type E_t. However, the identity of the patient to whom the two terms refer is different. In the posterior odds, it is the particular patient under review, whereas in the prior odds, it is a generic patient (perhaps the next patient) with the three defining characteristics M, D, and E_t. Thus, the prior odds can be regarded epidemiologically, as discussed below; on the other hand, the probabilities in the likelihood ratio involve thinking in terms of mechanism, arguing from cause to effect.

It is helpful to consider the information in C in chronological order. A typical chronological sequence is illustrated in Figure 1. The categories of case information include Hi, the patient's history antedating the onset of E; Ti, the timing of the onset of E in relation to the administration of D; Ch, characteristics of the event from time of onset to time of dechallenge, which can include information about duration, severity, evolution, and laboratory tests; De, response to dechallenge; and Re, response to rechallenge. The likelihood ratio (LR) is decomposed into factors corresponding to these chronological categories of case information:

$$LR = LR(Hi) \times LR(Ti) \times LR(Ch) \times LR(De) \times LR(Re) \qquad \text{Eq. 5}$$

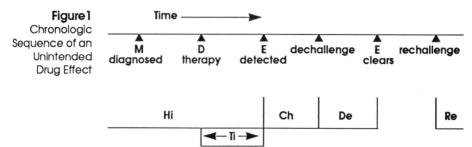

Figure 1
Chronologic Sequence of an Unintended Drug Effect

Ch = characteristics of E; D = suspected drug; De = dechallenge; E = unintended drug effect; Hi = patient's history; M = patient's condition; Re = rechallenge; Ti = timing of onset of E.

where, for example,

$$LR(Ti) = \frac{P(Ti \mid D \to E, B, Hi)}{P(Ti \mid D \nrightarrow E, B, Hi)}$$

Note that the probabilities that appear in each likelihood ratio factor are evaluated conditionally on B and all chronologically preceding case information.

In summary, then, the probabilistic approach to causality assessment is designed to calculate the posterior odds in favor of D-causation, by evaluating the subjective probabilities that appear in the prior odds and a series of likelihood ratio factors corresponding to chronological categories of case information.

Implementing the Probabilistic Approach

The probabilistic causality assessment outlined in this section is designed to elicit and process the opinions of assessors with medical or pharmacologic expertise. The method is illustrated by an analysis of a fairly simple case, based on assessments provided by Michael Kramer and Tom Hutchinson of the Departments of Pediatrics, Medicine, and Epidemiology and Biostatistics, McGill University. Further technical aspects of the method are discussed below. More details and examples can be found in Jones and Herman.[3]

EXAMPLE 3

On December 10, a 17-month-old boy who attends a daycare center developed signs and symptoms of an upper respiratory tract infection with rhinorrhea and cough, but without fever or gastrointestinal symptoms. On December 12, his temperature rose to 39.4 °C. He became irritable, and began to pull at his ears. He was seen by his pediatrician on that day and was diagnosed as having bilateral otitis media. Treatment was initiated with amoxicillin suspension 125 mg tid. Over the next 24 hours (December 13) the child had three watery bowel movements. By December 14, he was afebrile, and the diarrhea continued without exacerbation. The pediatrician suggested continuing the amoxicillin therapy as prescribed. From December 15 to 21, he remained afebrile and became less irritable and more playful, but the diarrhea persisted. On December 21, the amoxicillin was discontinued, and by December 23, the diarrhea had resolved.

IMPLEMENTATION STEP 1: DETERMINE THE CASE PARAMETERS (M, E$_f$, CAUSE LIST, TIME HORIZON)

The case parameters establish the context in which the assessment is carried out. M and E$_t$ create an epidemiologic reference set for the patient under consideration; the cause list specifies the alternative etiologic candidates; and the time horizon determines a period of time to which all considerations about drug-event connection are restricted.

M and E_t. E_t specifies the general type of the UDE E, and M abstracts out the most important aspects of the patient's condition that determine his risk for events of type E_t from causes other than the drug under consideration. It is important to define these parameters as explicitly as possible.

Sometimes there will be a question about whether to include certain aspects of the patient's condition or the event in the definitions of these parameters or in the appropriate chronological category of case information. The choice should be guided by the ease of the ensuing assessments and so depends on the assessor's experience and information. Roughly, the assessor should choose definitions for M and E_t that make it easiest to "think epidemiologically" about the class determined by these definitions. Consistency is essential in the course of the assessment: M and E_t are included in B, the background information, and are part of the reference set for every calculation.

Cause List. The cause list consists of a set of mutually exclusive propositions about the possible causes of E. Typically, there are a number of possible hypotheses specifying drug causal candidates (e.g., $D_1, \ldots ,D_n$) followed by a number of hypotheses specifying nondrug causes.

The requirement that the propositions on the cause list be mutually exclusive is somewhat artificial and requires a bit of care in defining and interpreting the propositions. For example, if the assessor believes that an interaction between drugs D_A and D_B may have caused E, he should have a separate entry on the cause list for this interaction. If he also believes that either drug alone also may have caused E, he must include entries for D_A alone (i.e., E would have happened as and when it did had D_A and not D_B been given, but not if D_B and not D_A had been given) and D_B alone. Similarly, there is an asymmetry between drug and nondrug causes: because of the definition of the proposition D caused E for a possible drug case D, if N is a possible nondrug cause, the proposition that N caused E implies that E would have happened as and when it did had none of the drugs mentioned in $D_1, \ldots ,D_n$ been given. Finally, since causality assessment focuses on the question of drug responsibility, it is possible to combine different nondrug causes, as long as they give the same probability to each case datum that distinguishes drug from nondrug causation.

Time Horizon. B includes the assertion that a patient with condition M experiences an event of type E_t. The time horizon puts an upper limit on the length of time after D-therapy begins in which it is asserted that the event occurs. To choose the time horizon, the assessor should think about the distribution for the onset of an event of type E_t that is caused by D; the time horizon should be about as long as the support of this distribution. It is easy to see that, for a coherent assessor, the exact value selected will not affect the resulting posterior odds. The reason for specifying a time horizon is that doing so increases the accessibility of some of the assessment tasks (especially the prior odds and likelihood ratio for timing).

Case Parameters for Example 3

M: upper respiratory infection and otitis media in a 12- to 24-month-old child

E_t: diarrhea

Cause list:

1. Amoxicillin (D)

2. Late-occurring gastrointestinal symptoms secondary to the original infection (M)

3. Coincidental infectious gastroenteritis (CG)

Time horizon: one week

IMPLEMENTATION STEP 2: COLLECT THE CASE INFORMATION

All the information that can differentiate between drug and nondrug causation should be listed in the appropriate chronological category.

Case Information for Example 3

Hi: 1. Occurrence in December (the incidence of infectious gastroenteritis fluctuates seasonally, with highest rates in winter)

    2. Daycare-center attendance (the incidence of infectious gastroenteritis is higher among daycare-center attendees)

Ti: Onset one day following initiation of D

Ch: Diarrhea persisted nine days until dechallenge

De: Diarrhea resolved within 48 hours after dechallenge

IMPLEMENTATION STEP 3: EVALUATE THE PRIOR ODDS

According to Equation 4, the assessor can determine his value for the prior odds by answering the following question: Consider a class of patients with condition M who receive D and subsequently (within the time horizon) experience an event of type E_t. In which proportion of these patients is the event caused by D?

Alternatively, the assessor can consider the same problem from a prospective point of view. Imagine a large class of patients with M. Suppose that half of them are selected at random and receive D, while the rest receive some alternative therapy with the same beneficial effects D, but which cannot cause events of type E_t. Let $P(E_t \mid D)$ represent the assessor's estimate of the proportion of the patients who receive D that experience events of type E_t, and $P(E_t \mid D^c)$, his corresponding estimate for the proportion of those who do not receive D. Then, for this assessor:

$$\text{prior odds} = \frac{P(E_t \mid D) - P(E_t \mid D^c)}{P(E_t \mid D^c)} \qquad \textbf{Eq. 6}$$

Thus, one strategy for assessing prior odds is to use what information is available to evaluate the two quantities $P(E_t \mid D)$ and $P(E_t \mid D^c)$ as defined above, and then use Equation 6 to determine the prior odds. Often, the assessor's uncertainty about the incidences in this imaginary clinical trial is sufficiently diffuse that it is best to assess her subjective distributions for these quantities, and then evaluate the means of these distributions to plug into Equation 6. These distributions also are helpful if the assessor should choose to carry out a sensitivity analysis at the conclusion of her assessment. Some other considerations bearing on the prior odds are discussed in the next section.

Evaluating the Prior Odds for Example 3. The assessors employed the strategy based on Equation 6, using observed frequencies obtained from a study monitoring antibiotic-associated gastrointestinal symptoms in pediatric outpatients in Montreal. Some results from this study, but not the raw data we use, are presented by Kramer et al.[9,15] In addition, we use data from diarrhea surveillance studies reported by Bartlett et al.[21,22]

To Evaluate $P(E_t \mid D)$: In the Montreal study about ten percent of more than 1300 patients receiving amoxicillin suffered from diarrhea within a week of beginning therapy. The assessors evaluated: $P(E_t \mid D) = 0.10$.

To Evaluate $P(E_t \mid D^c)$: The assessors estimated this quantity in two different ways. First, in the Montreal study, the lower incidence of diarrhea followed trimethoprim/sulfamethoxazole therapy, and was about 2.5 percent in the first week of therapy. This drug usually is not considered to be associated with diarrhea, but some of this incidence may represent drug-induced diarrhea, so the assessors considered it appropriate to adjust this figure downward slightly.

The assessors also developed a lower-bound estimate for the incidence of non-drug-induced diarrhea, by thinking about the spontaneous occurrence of diarrhea in children not taking drugs prior to their diarrhea. They assumed that one- to two-year-old children experience approximately one such episode per year on average,[21] equivalent to an incidence (per child) of about 0.019 per week. This must be increased somewhat, because it is not conditional on the children having an infection (M), which increases the probability of developing diarrhea.

So, their estimate for the incidence (per child) of nondrug-induced diarrhea among children with M, in the week following initiation of amoxicillin therapy, is between 0.019 and 0.025. They adopted a value of 0.022: $P(E_t \mid D^c) = 0.022$.

To Evaluate the Prior Odds by Equation 6:

$$\text{prior odds} = \frac{P(E_t \mid D) - P(E_t \mid D^c)}{P(E_t \mid D^c)}$$

$$= \frac{0.01 - 0.022}{0.022} \qquad \text{Eq. 7}$$

$$= 3.5$$

Here are some consequences of the assessments above that will be used below. Denote with $P(E_M \mid B)$ and $(E_{CG} \mid B)$ the assessments for the incidence of diarrhea caused by M and by coincidental gastroenteritis, respectively. Then, from the assessments above, one can conclude that:

$$0.022 = P(E_t \mid D^c) = P(E_M \mid B) + P(E_{CG} \mid B) \qquad \text{Eq. 8}$$

and assuming that having M does not affect the chance of contracting a coincidental gastroenteritis,

$$0.019 = \{P(E_M \mid B) \bullet P(M)\} + P(E_{CG} \mid B) \qquad \text{Eq. 9}$$

Because $P(M)$, the weekly incidence of M among one- to two-year-old children is relatively small (certainly less than 10 percent), the following relations hold (up to rounding error):

$$P(E_M \mid B) = 0.003, P(E_{CG} \mid B) = 0.019,$$

$$P(M \to E \mid B, D \not\to E) = \frac{P(E_M \mid B)}{P(E_t \mid D^c)} = 0.14 \qquad \text{Eq. 10}$$

IMPLEMENTATION STEP 4: EVALUATE THE LIKELIHOOD RATIO FACTOR FOR HISTORY, LR(HI)

Information in Hi differs from the data in the other chronological categories in that it antedates the UDE E and, frequently, the administration of D as well. Thus, it is easier to evaluate LR(Hi) as an adjustment to the prior odds (by restricting the relevant reference class) than to evaluate the probabilities for the data in Hi given the possible causes of E.

Evaluating LR(Hi) for Example 3. Basing their evaluation on data in Bartlett et al., the assessors estimated that daycare-center attendees are 1.4 times as likely to suffer from nondrug-induced diarrhea as the general pediatric population, because of their greater exposure rate to infections. On the other hand, they are at no greater risk for drug-induced diarrhea (given M). Also, again based on data in Bartlett et al. and general pediatric experience, the incidence of nondrug-induced diarrhea is approximately twice as high in the winter as the yearly average, while there should be no seasonal effects for drug-caused diarrhea (again, given M).[22]

To calculate LR(Hi), the assessors first modified Equation 6 by conditioning the data in Hi to compute the odds in favor of D-causation posterior to Hi. Neither the numerator, the incidence of D-caused diarrhea, nor $P(E_M \mid B)$ change, given M. However, $P(E_{CG} \mid B)$ increases by a factor of $2 \times 1.4 = 2.8$. Thus:

$$P(E_t \mid B, Hi) = (0.14)(0.003) + (0.86)(0.019)(2.8) \qquad \text{Eq. 11}$$
$$= 0.046$$

therefore,

$$\text{posterior odds given history} = \frac{0.10 - 0.022}{0.046} \qquad \text{Eq. 12}$$
$$= 1.7$$

Finally, we can compute LR(Hi) as the ratio of the posterior odds given history and the prior odds:

$$LR(Hi) = \frac{1.7}{3.5} = 0.5$$ **Eq. 13**

IMPLEMENTATION STEP 5: EVALUATE THE REMAINING LIKELIHOOD RATIO FACTORS

The probability for each piece of case information must be evaluated, given each possible cause and all preceding data. Even though only the probability for the data actually observed plays a role in these likelihood ratio factors, to ensure meaningful and reliable results, it is important to evaluate these probabilities in their proper context. For example, for information that refers to timing (time to onset of E, duration of E before dechallenge, time of disappearance of E after dechallenge), it is best to construct entire timing distributions for the relevant events, as illustrated in the example below. Similar considerations hold for probabilities about the results of laboratory tests. Some formulas and techniques useful in assessing likelihood ratio factors are presented in the next section.

Evaluating Likelihood Ratio Factors for Example 3. All the information in Ti, Ch, and De concerns timing. Moreover, to the assessors, all the relevant timing distributions were judged to be independent of one another (i.e., given the cause of the diarrhea, knowing how long it takes it to develop would not affect the assessor's opinions about how long it might persist) and to be independent of the information in Hi.

LR(Ti): To assess LR(Ti), the assessors evaluated their distributions for the time to onset of diarrhea given each of the three listed causes. Recall that they are conditioning on the facts that no diarrhea was present until the amoxicillin was first administered and that diarrhea then appeared sometime within the next week (the

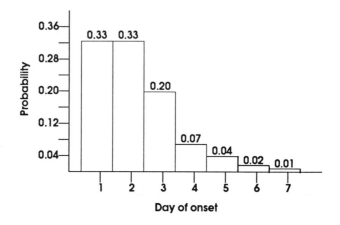

Figure 2
Time of Onset of
D-Induced Diarrhea

Probability

Day of onset

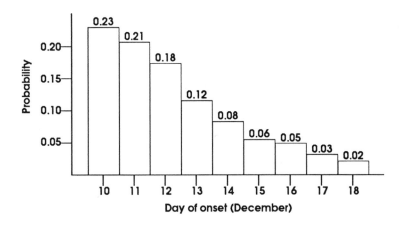

Figure 3
Time to Onset
of M-Induced
Diarrhea (from
December 10)

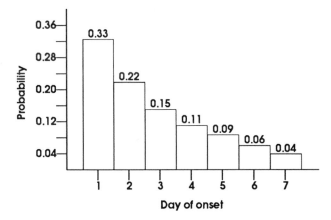

Figure 4
Time to Onset of
M-Induced Diarrhea

time horizon). Their timing distribution given drug causation is shown in Figure 2; it is based on the assumption that the mechanism for D-induced diarrhea is initiated by dose-dependent effects on gut flora and mucosal absorptive function.

The timing distribution for the onset of M-caused diarrhea is slightly more complicated to assess, because the reasonable time origin for such a distribution is the onset of M rather than administration of D. Thus, the assessors evaluated their distribution from this natural time origin (Figure 3), and then obtained the relevant distribution (Figure 4) by conditioning on diarrhea onset occurring after D-initiation (i.e., by truncating at December 12 and rescaling). The distribution for onset of diarrhea due to coincidental gastroenteritis is, of course, uniform over the relevant time period (Figure 5).

Using these distributions, LR(Ti) is evaluated as follows: Ti states that the diarrhea actually first occurred on the first day of D-therapy. So, $P(\text{Ti} \mid D \rightarrow E) = 0.33$.

By the law of total probability:

$$P(\text{Ti} \mid D \not\to E) = P(\text{Ti} \mid M \to E) \bullet P(M \to E \mid D \not\to E)$$
$$+ P(\text{Ti} \mid CG \to E) \bullet P(CG \to E \mid D \not\to E) \qquad \text{Eq. 14}$$
$$= (0.33)\,(0.14) + (0.14)\,(0.86)$$
$$= 0.17$$

Recall that the probability for M-causation given nondrug causation was calculated in the note following the evaluation of the prior. So:

$$\text{LR(Ti)} = \frac{P(\text{Ti} \mid D \to E)}{P(\text{Ti} \mid D \not\to E)} = \frac{0.33}{0.17} = 2 \qquad \text{Eq. 15}$$

LR(Ch): The information in Ch is that the diarrhea lasted until dechallenge (nine days). The assessors felt that most cases of D-caused diarrhea would last until the drug was withdrawn. More precisely, they evaluated $P(\text{Ch} \mid D \to E) = 0.70$. They also believed that the duration of nondrug-caused diarrhea would not depend on whether the diarrhea was a sequela to M or was caused by coincidental gastroenteritis, so they evaluated a single distribution for the duration of nondrug-caused diarrhea (based on their clinical pediatric experience), as shown in Figure 6. (*Note:* The assessors assigned a probability of 0.7 to the first week, but because to do so would be irrelevant to their analysis, they made no attempt to subdivide this probability further.)

The probability assigned by the distribution pictured in Figure 6 to a duration of nine or more days is 0.22. That is, $P(\text{Ch} \mid D \not\to E, \text{Ti}) = 0.22$.

Thus:

$$\text{LR(Ch)} = \frac{P(\text{Ch} \mid D \to E, \text{Ti})}{P(\text{Ch} \mid D \not\to E, \text{Ti})}$$
$$= \frac{0.70}{0.22} \qquad \text{Eq. 16}$$
$$= 3.2$$

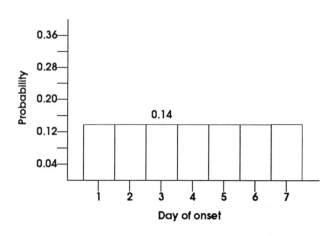

Figure 5
Time to Onset of Diarrhea Caused by Coincidental Gastroenteritis

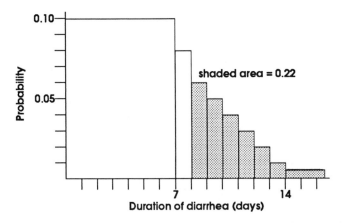

Figure 6
Duration of Nondrug-Induced Diarrhea

LR(De): The information in De is that the diarrhea resolved within two days of dechallenge (i.e., the drug was withdrawn on day 9, and the diarrhea resolved by day 11). The assessors believed that the time to resolution for D-caused diarrhea had the same distribution as the time to onset, because resolution is a matter of reversing the two processes that determine the onset time, namely the time to accumulation of D in the gut and the time it takes for change in the gut flora and gastrointestinal mucosal function corresponding to the new, D-enriched environment. Hence, $P(\text{De} \mid D \not\to E, \text{Ti}, \text{Ch}) = 0.33 + 0.33 = 0.66$. Ch is included in the conditioning statement because it states that the diarrhea persisted at least until dechallenge.

On the other hand, their assessment for the probability that resolution would occur within two days of dechallenge is determined by the distribution given in Figure 6: it is just the conditional probability of resolution on day 10 or 11 given that the diarrhea lasted at least nine days.

Thus, $P(\text{De} \mid D \not\to E, \text{Ti}, \text{Ch}) = 0.41$; therefore, $\text{LR(De)} = \dfrac{0.66}{0.41} = 1.6$

IMPLEMENTATION STEP 6: CALCULATE THE POSTERIOR ODDS FAVORING D-CAUSATION

This step is now automatic. The answer is obtained by multiplying together the prior odds and the likelihood ratio factors.

Calculating the Posterior Odds for Example 3

$$\text{posterior odds} = \text{prior odds} \times \text{LR(Hi)} \times \text{LR(Ti)} \times \text{LR(Ch)} \times \text{LR(De)}$$
$$= 3.5 \times 0.5 \times 2 \times 3.2 \times 1.6 \qquad \text{Eq. 17}$$
$$= 17.2$$

Equivalently, posterior probability of D-causation $= \dfrac{17.2}{18.2} = 0.95$.

Implementing the Probabilistic Approach: Some Technical Issues

MULTIPLE DRUGS

In Examples 2 and 3, there is only one drug on the cause list. As in Example 1, there often are many, and the problem of multiple drug causal candidates is one of the most difficult aspects of causality assessment. None of the SAMs deal with this problem in a satisfactory way; for example, most of them make it possible to report many probable drug causes of a single event E.

On the other hand, the problem is easily handled probabilistically, by means of the "one-drug-at-a-time strategy."[7] This strategy works as follows. Suppose that $D_1, \ldots, D_n$ are the drug hypotheses on the cause list and that N is the union of all nondrug causes. Let A_i represent "D_i or N" (i.e., A_i is the hypothesis that if E was caused by a drug, the drug cause was D_i). Also, let $PO(D_i)$ represent odds in favor of cause D_i, and $PO(D_i \mid A_i)$ the posterior odds in favor of cause D_i, given A_i. That is, $PO(D_i \mid A_i)$ solves the causality assessment problem for a case otherwise identical to the one under consideration, except that there is only a single drug causal candidate, D_i.

The following formula, which is a consequence of the rules of coherence, gives $PO(D_i)$ in terms of the conditional posterior odds:

$$PO(D_i) = \frac{PO(D_i \mid A_i)}{1 + \Sigma_{j \neq i} PO(D_j \mid A_j)} \qquad \text{Eq. 18}$$

Thus, when faced with a problem in which more than one drug candidate appears on the cause list, the assessor can solve the problem by first addressing a series of problems, each of which has only a single drug candidate, and then amalgamating the solutions to these problems using Equation 18. See Kramer for an example of the application of this strategy.[9]

It certainly is not necessary to use the one-drug-at-a-time strategy when carrying out a probabilistic causality assessment. However, assessors tend to become confused (and hence incoherent) when they try to directly compare the possible effects of many drugs. We have found that the strategy helps assessors achieve self-consistency by concentrating their attention on the effects of each drug candidate in turn.

MISSING INFORMATION

Physicians employed by pharmaceutical companies or national drug event monitoring agencies usually do not observe suspected UDEs, but instead rely for their base information on spontaneous reports submitted by attending clinicians. Such reports are notorious for the incompleteness of the information they contain. Thus, any causality assessment method should be able to take into account what information is available, as well as that which is not.

However, neither global introspection nor SAMs do well in this regard. Experts who are asked to carry out causality assessments based on spontaneous reports frequently say they cannot do so, without the results of this test or the exact time at which that occurred; others may base their assessments entirely on plausible but highly improbable scenarios that posit particular values to missing quantities and ignore the possibility that these assumptions are in error.[14] SAMs tend either to exclude missing information from consideration or to count it against the hypothesis of drug causation. How the probabilistic approach handles missing information will now be demonstrated, with respect to two important and common problems.

Noncompliance. A drug cannot cause an event if the patient did not take the drug. We generally know that a patient was prescribed a drug; our knowledge that he actually took the drug as prescribed usually is not so certain. Example 1 gives an extreme instance of this problem.

Here is the probabilistic solution to the problem of noncompliance, when only one particular administration of the drug is under consideration. Let Com be the proposition that the patient was compliant: she took drug D as prescribed. Let B be background information as defined previously; so B includes the statement that the patient took D (i.e., Com) and subsequently experienced an event of type E_t. Now, let B_0 consist of the noncase information in B, plus the information that a patient with condition M who was prescribed (but did not necessarily take) D experienced an event of type E_t. That is, B is the intersection of B_0 and Com.

The following can then be derived from the rules of the probability theory:

$$\frac{P(D \rightarrow E \mid B_0, C)}{P(D \nrightarrow E \mid B_0, C)} = P(\text{Com} \mid M) \times \frac{P(D \rightarrow E \mid B, C)}{P(D \nrightarrow E \mid B, C)} \qquad \text{Eq. 19}$$

In this expression, $P(\text{Com} \mid M)$ is the probability that a generic patient with condition M prescribed D will comply with his prescription; it is not calculated conditionally on the patient experiencing an event of type E_t.

Thus, Equation 19 can be read as follows. First, evaluate the chance that a patient with condition M who is prescribed D would comply with this prescription. Next, evaluate the posterior odds in favor of D-causation for the particular case under consideration, assuming that the patient actually took D as prescribed. Finally to calculate coherently the posterior odds that D caused E without assuming compliance, multiply the results of the previous two evaluations together.

For example, suppose that you believe, like Kramer,[9] that about 80 percent of the patients who undergo wisdom tooth extraction and are prescribed an analgesic to take as needed for postoperative pain will take the drug prescribed. Suppose that you would give 20:1 odds that the zomepirac killed the woman in Example 1, if you know she had taken the drug. Then, according to Equation 19, you should give 16:1 odds in favor of zomepirac, based on the actual information provided.

At the conference in which Kramer presented his findings,[9] some eminent experts in UDEs expressed the view that their posterior probability that zomepirac caused the woman's death could not exceed their probability that someone would take zomepirac after a wisdom tooth extraction.[3] Their error, put right by Equation 18, consists of mistaking $P(\text{Com} \mid M)$ for $P(\text{Com} \mid M, E_t)$. (In words, apparently healthy people who have their wisdom teeth extracted do not necessarily take a drug for pain; but almost no such people die suddenly—and for those who do, something had to kill them.) It is unrealistic to expect global introspection to produce coherent assessments, especially in the face of missing information.

Missing "Vital" Case Information. When an assessor must rely on second-hand case information (e.g., a spontaneous report), he may think of some item of missing information that, for him, would play a decisive role in his causality assessment were it available. In Example 1 there is no mention of whether or not the pathologist checked for a cerebral hemorrhage, which, if present, could provide a possible nondrug explanation for the woman's sudden death. Similarly, a spontaneous report of a case of suspected drug-induced pancreatitis fails to mention whether or not the patient was alcoholic or whether she was checked for gallstones (two of the most common causes of acute pancreatitis).[23]

To state the problem generally, suppose that A is a case information proposition which, if known, would have differential diagnostic significance for the causality assessment. How should the fact that neither A nor A^c is specified in the given data affect the resulting assessment? Let A* denote the information that neither A nor A^c is specified, and LR(A*) the contribution of A* to the posterior odds. The problem, then, is to evaluate the quantity LR(A*).

At first sight it might seem that negative information such as A* should have no effect on the causality assessment. However, the assessment would have a very different result if A were known to be true than if it were known to be false, and A* should affect the assessor's opinions about how likely A is to be true. For, if whoever submits the report has some chance of appreciating the significance of the truth of A and may therefore have sought to ascertain it, then the chance that the report is submitted and given that it is, that neither A nor A^c is mentioned in it, depends to some extent on whether A or A^c is true. Thus, A* should affect the overall causality assessment.

The quantitative effect of A* is given by the following formula, determined by the rules of coherence:

$$LR(A^*) = p + [(1-p) \times LR(A^c)] \qquad \text{Eq. 20}$$

where:

$$p = \frac{a}{a + bc}$$
$$a = P(A^* \mid A), b = P(A^* \mid A^c) - P(A^* \mid A) \qquad \text{Eq. 21}$$
$$c = P(A^c \mid B, D \nrightarrow E, S)$$

S is the case information chronologically preceding A. Now, c is just the denominator of LR(A^c), and hence would be evaluated in the course of assessing this likelihood ratio factor. The quantities a and b measure the assessor's opinion of the process, whereby the case information came to him; that is, for a, he has to decide how likely he thinks it is that the case report would not mention A, if A were actually true (and also, for b, if A were false).

Frequently, as in the two examples of missing case information cited above, A gives strong information in favor of one of the causal candidates (usually nondrug), while A^c gives weak evidence (by default) for the other candidates. In such cases it is reasonable to believe that the author of the case report is more likely not to mention anything about A when A is false than when it is true. From Equation 20 it then follows that $LR(A^*)$ can be regarded as an average of two components: 1, which is the appropriate likelihood ratio factor for information that does not discriminate between drug and nondrug causation; and $LR(A^c)$, the likelihood ratio factor that would be appropriate if A were known to be false. The more likely there is to be no mention of A when A is false than when it is true, the more $LR(A^*)$ will resemble $LR(A^c)$. Note that if A is always mentioned when it is true, then $LR(A^*)$ equals $LR(A^c)$ (because A^* then implies A^c); if there is no mention of A just as frequently when A is true as when it is false (so $b=0$, then $LR(A^*)$ equals 1 (i.e., there is no information in A^*).

In summary, to evaluate the likelihood ratio corresponding to the fact that a potentially vital piece of case information, A, is simply not mentioned, do the following:

1. Evaluate $LR(A^c)$ [and its denominator, $P(A^c \mid B, D \nrightarrow E, S)$].
2. Evaluate $P(A^* \mid A)$ and $P(A^* \mid A^c)$.
3. Calculate $LR(A^*)$ from Equation 20.

CONDITIONING AND DECOMPOSITION

Determining which probability assessment tasks are accessible is largely empirical and highly context dependent. Experts with some probability assessment experience can be queried to discover whether they feel comfortable carrying out particular types of assessment tasks. When they do not, they usually complain that they just do not know whether or not the proposition in question is true, rather than measure their uncertainty in it. Also, assessment tasks that pose questions that are insufficiently local often produce widely varying answers from assessors with similar expertise. It frequently is possible to probe for the sources of such disagreement in the form of information or posited mechanisms that some, but not all, of the disagreeing assessors have taken into consideration.

Once it is determined that an assessment task is too global, how can it be refined to increase accessibility? Two important techniques in this regard are decomposition and conditioning. Decomposition involves expressing a quantity as a series of component parts, each of which relates to a particular feature of the assessor's knowledge and experience. For example, the time to onset of a dose-dependent UDE often can be assessed more easily when it is decomposed into three components: T_1, the time it takes the drug or its relevant metabolite to build up to toxic concentrations in the target organ (which depends primarily on the pharmacokinetics of D); T_2, the time from onset of toxicity until the injury is clinically detectable (which depends primarily on the nature of the event type E_t); and T_3, the time from clinical detectability until detection (which depends on M and E_t and the intensity of surveillance, as well as personal attributes of the patients expressed on Hi). The assessor then must determine what dependencies, if any, there are between the distributions for the components. It is often the case, as in this example, that he can regard these distributions as independent (because they frequently depend on completely different aspects of the drug, event, patient, and surveillance system), in which case the distribution of their sum, the relevant time to onset, can be determined by convolution.

As an example of a situation in which conditioning is appropriate, suppose that an assessor wants to evaluate her distribution for time to onset of UDE, but is uncertain whether the mechanism for this reaction is immunologic or cytotoxic—and her timing distributions given these two possible mechanisms differ. She must then condition on each in turn, evaluate the relevant conditional distributions, determine her probability that each mechanism is actually the operative one, and then calculate the relevant timing distribution by the law of total probability.

To illustrate the use of both these techniques, here is the calculation for LR(Ti) in Example 1, with zomepirac as the drug causal candidate. As described in the preceding two subsections, for this calculation we may assume that zomepirac is the only drug candidate and that the woman actually took zomepirac. However, we do not know when she took the drug, and the only information in Ti is that the coroner placed the time of death at 4 pm ± 2 hours (recall that the surgery took place from 1 to 1:40 pm). Call this datum Ti.

To determine his probability for Ti, given that zomepirac was responsible for the woman's death, Kramer first decomposed the time of death into two components: the time at which the zomepirac was taken, and the time between taking

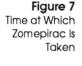

Figure 7
Time at Which
Zomepirac Is
Taken

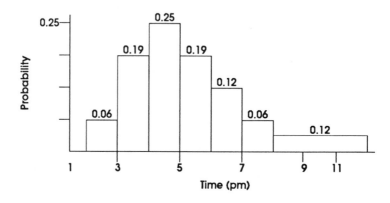

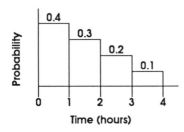

Figure 8
Time Between Taking
Zomepirac and
Zomepirac-Caused
Death

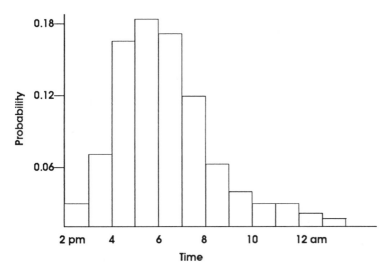

Figure 9
Time of
Zomepirac-
Caused Death

zomepirac and death.[9] Kramer's distributions for these quantities are given in Figures 7 and 8. The first of these depends on how long it would take the xylocaine to wear off and the patient's pain threshold, and the second depends on the absorption time of oral zomepirac and the mechanism of anaphylaxis. Hence, the distributions are independent, so their convolution, sketched in Figure 9, gives Kramer's distribution for the time of zomepirac-caused death.

Next, Kramer evaluated his probability for Ti, given that death actually occurred at hour j, for each possible hour j. He based the evaluation on the assumption that the coroner's stated time of death would be off by an hour in either direction with the probability 0.4, and would be off by two hours in either direction with probability 0.2.[2] This is, of course, a somewhat oversimplified summary of his opinions about the accuracy of pathological techniques for time-of-death determination.

From the evaluations reported in the preceding two paragraphs, the following calculation follows by the law of total probability:

$$P(\text{Ti} \mid D \to E)$$
$$= \sum_j P(\text{Ti} \mid \text{death at hour } j, D \to E) P(\text{death at hour } j \mid D \to E)$$
$$= \sum_j P(\text{Ti} \mid \text{death at hour } j) P(\text{death at hour } j \mid D \to E) \qquad \textbf{Eq. 22}$$
$$= (0.2)(0.025) + (0.4)(0.094) + (0.4)(0.169) + (0.2)(0.194)$$
$$= 0.15$$

On the other hand, because given nondrug cause, the woman was judged equally likely to die at any time in the period determined by the time horizon, which was taken to be 24 hours, $P(\text{Ti} \mid D \nrightarrow E) = \frac{1}{24} = 0.04$.

So with these assessments, $LR(\text{Ti}) = \frac{0.15}{0.04} = 3.75$.

THE PRIOR ODDS

Most serious UDEs are quite rare, with incidences in the range of 1 per 1000 to 1 per 1 million courses of therapy. As a result, few assessors can bring to bear much relevant personal clinical experience in assessing the prior odds. Moreover, there are not many reliable epidemiologic data on the incidence of UDEs. Consequently, the prior odds present the most challenging of the assessment tasks required by the probabilistic method.

The factors that are relevant to the assessment of the prior odds are listed below. The order of the factors is determined by how much information about the factor can sharpen an assessor's distribution for the prior odds. Much work remains to be done to develop techniques for converting information about these factors into usable probability distributions for the prior odds.

Frequencies. When epidemiologic data are available that allow the assessor to evaluate the quantities $P(E_t \mid D)$ and $P(E_t \mid D^c)$ reliably, as in the analysis of Example 3, the strategy based on Equation 6 is the best way to proceed. Usually, some subjective adjustments to published frequencies is necessary to accommodate these data to the appropriate reference set defined by M and E_t.

Sometimes only indirect frequencies are available. For example, in the analysis of the sudden death case (Example 1), we knew that about 30 cases of fatal anaphylaxis associated with zomepirac had been reported to the FDA prior to the receipt of the report on which this case was based. From sales data we estimated that at this time about 10 million patients had been exposed to the drug. To estimate $P(E_t \mid D)$ from these data, we only needed to estimate the reporting fraction: the proportion of such events that were actually reported to the FDA. This fraction depends on such factors as the seriousness and etiological specificity of the UDE, the amount of time the drug has been on the market, and the duration of the time interval between drug administration and event (i.e., exactly the factors that play a role in causality assessment). For this case, Judith Jones, who at the time this case was reported was in charge of the FDA's spontaneous reporting system, produced her distribution for the reporting fraction; this distribution had a mean of 20 percent. Thus, the estimate used for $P(E_t \mid D)$ used in the analysis was 1.5 cases per 100 000 patients exposed. A distribution around this figure (for sensitivity analysis) could be generated by our uncertainty distributions for the reporting fraction and the total number of exposures.

Drug Similarity. Are drugs that are similar chemically or pharmacologically to the drug associated with the event?

Event Similarity. Is the drug associated with UDEs that are predictably related to the event in question? (For example, the incidence of agranulocytosis caused by a drug may be predictable from the incidence with which it induces less severe neutropenia, which can be measured on a much smaller study population.)

Mechanism. How biologically plausible is the association?

Analogy of Uncertainty. How does the assessor's uncertain opinions about the strength of this drug-event association compare with his a priori opinions about other such associations, for which the risks have been qualified? Because zomepirac had been withdrawn from the market due to it association with anaphylaxis, the assessor in Kramer judged this association to be at least as strong as that of parenteral penicillin with anaphylaxis, which was reported to be 1:100 000.[9]

Appendix I
The Rules of Probability

Probability must satisfy the following relations:[19]

Relation 1. For every proposition A, $0 \leq P(A) \leq 1$; if A is certain, $P(A) = 1$.

Relation 2. For incompatible propositions A and B, $P(A \text{ or } B) = P(A) + P(B)$.

Relation 3. For any propositions A and B, with $P(B) > 0$,

$$P(A \mid B) = \frac{P(AB)}{P(B)}$$

There are three consequences of these rules:

Consequence 1. The law of total probability:
If $A_1, \ldots, A_n$ are incompatible, but one of them must be true, then for any other proposition B, $P(B) = \Sigma_1^n i\, P(B \mid A_i)\, P(A_i)$

Consequence 2. Bayes' Theorem:
By relation 3 above, $P(AB) = P(A \mid B)\, P(B)$ and also $P(AB) = P(B \mid A)\, P(A)$. Therefore $P(A \mid B) = P(AB) / P(B) = P(B \mid A)\, P(A) / P(B)$.
Using a similar expression for $P(A^c \mid B)$ (A^c is the denial of A) one obtains:

$$\frac{P(A \mid B)}{P(A^c \mid B)} = \frac{P(B \mid A)}{P(B \mid A^c)} \times \frac{P(A)}{P(A^c)}$$

Consequence 3. Odds Probability Transformation:
Suppose $\frac{P(A \mid B)}{P(A^c \mid B)} = C$, then $P(A \mid B) = \frac{C}{1 + C}$

Proof: by relations 2 and 3 above, $P(A \mid B) + P(A^c \mid B) = 1$. Therefore:

$$P(A \mid B) = \frac{P(A \mid B)}{P(A \mid B) + P(A^c \mid B)}$$

$$\frac{\dfrac{P(A \mid B)}{P(A^c \mid B)}}{\dfrac{P(A \mid B) + P(A^c \mid B)}{P(A^c \mid B)}} = \frac{C}{1 + C}$$

References

1. Venulet J, Berneker GD, Ciucci AG, eds. Assessing causes of adverse drug reactions. London: Academic Press, 1982.

2. Herman R, ed. Drug-event associations: perspectives, methods, and uses. *Drug Inf J* 1984;*18*.

3. Jones J, Herman R, eds. The future of adverse drug reaction diagnosis: computers, clinical judgment and the logic of uncertainty. *Drug Inf J* 1986;*20*.

4. Stephens M. The detection of new adverse drug reactions. London: Plenum, 1985.

5. Lane D. Causality assessment for adverse drug reactions: an application of subjective probability to medical decision making. In: Berger J, Gupta S, eds. Proceedings of the Fourth Purdue Symposium on statistical decision theory and related topics. 1987;*1*:235-50.

6. Auriche M. Approche Bayesienne de l'imputabilitie des phénomènes indésirables aux médicaments. *Therapie* 1985;*40*:301-6.

7. Lane D, Hutchinson T, Jones J, Kramer M, Naranjo C. A Bayesian approach to causality assessment. Tech. Rep. 472, Minneapolis: University of Minnesota School of Statistics, 1986.

8. Lane D, Kramer M, Hutchinson T, Jones J, Naranjo C. The causality assessment of adverse drug reactions using a Bayesian approach. *Pharmaceut Med* 1987; 2:265-83.

9. Kramer M. A Bayesian approach to assessment of adverse drug reactions: evaluation of a case of fatal anaphylaxis. *Drug Inf J* 1986;*20*:505-18.

10. Kahneman D, Slovic P, Tversky A. Judgement under uncertainty: heuristics and biases. Cambridge: Cambridge University Press, 1982.

11. Karch F, Smith C, Kernzer B, Mazullo J, Weintraub M, Lasagna L. Adverse drug reactions—a matter of opinion. *Clin Pharmacol Ther* 1976;*19*:489-92.

12. Koch-Weser J, Sellers E, Zacest R. The ambiguity of adverse drug reactions. *Eur J Clin Pharmacol* 1977;*11*:75-8.

13. Dangomau J, Begaud B, Boisseau A, Albin H. Les effets indésirables des médicaments. *Nouv Presse Med* 1980;*9*:1607-9.

14. Lane D. A probabilist's view of causality assessment. *Drug Inf J* 1984; *18*:323-30.

15. Kramer M. Assessing causality of adverse drug reactions: global introspection and its limitations. *Drug Inf J* 1986;*20*:433-8.

16. Stephens M. The diagnosis of adverse medical events associated with drug treatment. *J Adverse Drug React Acute Poison Rev* (in press).

17. Dukes M. Adverse reactions : a changing challenge. Proceedings of the Second World Conference on Clinical Pharmacology and Therapeutics. Bethesda, MD: 1984:223-32.

18. Hutchinson TA, Lane DA. Assessing methods for causality assessment of suspected adverse drug reactions. *J Clin Epidemiol* 1989;*42*:5-16.

19. de Finetti B. Theory of probability. New York: John Wiley & Sons, 1974.

20. Lane D. Coherence and prediction. *Bull Int Stat Inst* 1981;*49*:81-96.

21.Bartlett A, Moore M, Gary G, Starko K, Erben J, Meredith B. Diarrheal illness among infants and toddlers in day care centers: I. Epidemiology and pathogens. *J Pediatr* 1985;*107*:495-502.

22. Bartlett A, Moore M, Gary G, Starko K, Erben J, Meredith B. Diarrheal illness among infants and toddlers in day care centers: II. Comparison with day care homes and households. *J Pediatr* 1985;*107*:503-9.

23. Begaud B. Standardized assessment of adverse drug reactions: the method used in France. *Drug Inf J* 1984;*18*:275-82.

This chapter is an adapted and updated version of "Causality Assessment for Adverse Drug Reactions," which appeared in *Statistical Methodology in the Pharmaceutical Sciences*, D.A. Berry, Editor; Marcel Dekker, New York, 1990.

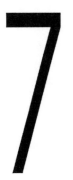

7

Drug Utilization Studies: Sources and Methods

Joaquima Serradell
Darrel C. Bjornson
Abraham G. Hartzema

Abstract

This chapter describes the history, development, and current status of drug utilization activities. Various methodologies employed in drug utilization studies are evaluated and presented along with a listing of principal drug databases available for drug utilization research. An analysis is presented comparing the validity of drug consumption rates based on individual patient usage or drug cost data as adopted in North America and the defined daily dose unit as originally developed in Europe. Drug utilization studies provide the methodological rigor for defining the denominator data needed in pharmacoepidemiologic research. Care is needed in interpreting drug utilization data. Geographic or time differences may be totally or partially explained, among other factors, by differences in the age and sex distributions, patterns of morbidity, diagnostic criteria, access to healthcare, the characteristics of drug supply (e.g., proportion of fixed-dose combinations), and the actual utilization of drugs (e.g., compliance, actual dose prescribed in selected indications). When appropriately used in conjunction with analytical studies on drug effects and other epidemiologic methods, drug utilization studies become a powerful scientific tool to aid drugs in becoming effective and safe.

Outline

This chapter discusses the units of measurement employed in drug use or utilization studies, describes the major sources of drug use data, reviews prescribing patterns based on national and international comparative drug use data analysis, and defines the contribution of drug utilization studies to pharmacoepidemiology.

Drug utilization has been defined as "the prescribing, dispensing, administering, and ingesting of drugs."[1] This definition recognizes that several steps and factors are involved in drug utilization and that, consequently, in each of these steps problems in drug use can arise. Factors that may contribute to these problems may have historical, social, organizational, political, economic, technologic, and physiologic or pharmacologic origins.

The World Health Organization (WHO) definition of drug utilization expands on this definition by including outcome variables in the definition. Drug utilization is defined by the WHO as "the marketing, distribution, prescription, and use of drugs in society, with special emphasis on the resulting medical, social, and economic consequences."[2] The WHO definition also includes the evaluation of the medical, social, and economic outcomes of drug therapy. Tognoni notes that if the emphasis of a study is on drug utilization, the point of observation is the act of prescribing the drug, and quantitative data need to be obtained on the extent and variability in usage and costs of drug therapy, from which medical and social qualitative consequences can be extrapolated.[3] In drug monitoring studies, the focus is on the observable effects of the drug which, depending on the specific aims of the method selected, are limited with the type and extent of drug exposure. The general goals of drug utilization studies, other than those describing drug use, include: (1) identification and definition of likely problems, (2) general analysis of the problem with regard to its importance, cause, and consequence, (3) establishment of a weighted basis for decisions on problem solving, and (4) assessment of the effects of the action taken.[4]

The users of drug utilization studies may include healthcare policy makers, the pharmaceutical industry, the academic and clinical health professions, social scientists, economists, and consumers. The complexity of the drug utilization process often calls for an interdisciplinary approach to methodology development and consequently fosters improved communication between the health science disciplines. This chapter focuses mainly on drug utilization research.

Defining the Unit of Measurement

Population-based drug utilization studies were pioneered in Europe during the late 1960s and early 1970s. The primary focus of these studies was determined by the needs of program administrators. Drug use statistics published in these studies were not linked to population data. However, in later studies, a shift toward a more epidemiologic approach occurred with the population denominator becoming increasingly important. In addition, more adequate measures for drug utilization data or numerator data were developed. Although drug utilization studies have employed different methodological approaches in quantifying drug use, three units for quantification of drug use are used predominantly. These three measures are cost data, prescription volume, and the defined daily dose (DDD).

In the early studies, gross drug sales data were the most commonly used indicator. This information is widely available and can be obtained from manufacturers or wholesalers. However, using data based on drug cost can introduce measurement errors, because differential pricing occurs according to distribution channels employed, quantity purchased, import duties and currency exchange rate differences between countries, and regulatory policies that affect pricing. These problems with the interpretation of drug cost data are compounded by the different classification systems used for drugs in different countries. Studies based on cost data do not allow for cross-national comparisons, for comparisons between different programs within one nation, or for longitudinal studies.[5] Consequently, cost data introduce considerable limitations in the interpretation of drug utilization studies.

The number of prescriptions written or dispensed for a particular drug product is used as a measure of drug use in drug utilization studies. Databases such as IMS America, LTD.'s National Prescription Audit, and P.D.S.'s Alpha System contain information compiled from prescription records. However, the quantity of the prescription items varies from prescription to prescription and the supply per prescription can be for any time period, with no adequate assessment provided of the amounts of drugs prescribed or dispensed. Drug use data based on prescription records are difficult to tabulate without the aid of computer systems. Thus, the main source for these data are computerized pharmacies, health maintenance organizations (HMOs), or third-party databases, (e.g., Medicaid in America and Sickness Funds in Europe).

Although drug utilization data based on prescription data are more accurate than cost data in estimating true drug utilization, the need to develop a more adequate index for drug utilization was felt necessary. To overcome the inherent shortcomings of drug utilization studies based on cost data or prescription volume, a new unit of analysis was developed, called the defined daily dose (DDD). The DDD was developed based on an assumed average dose per day for a drug product used for its major indication in everyday practice. The dosing levels have been defined according to recommendations in the medical literature and are thought to be the average maintenance dose when used for the major indication of a particular drug. The DDD is purely a technical unit of measurement and comparison and, as such, provides a rough estimate of the proportion of patients within a community who would receive that particular drug. Two basic assumptions underlie the use of DDD: first, that patients take the medication (in other words, the patients are compliant); and second, the doses used for the major indication are the average maintenance doses.

By applying such a measure to a defined population, it is feasible to: (1) examine changes in drug consumption over time, (2) make international comparisons, (3) evaluate the effect of educational programs directed either at the prescriber or the patient, (4) document the "relative therapy intensity" with various groups of drugs, (5) follow changes in the use of a class of drugs, and (6) evaluate regulatory change effects on prescription patterns.[6] A review of DDDs, with possible applications in the institutional setting and pharmacy and therapeutics committees, is provided by Wertheimer.[7]

To overcome limitations of the DDD, which is based on the standard doses for the major indication for the drug and does not reflect actual prescribing patterns, U.S. researchers have been using the prescribed daily dose (PDD). These researchers argue that the PDD reflects more accurately drug exposure in the U.S. population than the DDD, because the PDD is based on actual doses ordered by physicians for new prescriptions. PDDs can, for example, be derived from the IMS National Prescription Audit.[8]

Studies on the application of the DDD are confined mostly to the European literature. A number of significant qualitative and quantitative differences in drug prescription rates and therapy patterns between countries have been documented by these studies.[9-11] In addition, studies have employed the DDD for within-country comparisons of drug use and disease distribution.[12-15] The following is an illustration of the application of the DDD unit in a drug utilization study.

In 1979, Malmohus county in Sweden led the list of counties in the sales of hypnotics, sedatives, and minor tranquilizers, with sales of 82.9 DDD/1000 inhabitants/day. In comparison, the national mean was 64.4 DDD/1000 inhabitants/day. This observed difference led to an investigation in which prescriptions for hypnotics, sedatives, and minor tranquilizers dispensed at pharmacies in the city of Malmo were further analyzed.[16]

Ten to 15 physicians accounted for a very high prescription volume in psychotropics; the remaining physicians were responsible for only a moderate number of prescriptions. These findings led to a consensus conference at which guidelines for the prescribing of hypnotics, sedatives, and minor tranquilizers were established. An information letter containing these guidelines was sent by the local medical association to all physicians in the area, including the indications for and the precautions to be taken in the prescribing of these drugs. In a follow-up study done in 1981, the consumption in DDD units for Malmohus county had decreased to 76.8 DDD/1000 inhabitants/day. The provision of prescribing information proved to be effective even though the consumption of hypnotics, sedatives, and minor tranquilizers in Malmohus county was still above the national mean.[16]

Major Sources of Drug Utilization Data

Pharmacoepidemiologic databases, including drug utilization databases, can be ordered using the following taxonomy: (1) population databases including both drug and diagnostic data, (2) population databases including only diagnostic data, and (3) population databases with only drug data. Population databases with both drug and diagnosis data can be divided into outpatient databases (e.g., Medicaid MMIS or the COMPASS databases), and inpatient databases (e.g., the Boston Collaborative Drug Study Program). Further, in population databases with diagnosis and drug data, diagnosis-specific population databases (e.g., the American Rheumatism Association Medicaid Information System), drug-specific population databases (e.g., Smith, Kline & French Cimetidine Cohort Database), and spontaneous drug event reporting systems (e.g., the FDA Spontaneous Drug Event Reporting System and, more specifically, the National Registry of Drug Induced Ocular Side Effects) are included.

Examples of the other two main categories of databases are the Population Database Diagnosis Data Only, an example being the Framingham Study; and Population Databases Drug Data Only, examples including IMS or the Prescription Data Services databases.

A commercially available compendium containing descriptive information on drug and diagnosis databases is the "International Drug Benefit/Risk Assessment Data Resource Handbook," prepared under the auspices of Ciba-Geigy. Separate volumes of the compendium have been prepared for data sources in North America, the United Kingdom, Japan, West Germany, the Netherlands, and Switzerland.[17]

Four major sources of drug utilization data which are the major vehicles for drug utilization studies will be discussed in more detail. These sources are: (1) market surveys primarily based on sales data or prescription volume data, (2) third-party payers or HMOs, (3) institutional and ambulatory settings, and (4) pharmacoepidemiologic studies designed for monitoring and evaluating exposure-related outcomes.

MARKET SURVEYS

These data often are collected by commercial database vendors who will resell the aggregate data to pharmaceutical firms for marketing studies. Commercial vendors include IMS American, Ltd., which surveys physician-patient contacts for diagnoses and therapies, monitors prescriptions dispensed in pharmacies, and collects sales data from hospitals and drug stores.

IMS provides the following specific information:[18]

National Prescription Audit. The NPA, based on a panel of 1400 computerized pharmacies and 600 noncomputerized pharmacies, measures the prescription volume that moves out of pharmacies into the hands of the consumers. These data are derived only from retail pharmacies; however, it is estimated that retail pharmacies account for 90 percent of the prescriptions dispensed in the U.S. The unit of measurement is the prescription; thus, the data obtained do not reflect an exact dollar amount or units of medication, because prescription size fluctuates.

National Disease and Therapeutic Index. The NDTI uses an office-based physician panel and measures drugs mentioned during physician-patient contact. It captures drugs administered directly by physicians and includes hospital drug use, but excludes refill prescriptions that do not involve patient contact with a physician. The unit of measurement is the prescription.

U.S. Pharmaceutical Market–Drugstores. This source uses drugstore invoices to assess the flow of both ethical and proprietary drugs into pharmacies. It collects financial data from retail pharmacies, proprietary drug stores, and discount houses.

U.S. Pharmaceutical Market–Hospitals. The data are generated from non-federal hospital drug purchase invoices.

A second commercial data course is the Prescription Card Service (PCS). The PCS, through its subsidiary Pharmaceutical Data Services (PDS), provides data on third-party paid prescriptions and tabulates national estimates. PDS Alpha system has access to the statistical information within the National Data Corporation computer system, which contains current drug sales data from 839 pharmacies in 42 states. Approximately 300 of the pharmacies included in the sample are used for the PDS Alpha audits, and data on all pharmacies are used for customized studies for individual clients. An estimated 4 million prescriptions per month are entered into the database, providing information on inventory statistics, and the prescribing rates of physician specialty groups including dentists, podiatrists, and veterinarians. In addition, the structure of the database allows the researcher to follow drug utilization and compliance rates for individual patients.[19]

Other sources of data are available to the researchers and policy makers. These sources often are required to assemble and integrate data from different databases. For example, the U.S. Department of Health and Human Services conducts a continuing National Health Care Expenditure survey which has data on drug use as well as the utilization of other health and social services.

Further, the Retired Persons Services organization, which operates approximately one dozen pharmacies throughout the U.S. on behalf of the American Association of Retired Persons, has an extensive drug utilization database. Other important sources are special registries established for groups of patients thought to be at higher risk, including the National Registry of Drug-Induced Ocular Side Effects, Registry of Tissue Reactions to Drugs, Dermatological Adverse Reaction Reporting System, Hepatic Events Registry, and the International Registry of Lithium Babies. These registries are particularly important as spontaneous drug-event reporting systems.

THIRD-PARTY PAYERS/HMO/MEDICAID

Noncommercial national and international drug utilization sources include the FDA's Post-Marketing Surveillance (PMS) system and the Swedish Diagnosis and Therapeutics system. Drug utilization information originating from the FDA includes drug utilization trends over time, by age and sex distribution, and by drug category. The primary focus of the FDA's PMS system has been capturing information on unintended drug effects (UDEs) to assess risks. Much of these data come from various group health organizations in which the continuity of care of an enrolled captive population allows for the linkage of pharmacy records with medical charts. Clinical databases that allow for record linkage are discussed in greater detail in Chapter 20. Appendix I summarizes several of the national databases presently used for pharmacoepidemiologic studies.

The Medicaid health insurance system in the U.S. is a computerized medical and pharmaceutical care billing system of which selected data items from the computerized files have been used for pharmacoepidemiologic studies. For example, one combined database of such data from several states is the Computerized On-Line Medicaid Pharmaceutical Analysis and Surveillance System.[20] State Medicaid programs make data available without patient identification to researchers at a nominal cost. Although Medicaid data reflect consumption of a changing and non-random patient population skewed to lower income groups, it can have value, especially for identifying trends of utilization.

Medicaid databases have been employed for drug utilization studies to examine the effects of formulary restrictions on drug expenditures and drug usage, to provide cost analysis of specific disease states, and to assess the influence of demographic variables on prescription drug use.[21-23]

In Sweden, the prescribing of medicines in ambulatory care patients has been collected in the Diagnosis and Therapy Survey since 1978. Prescription copies, containing not only drugs but also diagnosis and/or symptoms, are collected from a stratified, randomized sample of physicians. This survey connects the diagnosis/symptoms for which the drugs are prescribed and allows for the important diagnosis-therapy link.[16] Appendix II provides an overview of the international drug utilization databases available for pharmacoepidemiologic research.

INSTITUTIONAL/AMBULATORY SETTINGS

It is important for administrators and health professionals to know patterns of drug use along with population changes and disease prevalence. As shown earlier, descriptive data are readily available on the extent of drug use, where drugs are used, local differences in choice of drugs, use in various groups, and changes over time. However, there is a need for information on the outcomes of treatments, real drug intake, and prescribing patterns for different indications. These factors require in-depth studies using individualized data on a longitudinal basis correlated with healthcare utilization data.[24] Patterns of drug use data are the primary source of information on how the effects of drugs, as predicted from clinical trials and from known prescribing practice, are related to recommended treatment regimens.[25] Drug utilization review (DUR) studies are the major source of this information in institutional settings, and the term DUR is the common nomenclature for all quality assurance studies examining the relationship between diagnosis and drug therapy.

In the U.S., DUR activities generally are mandated by the Professional Review Organizations (PROs) and by institutional accrediting bodies, such as the Joint Commission on the Accreditation of Healthcare Organizations.[26] PROs were initiated to help the federal government curb its expenditures for Medicaid recipients while ensuring quality of care. The PROs include peer review in the use of services, quality assurance activities, and credentialing, with its emphasis primarily focused on hospital-oriented activities.[27] An extensive amount of literature on DUR studies in institutional care has been published providing the researcher access to data on the use of drugs in the clinical practice setting.[28-31]

Different methods to interpret drug use data have been developed:

Medical Audit. Drug utilization data provide information about drug patterns, prescriber's performance, and patient contacts with the healthcare system. Therefore, drug utilization data can be used as an indicator to evaluate, at the macro level, the functions of the healthcare system. The medical audit concept serves to evaluate differences in prescribing between individual prescribers or between groups. Medical audits examine differences between institutional and community prescribers at the local or national level or across countries.

The objective of a medical audit is to identify problems associated with prescribing and to be able to provide recommendations leading to a solution for the problems identified. This then facilitates appropriate prescribing to maintain high standards of care.[32] Two types of medical audit can be distinguished. First, in the self-audit, the initiative for the audit comes from oneself. Personal activities toward updating knowledge about new therapies, concepts regarding drug policies, and diagnostic techniques are related to expectations to maintain high standards of care. Moreover, medical training, including the abilities to endure criticism and learn from mistakes, is of interest to those who want to ensure appropriate standards of care.[32] Although the self-audit has value, such data must be questioned with regard to validity and reliability.

Another approach to medical audits is to study prescribing patterns of care given at community, state, or national levels. This often is called peer audit. Thus, studies can be conducted not only in institutions, but also in the community where most of the drugs are used.

The advantages of medical audits over other types of available drug use data is that they provide the diagnosis on which the prescribing has taken place, thus providing documentation for the diagnosis-therapy relation. Some studies have suggested that the medical audit may threaten the physician's ability to change prescribing behavior.[24,33] It therefore is important to perform medical audits objectively and with physicians' input. In this way, rational drug prescribing can be enhanced.

MONITORING AND EVALUATING EXPOSURE-RELATED OUTCOMES

A fourth source of information on drug use and performance is specific studies designed to address pharmacoepidemiologic questions. This type of drug utilization research involves epidemiologic methodologies, such as case-control and co-hort studies.[34,35] Herbst et al., for example, demonstrated that with only eight cases and four controls per case, a significant association between diethylstilbestrol ther-apy and vaginal and cervical adenocarcinoma in young women could be estab-lished.[36] Case-control studies usually are not designed as drug utilization studies, but instead are designed to test hypotheses. In fact, they generally are used to con-firm or refute reported UDEs associated with a defined pharmacologic agent in postmarketing surveillance.

Another epidemiologic design, the cohort study, follows a cohort of individ-uals over time who have been exposed to a drug thought to be a potential risk fac-tor for an adverse outcome. An example of a cohort study is one performed by Jick et al., which showed an association between replacement estrogens and endome-trial cancer.[37] Case-cohort and cohort designs, which are appropriate for postmar-keting surveillance, are not ideally suited for drug utilization studies. Pharma-coepidemiologic methodologies used in postmarketing studies are discussed in Chapter 8.

Drug utilization data obtained by the methodologies discussed under the four major data sources reviewed above are used for a wide variety of inquiries. Phar-macoepidemiologic inquiries range from what the utilization rate for a class of drugs is, estimates of the population at risk for the use of a defined causal agent, prescribing rates as an indicator for the prevalence of a nonreportable disease,[38] quantification of the incidence of a UDE, evaluation of shifts in prescribing patterns to document secondary indications for labeling purposes, and the establishment of causality between a reported event and a pharmacologic agent. The nature of the inquiry determines the appropriate drug utilization data course and the phar-macoepidemiologic method. An understanding of the validity of drug use data and the methodology by which these data are obtained is important in examining any of these inquiries.

Approaches to Comparative Drug Utilization Analyses

Drug utilization studies explore what drugs are used, in what quantity, by whom, how they are used, and the context in which they are used. These studies also may examine why patient outcomes vary with drug use. Descriptive data on patterns of drug use by gender, age group, and other demographic information are available from sources described earlier. Drug utilization studies have reviewed drug use in specific populations, which may be the young, the old, or others de-fined by the aims of the study. Olubadewo et al. surveyed outpatient drug use in a pediatric population and found that three pharmacotherapeutic categories con-stituted 78 percent of all prescribed medications. These categories were antiinfec-tives/chemotherapeutics, central nervous agents, and respiratory agents. Amoxicillin, aminophylline, and acetaminophen were the most frequently prescribed drugs in each category.[39] Stoller examined the use of prescription and over-the-counter (OTC) medication use among the ambulatory elderly. She showed that health-status indicators are better predictors of the use of prescription than OTC medications, suggesting that self-medication with OTC drugs may be a first step in illness behavior rather than a substitute for physician consultation. The most frequently prescribed medications are antihypertensives (30.5 percent), cardiac agents (20.8 percent), and antihistamines (16.4 percent). The most frequently reported OTCs are analgesics (38.6 percent) and laxatives (16.9 percent).[40] Although most studies are incidental, providing a cross-sectional view of drug utilization for one period in time, valuable information also is provided by longitudinal studies.

A major source of information on drug use patterns in the U.S. is the FDA's annual review of national outpatient drug use. These reports provide an overview of the most widely used drugs in current practice. They also provide data for comparative analysis of classes of drugs and by geographic region. Because many combination drug products contain multiple pharmacologically active agents, a listing of the active ingredients is provided in the review.

Even though the elderly constitute only 11 percent of the population, they consume 30 percent of the prescription and OTC drugs, accounting for more than 20 percent of the nation's total expense on drugs. As a group, the elderly make substantially more physician visits than younger people, use the hospitals twice as often, and stay twice as long.[41]

Data published in the FDA's 1985 review summarized the following trends in overall drug use. From 1971 to 1985, both the number of prescriptions dispensed and the population size increased by 16 percent, while the prescription size increased by 29 percent. Consequently, population exposure to prescription drugs increased 29 percent over this time period.[8,42]

In major therapeutic classes, cardiovascular drugs held 15 percent of the 1985 prescription drug market and were the most frequently dispensed, followed by antiinfectives (13 percent of the market), and psychotherapeutics (9 percent). These categories, including analgesics and diuretics, accounted for 50 percent of the prescriptions dispensed.[8,42]

The most frequently dispensed drugs (based on dispensing volume) in 1985 were: (1) Dyazide, (2) Lanoxin, (3) Inderal, (4) Valium, and (5) Tylenol with Codeine.[8]

A valuable approach to drug utilization studies is comparative analyses of factors explaining drug use levels across different countries. Kohn and White reported on an international comparative analysis of medication consumption by 48 000 respondents representing 15 million persons in 12 study areas (6 areas in North America, 2 in Yugoslavia, and 1 each in Buenos Aires, Poland, Liverpool, and Helsinki). This study showed that women are generally more likely than men to use medicines for every age group, and in all the study areas one exception was found for men aged 65 and over residing in Yugoslavia.[43]

Kohn and White also found that drug use rates increase with age, except for women in the six North American study areas where women of reproductive age (15–44) showed a slightly higher usage rate than those aged 45–64, which can be explained by the use of oral contraceptives.[43]

Analyzed by therapeutic class, antiinfectives administered for systemic effects were the most frequently mentioned products, followed by cardiovascular drugs. Diuretics were classified separately from cardiovascular drugs and showed usage rates consistently higher for the six North American study areas, intermediate in Liverpool, Helsinki, and Buenos Aires, and low in Poland and the two Yugoslavian study areas.[43]

A comparative analysis of descriptive data on drug use in several countries provides a first insight that the drug utilization rates are rather similar. Does this indicate that disease prevalence has the same magnitude? Are medical prescribing patterns similar? Are peoples' beliefs in medicines the same across these countries? Does it indicate that sociodemographic population parameters are equal? Descriptive data do not provide us with an explanation for the observed data distributions, but provide the qualitative information from which hypotheses can be generated to be tested in pharmacoepidemiologic studies.

Patterns of drug use in different countries can be found in the drug utilization literature; these consumption patterns often provide clues to the cause of the observed differences. Baksaas, studying antihypertensive consumption in the Nordic countries using 1980 sales figures for Sweden and Denmark, found that 10 percent of the population received antihypertensive drugs on a chronic basis. Because beta-blockers and diuretics are used for other indications as well, sales figures may give a distorted view of the prevalence of the primary disease indication. Statistics linking prescribing to diagnosis indicated that about 75 percent of the beta-blockers and 85 percent of the thiazides were used in the treatment of hypertension in Sweden. In Norway, 50 percent of hypertensive patients used more than one drug. Therefore, only 4–5 percent of the population in the Nordic countries might receive antihypertensives as long-term treatment. The drug of choice to treat hypertension varies from country to country, but diuretics are the most widely used, with Danish physicians being especially high prescribers of thiazide diuretics.[10]

Another study comparing drug use for hypertension in Spain with the Nordic countries showed that the consumption of antihypertensive drugs measured in DDDs was much lower in Spain than in the Nordic countries. The use of beta-blocking agents, synthetic hypotensives, and diuretics was also lower in Spain than in the Nordic countries. Only rauwolfia preparations, including combinations with other antihypertensives, were more commonly prescribed. However, thiazides and other diuretics were the most commonly prescribed drugs for hypertension.[44]

Other approaches to comparative analysis of drug utilization patterns are possible. It is not the purpose of this section to review the drug utilization patterns or comparative analytical strategies as contained in the medical and pharmaceutical literature. This would be impossible to achieve. For example, the World Health

Organization publishes a comprehensive bibliography of all drug utilization studies published between May 1981 and January 1990. This publication contains 1018 references to drug utilization studies. It is available from the WHO Collaborating Centre for Drug Statistics Methodology, P.O. Box 100, Veitvet, 0518 Oslo 5, Norway.[45]

Drug use patterns are influenced by patient characteristics, diagnosis, disease severity, related physical conditions, and age; prescribing and consumption are impacted and protected by national and regional prescribing norms, traditions, economics, payment systems, number of physicians, the role of advertising, patient educational levels, and other healthcare system variables. Moreover, it appears that these patterns evolve regularly and continuously. Therefore, drug use data cannot be used without consideration of these and other confounding variables. Further studies are necessary to evaluate methodologies to quantify the different factors discussed above as they impact on drug utilization.

Summary

There are more and more effective drugs on the market today than ever before. Variation in the utilization of drugs and prediction of that utilization together with the generation of hypotheses exploring that variation is the object of pharmacoepidemiology. Patients are better educated, have greater expectations from healthcare, and frequently use multiple sources of care.[33] A high correlation between the use of healthcare services, particularly physician contacts, and the use of prescribed drugs can be observed. However, all prescribing is not based on patient needs and all patient needs are not met with drug therapy. Consequently, there is as much concern about inappropriate and expensive prescribing as there is about underprescribing.

The assessment of the rationality of drug therapy through drug utilization studies is of particular interest in some of the developed countries.[46] For instance, in Sweden there are several reasons for this interest. The three major reasons are (1) the population in general feels there is an imbalance between the beneficial effets and the UDEs of drug therapy and between the importance of pharmacologic and nonpharmacologic treatment, (2) primary care physicians are mandated to have better knowledge of the sociomedical status of patients in their practice areas including prescription drug use patterns, and (3) limited resources available in the healthcare system necessitate the review of drug therapy outcomes.

The assessment of the rationality of drug use in less-developed countries continues to be an issue.[47] These issues are related to four major areas. First, national drug policies have been established without referring to the need for assessing drug utilization. Second, healthcare practices and services suffer from communication problems, lack of guidelines, and poor control over the introduction of new medications in the market. Third, education and training programs for healthcare professionals have generally lacked emphasis to newer medical care concepts and, in particular, pharmacology and pharmacotherapy.

Also, major changes are underway in the U.S. that will impact prescribing practice and, consequently, drug utilization in the near future. The prepaid care practice format referred to as "managed care" is making a profound impact on patterns of drug use in the U.S. Managed care organizations including HMOs, preferred provider organizations, and health insurers will play an aggressive role in directing and controlling the utilization of services. Examples include directing patients to specified hospitals, clinics, and specialists; and implementing formularies with a focus on generic (multisource) products. All this will influence established drug utilization trends. Moreover, buying arrangements with selective manufacturers will direct demand for products made by those manufacturers, which sometimes may be very different from local trends and prescribing patterns. Managed care organizations, through the use of payment sanctions to prescribers and dual copayment levels to patients, will succeed in modifying previous drug use patterns.

The interpretation of drug utilization data is essential for clinical researchers, regulatory agencies, and manufacturers to evaluate marketed drugs for both therapeutic efficacy (primary and secondary effects) and unexpected reactions not identified during Phase I, II, and III premarketing studies. These data are needed in an effort to endorse the selection of efficacious and comparatively less toxic drugs based on the incidence of UDEs in larger populations.

The population at risk for a given medical condition must be known to justify the level of drug use for that specific diagnosis in the defined population. Descriptive data on drug use are easy to obtain and provide the most common information originating from drug utilization studies. Drug utilization data have important applications in pharmacoepidemiology, with each of these applications putting different demands on the methodologic rigor with which the data are collected. Drug utilization frequencies provide information on the use of classes of drugs or the use of drugs over time. Utilization frequencies also define the sample frame of the population at risk for a UDE. Used in rates, drug utilization data can provide the numerator data to assess drug utilization per population unit, or patient population with a defined diagnosis. Used as denominator data with the incidence of UDEs defining the numerator, drug utilization data can be used to calculate the incidence rate and the relative risk of a UDE for the drug under investigation. Each of these applications of drug utilization data requires the correct unit of measurement, which can be sales data, prescription volume, or defined daily dose.

Care is needed in interpreting drug utilization data as a health indicator. Discrepancies between geographic patterns of morbidity and drug sales can be attributed to factors such as diagnostic criteria, differences in the age distribution of the population, access to healthcare, and prevalence of the disease.[48,49] Moreover, drug sales do not necessarily equate with drug intake. The confounder drug compliance needs to be addressed; it often is assumed in drug utilization studies that all drugs are being taken as directed by the physician. Drug utilization studies provide the necessary denominator data to be used in more pharmacoepidemiologic research. Drug utilization methods used in conjunction with in-depth observational studies (cohort, case control) and other surveillance methods can ensure that future drug use will become more rational, safe, and efficacious.

Appendix I National Databases for Pharmaco- epidemiologic Research	**Name**	**Group Health Cooperative of Puget Sound**
	Population	HMO in Seattle area 280 000–300 000 members
	Characteristics	Boston Drug Surveillance Programs use the database for cohort studies, prepaid group HMO.
	Advantages	drug costs covered by membership fee, assumes complete drug use data in members pharmacies fully automated since July 1976 complete record of all prescriptions filled by 28 000 people for a period of eight years hospital discharge diagnosis available dating back to 1972 95 percent of patients with a prescription will have it filled at an HMO pharmacy. validity of data high (reported to be >99 percent through interviews and record searches)
	Disadvantages	population served is primarily young, employed; excludes elderly
	Name	**Kaiser Foundation Health Plan: Southern California**
	Population	~ 1.8 million in southern California
	Characteristics	prepaid group HMO
	Advantages	age, gender, and sex distribution is similar to general population all areas have computerized pharmacies effective 1984 basic descriptive and demographic data on hospital discharges are stored on computer files
	Disadvantages	outpatient encounters and details of hospital episodes available only by manual review
	Name	Medicaid
	Population	primarily needy, indigent, disabled
	Characteristics	programs are designed for states to provide needed medical care to defined population
	Advantages	temporal associations between drug and diagnostic events can be examined longitudinal medical histories data collection is continuous for several years in most states fairly rapid retrieval and relatively inexpensive reliable denominator data absence of classic biases (e.g., interview, recall, reporting)
	Disadvantages	data validity database is a medical billing database rather than medical records

Disadvantages cont'd. — loss to follow-up because of eligibility changes
skewed population with respect to demographics, income, and social factors.
state-to-state variations in eligibility and treatments covered
potential confounders not documented (e.g., smoking, alcohol consumption, parity)

Name — COMPASS (Computerized On-Line Monitoring)
Population — a compilation of billing information submitted by Medicaid in ~10 states
Characteristics — database run by Health Information Designs, Arlington, Virginia 22209
Advantages — dates back to 1980
very large, comprehensive data collection
(see Medicaid advantages)
Disadvantages — (see Medicaid disadvantages)

Name — The Saskatchewan Database
Population — ~1 million people in the province of Saskatchewan
Characteristics — drug plan database has accumulated 37 million prescriptions since 1975
1600 formulary products covered
Advantages — drug database linkable to: separation data from hospitals, physician services, psychiatric services, cancer foundation, and vital statistics
Disadvantages — none

Name — ARAMIS (American Rheumatism Association Medical Information System)
Population — tracks 22 000 patients from 17 centers
Characteristics — national arthritis data resource
prospective protocol assess routine clinical data, mortality, disability, discomfort, UDEs, and economic impact
Advantages — can investigate: comparative toxicity of drugs, long-term drug effects, effects of drug combinations, effects of comorbidity, generalizability of premarketing estimates, clinical characteristics of those with UDEs
Disadvantages — focused population

Name — The Boston University School of Medicine Slone Epidemiology Unit (SEU)
Population — over 50 000 cases studied, including 11 000 with cancer and 5500 children with congenital malformations
Characteristics — goal is to quantify the serious unintended effects of drugs
chief strategy is case-control approach
22 collaborating hospitals
Advantages — information is collected by personal interview
information is gathered on both prescription and nonprescription medications
Disadvantages — normal biases when using interview techniques (e.g., recall, interviewer)

HMO = health maintenance organization; UDE = unintended drug effects.

Appendix 2
European Databases for Pharmacoepidemiologic Research

England and Wales	Prescription Pricing Authority (PPA) collects all prescriptions within the National Health Service for reimbursement to pharmacies. Specialized studies can be made with this material based on PPA's limited resources.
Finland	Finnish Committee on Drug Information and Statistics. Finnish Statistics on Medicines. Wholesale figures by drug classes following the Anatomical Therapeutic Chemical Classification (ATC). Sources of data are wholesaler sales to pharmacies and hospitals provided in DDD as unit of measurement.
Northern Ireland	Department of Therapeutics and Pharmacology, Queen's University of Belfast, has received information from the National Health Service prescription database since 1962. Provides drug-prescribing frequencies for each drug and prescribing profiles for each physician.
Norway	Norwegian Wholesalers' Monopoly, Norsk Medicinal Depot (NMD) publishes sales statistics for drugs in Norway, monitors drug utilization in the country, and makes data available on request.
Sweden	National Corporation of Swedish Pharmacies (Apotheksbolaget). Sales statistics in monetary units and in DDDs, regional and for the whole country (Svensk Lakemedel Statistik).
	Diagnoses–Therapy Survey. A sample of doctors deliver prescription copies with the diagnoses that caused prescribing. Sample of 1 prescription out of 25 dispensed in computerized pharmacies provide age and sex distribution of prescription drug users.
	The Jam Hand Study. 17 600 inhabitants of the county of Jam Hand are followed continuously with regard to drug prescriptions.
	The Tierp Study: Department of Social Medicine, University of Uppsala. 22 000 inhabitants in the community of Tierp are monitored for all health-related events. Includes physician visits and prescriptions filled.
	Swedish Data Bank at the Department of Health and Welfare. Based on sales statistics.
	Nordic Council of Medicines. Monitors drug utilization in the Nordic countries. Publishes DDDs for all drugs, including revisions.

DDD = defined daily dose.

References

1. Brodie DC. Drug utilization and drug utilization review and control. In a study supported by National Center for Health Services Research and Development. Health Services

and Mental Health Administration, Department of Health, Education, and Welfare, 5600M Fisher's Lane, Rockville, MD 20852 (NCHS-RD-70-8).

2. World Health Organization. The selection of essential drugs. Report of a WHO expert committee. Geneva: Technical report. Ser. no. 615, 1977.

3. Tognoni G. Drug use and monitoring. In: Holand WW. Evaluation of health care. Oxford: Oxford University Press, 1983:207-25.

4. Lunde PKM, Baksaas I. Epidemiology of drug utilization—basic concepts and methodology. Acta Med Scand 1988;721(suppl):7-11.

5. Scruba TJ. International comparison of drug consumption: impact of prices. Soc Sci Med 1986;22:1019-25.

6. Lunde PKM. Drug statistics and drug utilization. In: Columbo F, Shapiro S, Slone D, Tognoni G, eds. Epidemiologic evaluation of drugs. Littleton, MA: PSG Publishing, 1977.

7. Wertheimer AI. The defined daily dose system (DDD) for drug utilization review. Hosp Pharm 1986;21:233-41, 258.

8. Baum C, Kennedy DL, Knapp DE, Faich GA. Drug utilization in the U.S.—1985: seventh annual review. Rockville, MD: Food and Drug Administration, December 1985.

9. Bergman U, Wessling A, Sjoqvist F. Validation of observed differences in the utilization of antihypertensive and antidiabetic drugs in Northern Ireland, Norway, and Sweden. Eur J Clin Pharmacol 1985;29:1-8.

10. Baksaas I. Patterns in drug utilization—national and international aspects: antihypertensive drugs. Acta Med Scand 1984;683(suppl):59-66.

11. Aquilonius SM, Granat M, Hartvig P. Utilization of antiparkinson drugs in Norway, Sweden, Denmark and Finland 1975-1979. Acta Neurol Scand 1981; 64:47-53.

12. Bjelle A, Mjorndal T. Drug prescription patterns for rheumatic disorders in Sweden. J Rheumatol 1984;11:493-9.

13. Jakovljevic V, Stanulovic M. Extremes in drug utilization patterns. Low prescribing of antihypertensives in the district of Novi Sad, Yugoslavia. Acta Med Scand 1984;683 (suppl):67-9.

14. Gustafsson LL, Boethius G. Utilization of analgesics from 1970 to 1978. Prescription patterns in the county of Jamtland and in Sweden as a whole. Acta Med Scand 1982;211:419-25.

15. Bergman U, Sjoqvist F. Measurement of drug utilization in Sweden: methodological and clinical implications. Acta Med Scand 1984;683(suppl):15-22.

16. Westerholm B. Drug utilization studies—a valuable tool for optimization of drug therapy and drug control. J Soc Admin Pharm 1981;1:1-8.

17. International drug benefit/risk assessment data resource handbook. Vol. 1. North America. Prepared by Pharma Corporation and the Degge Group Ltd. Basel, Switzerland: CIBA-Geigy, 1988.

18. Baum C, Kennedy DL, Forbes MB, Jones JK. Drug use and expenditures in 1982. JAMA 1985;253:382-6.

19. An introduction to the PDS Alpha system. Phoenix, AZ: Pharmaceutical Data Services, 1981.

20. Strom BL, Carson JL, Morse ML, et al. The computerized on-line Medicaid pharmaceutical analysis and surveillance system: a new resource for post-marketing drug surveillance. Clin Pharmacol Ther 1985;38:359-64.

21. Kreling DH, Knocke DJ, Hammel RW. The effect of an internal analgesic formulary restriction on Medicaid drug expenditures in Wisconsin. *Med Care* 1989; 27:34-44.

22. Jacobs J, Keyserling JA, Britton J, et al. The total cost of care and the use of pharmaceuticals in the management of rheumatoid arthritis: The Medi-Cal Program. *J Clin Epidemiol* 1988;41:215-23.

23. Kotzan L, Carroll NV, Kotzan JA. Influence of age, sex, and race on prescription drug use among Georgia Medicaid recipients. *Am J Hosp Pharm* 1989; 46:287-90.

24. Westerholm B. Data collection in Sweden. In: Bergman U, Grimsson A, Wahba AHW, Westerholm B, eds. Studies in drug utilization. Methods and applications. WHO Regional Publications. European Series No. 8. Copenhagen: World Health Organization Regional Office for Europe, 1979:63-82.

25. Tognoni G, Liberati A, Pello L, Sasanelli F, Spagnoli A. Drug utilization studies and epidemiology. *Rev Epidemiol Sante Publique* 1983;31:59-71.

26. Accreditation manual for hospitals. Chicago: Joint Commission on the Accreditation of Hospitals, 1978.

27. Sheldon G. Self-audit of prescribing habits and clinical care and general practice. *J R Coll Gen Pract* 1979;29:703-11.

28. Brodie DC, Smith WE Jr, Hylnka JN. Model for drug usage review in a hospital. *Am J Hosp Pharm* 1977;34:251-4.

29. Olson DC. Guidelines for PSRO review of prescription drugs in acute care hospitals. HEW contract report no. 240-75-0015, Ambler, PA, 1977.

30. Reilly MJ. Drug utilization review by pharmacy and therapeutics committees. *Am J Hosp Pharm* 1973;30:349-50.

31. Department of Health, Education, and Welfare. Guidelines for PSRO long-term care review. PSRO transmittal no. 62, Washington, DC, Feb. 28, 1978.

32. Crooks J. The concept of medical auditing. *Acta Med Scand* 1984;683(suppl):47-52.

33. Reilly PM, Pattern MP. An audit of prescribing by peer review. *J R Coll Gen Pract* 1978;28:525-38.

34. Sartell PE. Retrospective studies: a review for the clinician. *Ann Intern Med* 1974;81:381-7.

35. Jick H, Vessey MP. Case control studies in the evaluation of drug-induced illness. *Am J Epidemiol* 1978;107:1-7.

36. Herbst AL, Ulfelder H, Poskanzer DC. Adenocarcinoma of the vagina: association of maternal stilbestrol therapy with tumor appearance in young women. *N Engl J Med* 1971; 284:878-81.

37. Jick H, Watkins RN, Hunter JR. Replacement estrogens and endometrial cancer. *N Engl J Med* 1979;300:218-22.

38. Anderson DW, Bryan FA, Harris BSH III, Lessler JT, Gagnon JP. A survey approach for finding cases of epilepsy. *Public Health Rep* 1985;100:386-93.

39. Olubadewo J, Ikponmwamba A. Profile of prescription medications in a pediatric population. *Drug Intell Clin Pharm* 1988;22:999-1002.

40. Stoller EP. Prescribed and over-the-counter medicine use by the ambulatory elderly. *Med Care* 1988;26:1149-57.

41. Vestal R. Drugs and the elderly. Washington, DC: National Institutes of Health. U.S. Government Printing Office, 1978.

42. Baum C, Kennedy DL, Knapp DE, et al. Prescription drug use in 1984 and changes over time. *Med Care* 1988;26:105-14.

43. Kohn R, White K. Health care on international study. Oxford: Oxford University Press, 1976.

44. Capella D, Porta M, Laporte JR. Utilization of antihypertensive drugs in certain European countries. *Eur J Clin Pharmacol* 1983;25:431-5.

45. Drug utilization bibliography. Copenhagen: World Health Organization Regional Office for Europe, 1989.

46. Boethius G. Approaches to assessing the rationality of drug usage in a developed country. *Acta Med Scand* 1988;721(suppl):21-6.

47. Ali HN. Problems in assessing rationality of drug utilization in less developed countries. *Acta Med Scand* 1988;721(suppl):27-30.

48. Hjort P, Holmen J, Waaler H. The relation between drug utilization and morbidity pattern: antihypertensive drugs. *Acta Med Scand* 1984;683(suppl):89-93.

49. Westerholm B, Dahlstrom M, Nordanstam I. Relation between drug utilization and morbidity patterns. *Acta Med Scand* 1984;683(suppl):95-7.

8 Postmarketing Surveillance Methodologies

Stanley A. Edlavitch

Abstract

Chapter 5 describes and discusses the strengths and limitations of the major pharmacoepidemiologic methodologies employed in postmarketing drug surveillance and describes the current status of the U.S. surveillance system. Special attention is given to study design considerations to permit causal inferences to be made. The main methodologies employed in postmarketing drug surveillance include controlled clinical trials, observational epidemiologic studies (cohort, case-control, cross-sectional), demographic methods, drug utilization surveys, spontaneous reports of unintended drug effects, and automated databases linking medications and diseases. Examples of pharmacoepidemiologic studies using each of these methodologies are presented. When a question arises about the efficacy and/or safety of a marketed drug, typically a mixture of these study methodologies is employed. The chapter also provides a brief discussion of the roles of the Food and Drug Administration, pharmaceutical manufacturers, and academic institutions in initiating and conducting postmarketing drug studies. Finally, the author suggests that critical factors for the growth of pharmacoepidemiology as a scientific discipline include the value society places on the questions addressed by this discipline, the availability and use of high-quality data to pursue the answers, the development of training programs to prepare pharmacoepidemiologic scientists, and the expansion of currently existing forums for exchanging knowledge.

An increased awareness of the potential of drugs for preventing and treating disease, coupled with an awareness of the potential for some drugs to cause unwanted adverse effects, has led to the emergence of a challenging new scientific discipline, pharmacoepidemiology. This chapter discusses the major pharmacoepidemiologic methodologies employed in postmarketing drug surveillance, and describes the status of the U.S. surveillance system. In Chapter 1 Porta and Hartzema list the main questions that should be addressed by postmarketing drug studies. These include discovery of chronic or latent effects of a drug, discovery of rare effects, determination of efficacy in customary practice as well as in new indications, and identification of modifiers of a drug's efficacy.

Because there are more than 30 000 different prescription drugs (more than 2000 different molecular entities) and 300 000 over-the-counter (OTC) products (800 active ingredients) on the market, it is impossible to conduct individual, continuous, formal studies for each marketed drug. To further complicate the scientific challenge, our knowledge and questions are not static. We continuously develop questions about a drug's efficacy and safety for current and new indications and either formally or informally we evaluate the drug's efficacy and toxicity in comparison to alternative therapies. Furthermore, the manufacturer may change the drug's formulation and, once the patent for the innovator drug expires, a number of generic versions with similar, but not exact, bioavailability may be marketed.

Issues surrounding postmarketing surveillance (PMS) have generated vigorous, healthy, and sometimes heated scientific debate.[1-6] Somewhat esoteric discussions of study design, statistical significance, and comparison of diagnostic algorithms have dominated these debates, but almost all parties agree on a few principles. These include: (1) Premarketing clinical evaluations of a new drug may leave unanswered important questions about its optimal use. The limitations of premarketing studies include relatively small numbers of patients, short duration of therapy, highly screened volunteers, and exclusion of children, pregnant women, and the elderly, are addressed in Chapters 4 and 7. (2) The number of "unsafe" drugs that have reached the market is relatively small compared with the total number of marketed drugs. The manufacturers' caution during pharmaceutical development; Food and Drug Administration (FDA) enforcement of federal drug regulations and the vigilance of physicians, nurses, pharmacists, other health practitioners, and the public have all contributed to the presence of relatively few medical disasters in the marketing of drugs. (3) U.S. standards for medical care are very high. As a society, we exhibit very low tolerance when pharmaceutical manufacturers or the FDA permit the marketing of unsafe or ineffective drugs. (4) Physicians and patients have different perspectives on drug effectiveness and safety. Physicians and pharmacists are advised to consider the efficacy, cost-effectiveness, and benefit-to-risk ratio of one drug versus another or of various regimens; the patient is concerned primarily with whether the drug is effective and affordable (or covered by insurance) and whether the unintended drug effects (UDEs) that the patient associates with the drug are tolerable. (5) There is no simple single approach to postmarketing drug surveillance. Some postmarketing discoveries of UDEs and new indications have been serendipitous, but drug surveillance cannot rely on chance alone.[7-10] The complexity of monitoring the efficacy and safety of all drugs and the desire to identify rare events require the use of modern population methods, in particular, the use of epidemiology and biostatistics.[11-14] (6) A PMS system must involve pharmaceutical manufacturers, the FDA, physicians, nurses, pharmacists, third-party payers, the academic community, the general public, legislators, and the legal community. (7) A PMS system should provide quantitative data to aid in making therapeutic and regulatory decisions. These data must be adequate to measure both the beneficial effects and the risks associated with drugs.

Unintended Drug Effects

A UDE can be defined as a noxious and unintended response to a drug in humans that occurs at usually recommended doses.[15] In Chapter 5, Rogers discusses the distinction between the pharmacologic categories of UDEs and the importance of considering the impact of the reaction on patient morbidity and mortality. The effects on physical, mental, and social functioning and on the quality of life are difficult to measure and evaluate, but definitely have an impact on health professionals as they relate to patients and their families. Rawlins and Thompson proposed a useful dichotomy of UDEs (adverse drug reactions) into two broad classes, type A reactions and type B reactions. Type A reactions result from exaggerated pharmacologic effects, and type B reactions are rare, unpredictable, and often more serious. Improvement in premarketing pharmacokinetic and pharmacodynamic studies, physician prescribing, and patient compliance could reduce the incidence of type A reactions. However, type B reactions can only be discovered through PMS.[16]

The foundation to any PMS system is the quality of information available for decision-making. Therefore, the most important roles played in PMS are those of the healthcare professionals who are relied on to correctly identify and report unusual or unwanted life events as well as therapeutic successes.

A critical role belongs to patients who best know how they are feeling, but have not traditionally been encouraged to recognize and report adverse events. Frequently the physician or pharmacist chooses not to report patients' complaints about drugs to the drug regulatory authority. In the U.S., the FDA, which for practical reasons returns patient-initiated reports and requests that patients ask their physicians to resubmit the report, reinforces the message that only health professionals can objectively identify the symptoms of drugs not working as expected.

It is beyond the scope of this review to do more than mention the importance of the pharmacist in educating patients on proper administration of medications and about potential UDEs and drug interactions.

Major Methodologies Employed in Postmarketing Surveillance

CLINICAL TRIALS

Many scientists believe controlled clinical trials are the "gold standard" for establishing the effectiveness of various therapeutic regimens.[11,12,17,18] This is particularly true when the trial is a randomized, double-blind, or triple-blind design.

A controlled clinical trial is a prospective study that involves two or more treatment groups and controls who may be treated with an active drug, a placebo, or both. The purpose of conducting a controlled clinical drug trial is to assess the effectiveness of drug therapy in either preventing disease (prophylactic trials) or treating established disease (therapeutic trials).

A randomized, controlled, clinical trial is characterized by assignment of participants to treatment of control groups in a random, unbiased fashion. The most stringent clinical trial methodologies involve double-blind techniques where neither the patient nor the physician knows which therapy the patient is receiving, and triple-blind techniques where the epidemiologist/statistician also is unaware of the patient's therapy. (Frequently, the pharmacist is the only professional involved in the treatment process who has regular access to therapy information during the trial so that dispensing accuracy can be checked and emergency intervention is possible.)

Clinical trials are scientifically acceptable as the primary study design to control for a number of biases inherent to observation and the findings of well-designed clinical trials are generally widely accepted. Foremost in these potential biases is protection against patient selection for a particular therapy based on subjective factors or judgmental factors related to the outcome of interest. Clinical trials also permit a direct estimate of efficacy and risk of developing an adverse event. When the trial fails to demonstrate a difference between therapies, it is possible to evaluate the probability that this lack of difference is an error and may be due to variation alone (power of the trial).

Clinical trials have some inherent limitations. They require extensive planning and cannot be quickly initiated. They are not exploratory, but usually are tailored to evaluate single diseases and treatments, and tend to concentrate on expected therapeutic effects and adverse reactions. Because of sample size, clinical trials cannot be expected to discover rare adverse reactions and they take a long time to complete (depending on the acuteness of the condition being treated, the length of time it takes for the drug to have its desired effect, and the anticipated latency period).[17,19]

Although such studies far exceed the extremely limited follow-up (average six months) of premarketing trials, postmarketing trials rarely extend longer than five to seven years. They are, therefore, limited in measuring the effects of prolonged drug use and of latent effects.

Another potential limitation of clinical trial results is their extrapolation to the total population who may be treated with the study drug. As in premarketing studies, the population of volunteers willing to participate in a clinical trial is a subset of the general population. This is true no matter how carefully the trial attempts to enlist a "representative" sample of the population.[20]

Other advantages and limitations of postmarketing clinical trials were discussed earlier in this book.[1] Excellent references on clinical trial design, conduct, and interpretation are available.[21-23]

Major postmarketing clinical trials have been conducted to study the effectiveness of drug therapy in reducing the consequences of disease, such as the Aspirin Myocardial Infarction Study (AMIS) and the Veterans Administration and U.S. Public Health Service trials of the treatment of mild hypertension: the Hypertension Detection and Follow-up Program (HDFP), the Multiple Risk Factor Intervention Trial (MRFIT), the Lipid Research Clinicals (LRC), and Systolic Hypertension in the Elderly Program (SHEP).[24-31]

Senior researchers have debated whether placebo-controlled or randomized clinical trials are ethical and necessary.[14,32,33] To avoid assigning patients to placebo therapies, suggestions for alternative study designs (e.g., historical controls) may be appropriate in special situation. Dropouts and patient-elected crossovers from placebo to treatment therapy frequently confuse interpretation of the trial findings.

Strom et al. have published very provocative articles on the necessity of conducting experimental studies (e.g., randomized clinical trials) to study a marketed drug's efficacy.[12,13] The essential idea is that we conduct randomized studies to protect against selection bias when the efficacy of a drug on a particular outcome can be confounded by the health status of the patient when the drug was prescribed. For example, confounding occurs if patients with more severe diseases receive the drug, and patients with better prognoses do not receive the drug so that the drug appears less effective than it actually is. Randomization is helpful in solving the problem because it helps produce two groups with comparable baseline states. When the indication for treatment can be fully characterized, randomization may not be essential. When Strom et al. applied these criteria to the 100 most recently approved drugs (since 1978), representing 131 potential drug uses, they found that the efficacy of 68 percent of the drugs could be evaluated from clinical observations, 10.7 percent could be evaluated by experimental or nonexperimental studies, 4.6 percent only by experimental studies, 8 percent only by nonexperimental studies, and 22.1 percent "could not be studied by either technique."[12,13,34] Another interesting approach for optimizing therapy for an individual patient is the N of 1 randomized clinical trial proposed by Guyatt et al. The patient serves as his own control in a crossover design.[35]

OBSERVATIONAL EPIDEMIOLOGIC SURVEYS

Observational studies are those in which the investigator has no control over who receives what kind of drug.

Cohort Studies. The observational study design that most closely resembles the controlled clinical trial is the controlled cohort study. In this type of study, groups of individuals (cohorts) are identified, characterized, and followed over time to determine the incidence of some predetermined event or outcome. Controlled cohort studies with one cohort characterized by exposure to the drug being evaluated and a second cohort untreated or exposed to an alternative drug are scientifically preferable to uncontrolled cohort studies in which there is no control group. Cohort studies may be conducted either prospectively (concurrent) or retrospectively (nonconcurrent).[17]

In a prospective cohort study, a cohort may be selected for reasons of convenience (e.g., medical records are available, volunteers) or because the group is known to have experienced an exposure of interest (e.g., the first 1000 people to receive a prescription for a newly marketed drug). The major advantages of the prospective cohort study are that the cohort is chosen, and that characteristics of the cohort can be determined (e.g., drug exposure, smoking, compliance) prior to knowing whether a disease outcome or a UDE has occurred. The investigator can determine in advance what information to collect. Prospective cohort studies also permit calculation of UDE incidence rates and comparison of the difference of incidence in rates between cohorts (attributable risk).

The main disadvantages of cohort studies are their cost and the difficulty of guarding against inherent biases (e.g., physician and patient selection of treatment, selection of alternative therapies, and of enrolling representative volunteers). In addition, prospective cohort studies typically are not large enough to detect rare adverse reactions and large cohorts are required when the disease of interest has a low incidence.

Large prospective postmarketing cohort studies (7607–22 653 people) were reviewed by Rossi et al. for cimetidine hydrochloride, cyclobenzaprine hydrochloride, and prazosin hydrochloride. The authors expressed specific concerns about the designs of these studies, each of which was very expensive and failed to discover adverse reactions that were not already known from premarketing trials. They also found that reporting of adverse reactions occurred at substantially lower rates in postmarketing versus premarketing studies.[36] Frequency of reporting decreased with the length of the study, and despite the fact that the practitioners were very willing to agree to participate in these studies, compliance with the protocol was found to be poor.[36,37]

There are also numerous reports of successful prospective cohort studies, both uncontrolled and controlled.[13,38,39] A large successfully conducted multicenter prospective cohort study was the Collaborative Perinatal Project, sponsored by the National Institute of Neurological and Communicative Disorders of the National Institutes of Health. Between 1959 and 1965, it enrolled 50 282 mother-child pairs in 12 medical centers. Although this study did not identify any "new thalidomides," new methods to analyze the enormous amount of information that is collected in large prospective cohort studies were developed. In addition, reference data on the expected incidence of various types of malformations helped in the design of future studies.[40]

Historical Prospective Studies. These are similar to other prospective cohort studies except that cohorts are constructed retrospectively from existing records. This is possible only when existing clinical records permit correct classification of the individual's past exposures. The longitudinal information characteristic of these studies covers time intervals from the past to the present or to the future. The integrity of this study design depends on the completeness of the recordkeeping system that is being relied upon to provide data from the past.

The Mayo Clinic provides an ideal environment for such a study design. Since 1907, it has kept complete records, including prescriptions written for outpatient visits and hospitalization for Olmsted County patients.[41]

CASE-CONTROL STUDIES (CASE-REFERENT STUDIES)

Probably the least expensive, the simplest, and often the most controversial design to implement and interpret is the case-control study.[5,11,17,20,42-47]

In a case-control study, patients are selected according to carefully defined criteria and compared with controls who do not have the disease being studied. Existing medical records and/or interviews and surveys are used to determine past exposure in both case and control groups to some characteristic of interest (e.g., past use of a drug).

To ensure that differences in the experiences of cases and controls can be attributed to the drug or risk factor being studied, the study design must incorporate the following considerations: (1) Diagnoses for both case and control groups must be defined as accurately as possible. (2) The investigator should be aware of the possibility of confounding the progression of the illness under study with exposure to the drug of interest. (3) Patients included for study should have a reasonable probability of having been exposed to the drug of interest (men with breast cancer have almost zero chance of being previously exposed to oral contraceptives). (4) It is important to guard against selection biases in cases and controls. Preferably only newly diagnosed patients will be included so that patients who died immediately from the disease or were cured quickly are not excluded. (5) The same eligibility criteria should apply to both cases and controls. (6) Control subjects should be comparable to patients in all relevant ways except they should not have the disease under study, nor should they be more or less likely than those with the disease to take the drug under question (protopathic bias). Patients with conditions that are indications for drug use or contraindications for the drug must be excluded, as must patients with conditions known to be caused by or prevented by the drug. For example, in a study of the relationship of salicylates to Reye's syndrome, you would want to exclude hospitalized children with rheumatoid arthritis or other rheumatic diseases because hospitalized children have an increased propensity to use aspirin for rheumatoid conditions.[48]

An important assumption underlying the validity of case-control studies is that controls are just as likely as cases to be exposed to the drug under study. Miettinen suggests that the appropriate strategy for case-control studies is to identify the study base represented by cases and controls or your referent series.[44] If the study base is defined a priori, it will be easier to ensure that the controls are representative of that referent base and to control for covariates that could act as confounders.

The major advantages of the case-control design are that it can often be used with study populations of relatively smaller size than prospective cohort studies or clinical trials, and at a somewhat lower cost. This efficiency of size and cost is particularly advantageous for studying rare conditions or conditions that appear after long latency periods. A classic small, definitive case-control study consisting of only 8 cases and 32 controls was responsible for definitively establishing the link between maternal diethylstilbestrol therapy and adenocarcinoma of the vagina in daughters.[49]

The major problems in conducting a case-control study relate to selecting cases and controls, collecting valid retrospective data from records or relying on recall, and interpreting the results to remove the effects of confounding factors (factors associated with exposure to the drug and with the disease or UDE under study); sex, age, educational level, and socioeconomic status are often related to drug selection and access to medical care.

Another analytic disadvantage of case-control studies is that they do not permit a direct estimate of UDE incidence rates. In a cohort study, the incidence of an event (e.g., UDE, disease, death) can be calculated directly for exposed and unexposed groups. The ratio of these rates is called the relative risk. In a case-control study, the size of the underlying exposed and unexposed populations usually is unknown. The probability of drug exposure in cases can be compared with the probability of drug exposure in controls. The ratio of these probabilities is called the odds ratio, which is a good estimate of relative risk when the outcome of interest (e.g., UDE) is rare. Even so, the concept of relative risk is intuitively easier to understand than the odds ratio.

Examples that illustrate the difficulties in designing and interpreting case-control studies are the controversies generated by the studies linking endometrial cancer with estrogen use, Reye's syndrome to aspirin, and breast cancer to reserpine.

Hundreds of investigations of drug-disease relationships were conducted using case-control methodologies by the Boston Collaborative Drug Surveillance Program (BCDSP) and the Slone Epidemiology Unit (SEU), formerly the Drug Epidemiology Unit. BCDSP and SEU have maintained in-hospital monitoring studies that identify patients hospitalized with diseases that are potentially drug-induced and sufficiently serious to warrant ongoing drug surveillance efforts. General cautions concerning confounding, patient deficiencies in drug recall, and difficulties with assessing the validity of medical records apply to these databases.[4,50]

The BCDSP effort collected information in seven countries on over 35 000 medical inpatients and on regular outpatient drug use in over 40 000 medical and 5000 surgical inpatients. Now, major energies of the BCDSP research program are oriented toward automated databases. However, limited hospital surveillance continues under their auspices.

The largest current ongoing in-hospital monitoring studies are conducted by the SEU. Histories of drug use and current medical status are collected for patients hospitalized with targeted conditions. These include myocardial infarction, agranulocytosis, peptic ulcer, various cancers, and hepatic diseases. Over 40 000 hospitalized patients have been interviewed by nurse abstractors in hospitals in Boston, Baltimore, New York, Tucson, Philadelphia, Kansas City, and London, Ontario.

CROSS-SECTIONAL STUDIES

A cross-sectional study or survey is an observational study in which drug exposure and disease status or symptoms are determined at the same point in time. A cross-sectional survey may be launched to gather only a few pieces of information or a more elaborate survey might include quite extensive interviews and well developed procedures and instruments for data collection. The U.S. census is probably the best known cross-sectional survey.

Cross-sectional studies are most useful for describing current practice or generating hypotheses that must be validated using other study designs. Cross-sectional studies are not conducted to provide estimates of events following an exposure; therefore, associations observed may not be causal.

The most extensive cross-sectional health study undertaken in this country is the National Health Survey, which has been conducted for over 20 years by the National Center for Health Statistics (NCHS). The Health Survey collects data periodically through a number of programs, including Health Interview Surveys of 40 000 households, Health Examination Surveys of people aged 1–74 years, the National Discharge Survey, the National Nursing Home Survey, and the National Family Growth Survey. Of particular interest to pharmacoepidemiology is the ongoing National Ambulatory Care Survey which asks physicians to report on medical conditions and drugs prescribed (restricted almost exclusively to prescription drugs) during one week of practice. Aside from providing valuable information on health and health practices, NCHS has made major contributions to survey and biostatistic methodologies. In addition to numerous publications, another source of NCHS survey data is "public user" tapes which can be purchased at nominal charges through the Scientific and Technical Information Branch, NCHS. The Center is also currently putting much of the raw survey data on floppy diskettes formatted for IBM personal computers.[51]

On a much smaller scale than NCHS surveys, surveillance data are collected in large research programs. One such example is the community survey data from the Minnesota Heart Survey which collects information on prescription and OTC medications and health histories, and measures cardiovascular risk factors for a sample of 5000 Minneapolis-St. Paul residents.[52]

DEMOGRAPHIC STUDIES—VITAL STATISTICS

The health of a population can be studied by evaluating its vital statistics. Vital statistics data collected from ongoing recording or registration of vital events include births, adoptions, deaths, fetal deaths, marriages, divorces, legal separations, and annulments.[17] The Centers for Disease Control (CDC) keeps records of abortions, congenital malformations, rubella, nosocomial infections, tuberculosis, and other conditions that may have a preventable component. All states have a common list of over 45 reportable diseases that physicians are asked to report to their state health departments, which in turn forward the information to CDC.

Studies of vital statistics have prompted many investigations and helped formulate a number of important questions about disease incidence and mortality. For example, why have stomach cancer rates decreased so dramatically in this century? Why has there been a linear decrease in stroke rates since the mid-1900s (which is prior to the introduction of antihypertensive medications)? Why was there an increase in coronary heart disease mortality rates until 1968, but a steady decrease since then?

Vital statistics also have influenced drug monitoring safety by exposing links between drugs and disease. For example, vital statistics provided evidence that the introduction of oral contraceptives may be related to thromboembolism and pulmonary embolism, and that large doses of halogenated hydroxyquinoline may be related to subacute myelo-optic neuropathy in Japan. In the U.S., vital statistics also provided evidence that methyldopa was strongly implicated as a cause of cancer of the biliary ducts and that saccharin use is not closely related to bladder cancer.[53]

DRUG UTILIZATION SURVEYS

Drug utilization methods are reviewed in some detail in Chapter 7. The authors categorized drug utilization data according to the three sources of information: drug consumption data based on gross sales and distributions, physician prescriptions either in institutions or ambulatory care settings, and specific drug monitoring studies.

One of the major sources of drug utilization data in this country is IMS America, Inc. IMS conducts a number of ongoing cross-sectional surveys. The one referred to most often is the National Prescription Audit, which is based on a panel of 1200 computerized retail pharmacies.[54,55] Obtaining access to IMS data and methodologies has been a problem in the past for researchers not working through a pharmaceutical manufacturer or employed by the FDA.

SPONTANEOUS REPORTS

The U.S. Government's system is operated by the FDA and the FDA's Drug Experience Report form (GPO number 1639) has become synonymous with UDE reporting. Although physicians and other health professionals are encouraged to report new and unusual UDEs to the FDA, the system relies heavily on pharmaceutical manufacturers, whose field representatives and headquarters regulatory personnel are often the first to identify a potential reportable event. The pharmaceutical manufacturer is legally required to report serious unlabeled UDEs to the FDA within 15 working days of learning of the UDE.[55] More than 80 percent of spontaneous reports about UDEs come to the FDA through drug companies.[56]

UDE reporting fluctuates with the length of time the drug has been on the market and peaks with positive or negative reports published in major journals. Even given the above considerations, these spontaneous reporting systems are valuable. They monitor an enormous number of drugs (potentially all those marketed) over all patient categories, and at a relatively low cost. Voluntary reporting systems have the potential to capture rare, unexpected UDEs more quickly than other study designs. Because, in theory, these systems cover all drugs and are managed by relatively few personnel, they have a certain amount of appeal and cost-effectiveness.

It is impossible to determine rates of under- or overreporting, or to determine the validity and reliability of information supplied. Other stumbling blocks include establishing the nature of the population at risk of receiving the drug, the number of people already exposed to the drug, the accuracy of diagnoses provided, and the final disposition of the patient. Venning reports that none of the 18 UDEs United Kingdom physicians identified as most important were discovered through the spontaneous reporting systems of regulatory agencies.[8,9]

Medical Literature. One of the most important sources for identifying new and unsuspected serious UDEs is the worldwide medical literature.[7] Manufacturers maintain their own reference libraries of all published articles relating to their products, and often subscribe to various clipping services. For example, the Burroughs Wellcome database includes company-generated information and references obtained from their scanning of current journals, the National Library of Medicine computerized searches (e.g., MEDLINE, TOXLINE), Biological and Chemical Abstracts, Alerting Service from Wellcome, UK, Excerpta Medica, and their own internal files.There are, however, also problems with using reports from the medical literature to interpret the incidence of UDEs. Such reports often do not contain the information necessary to interpret the impact or the validity of the findings. In addition, it is often not possible to calculate an incidence rate for a population at risk from information provided. Therefore, practitioners have no way of knowing whether their patients are at a high risk of developing a similar reaction. Recent attempts to establish guidelines for publishing UDE reports may help to rectify these problems. These guidelines ask authors to identify age and sex of patients; to identify cases that have been previously reported; and to specify why the drug was given; its route, dose, and timing relative to the UDE; blood concentrations; and outcome.[57]

Determining whether a UDE has occurred is often difficult and a number of reports demonstrate substantial disagreement among experts in the assessment of UDEs.[56,58-61] In an effort to capture all UDEs of a study drug, Inman developed a new system called Prescription Event Monitoring, which identifies all prescriptions for a selected drug issued through the Prescription Pricing Authority. He enlists all general practitioners who have issued a prescription for the drug and requests they report "any new diagnosis, any reason for referral to a consultant or admission to a hospital . . . any unexpected deterioration (or improvement) in a concurrent illness, any suspect drug reaction, or any other complaint which was considered of sufficient importance to enter into the patient's notes." This system has not yet demonstrated its effectiveness at discovering rare events or quantifying known reactions.[62]

Lane et al. suggested an alternative to the above methods that uses Bayesian statistical approaches to assess causality for suspected adverse reactions.[63,64] Their pilot studies have been promising, but to use the technique it is necessary to establish a number of probabilities about symptoms and outcomes based on either expert opinion or prior experience with the drug. The approach is not easily implemented in present form, but the authors are optimistic that it can be made readily applicable.

AUTOMATED DATABASES

The most promising new technology for conducting observational studies is the use of large automated databases. Computerized databases that link drug histories with medical care records allow pharmacoepidemiologists to design and implement cost-effective studies.

In general, the strengths of these databases are their efficiency in identifying large numbers of people who were exposed to a drug or who developed a disease and in providing additional information to analyze the temporal relationship between these events. The ideal computerized database links drugs, disease occurrence, and symptoms, and provides pertinent laboratory values. It relies on data collection procedures that are part of normal medical care documentation and does not add to the cost of providing care. Table 1 from Jones et al. presents one set of ideal scientific criteria for one or a combination of such databases.[65]

The primary limitations of these databases are that the investigator does not know what factors may have affected the physician's decision to prescribe a drug or whether the diagnosis was accurate and complete. The accuracy and completeness of drug data may also influence the findings. Issues such as physician and patient selection of drugs and therapies are beyond the control of the research. Access to the patient, the physician, and existing medical records becomes essential to evaluating the impact of variables that may affect the outcome of interest.

When patients and/or medical records are accessible, large automated databases provide a cost-effective ideal method for identifying patients of interest for either case-control or cohort studies. Case-control and cohort studies may still be conducted when direct access to medical records is impossible, but conclusions from these studies may be greatly limited due to the inability to control for confounding factors. Under such circumstances, the safest studies to conduct are ecological, i.e., studies that measure the impact on groups of individuals, but do not report conclusions based on the experience of individual participants.

Computerized databases that are useful for pharmacoepidemiologic studies fit into three broad categories: databases containing information on disease only, databases including information on drugs and disease, and clinical databases that contain drug and disease histories and pertinent laboratory values. To evaluate the usefulness of a particular database, it is imperative to know whether both inpatient and outpatient morbidity and mortality outcomes are available, and whether the original medical record is accessible.

Some examples of computerized databases useful in pharmacoepidemiology follow.

Table 1
Postmarketing Surveillance Databases: Evaluation Criteria for the Value of a Data Resource for Detection of Risk to Drugs[65]

Criteria	Ideal Source or Group of Sources
Drug coverage	covers all drugs used by U.S. population
Denominator	provides actual concomitant or linked denominator (or estimate) of use of drugs (prescriptions or prescriptions dispensed)
Extent of population coverage	covers a sufficient population base to detect "rare" events either acute and/or chronic and allow control or potential confounding factors
Comprehensiveness of population coverage	covers all major representative population subgroups to allow identification of high-risk age, sex, and other subgroups
Diagnosis coverage	detects acute, subacute, and long-term effects of drugs, including both signs (diagnosis codes) and symptoms (subjective terms)
Diagnosis validity	coded diagnosis representative of actual clinical condition in high percentage and/or data contain verifying information (procedures, laboratory data)
Detection sensitivity	has a uniformly high percentage of detection of the total number of unintended drug effects of all types (acute, subacute, long-term)
Pathological comprehensiveness	detection covers all body systems, including birth defects, and includes laboratory data

Computerized Coding of Disease Only. The research group at Kaiser Permanente, Oakland, identifies patient records of interest using computerized database discharge diagnoses. Drug information is not currently captured. To obtain prescription information, medical records must be pulled and orders abstracted. Because patients are required to make copayments for prescription and OTC products, they often are not purchased through Kaiser, and hence the drug histories are not always complete.[66,67]

The Epidemiology Section at Mayo Clinic records ICD codes for all outpatient and inpatient diagnoses in a computerized master file that extends back to 1950. The Mayo Clinic estimates that residents of Olmsted County, Minnesota (population 250 000) use Mayo Clinic or affiliated clinics and hospitals for over 90 percent of their medical care. Again, prescription drug information must be abstracted in a manner similar to the Kaiser system.[40]

The Manitoba Health Plan contains an extensive automated database with data on healthcare utilization and diagnoses for all residents of Manitoba. Prescription data are currently unavailable, but it is possible to identify potential participants for case-control studies or cohort studies or particular types of patients (e.g., patients with diabetes).[68]

Computerized Capture of Drugs and Disease. The Group Health Cooperative (GHC) contains information on outpatient prescriptions filled in the health maintenance organization's (HMO) pharmacies and on hospital discharge diagnoses since 1976. Currently GHC has over 300 000 members. Information on outpatient diagnoses and OTC drug use is not captured. One of the principal advantages of this database is that copies of the discharge summaries and, where appropriate, complete medical records have been available for pharmacoepidemiologic studies.[69]

In the past ten years, the Health Care Finance Administration (HCFA), the FDA, and individual states have recognized the potential power of the Medicaid database for providing meaningful information on drug utilization and on the relationship of drugs to disease development or progression. Two of the largest efforts to tap this source of information are HCFA's Tape-To-Tape project, which creates longitudinal records for Medicaid beneficiaries in five states, and the COMPASS system developed by the FDA in collaboration with Health Information Designs. COMPASS contains longitudinal records beginning in 1980 from 2 states and anticipates expanding it to include 12 states in the near future.

Medicaid's primary beneficiaries are persons of low socioeconomic status, the disabled, the elderly, and the single-parent family. Preliminary work has been completed to validate this data source, but additional studies are warranted.

All 1.1 million residents for the province of Saskatchewan are covered by the Saskatchewan Health Prescription Drug Plan, which captures drug prescriptions and in- and outpatient diagnoses on its database. Preliminary studies suggest that this is a valuable resource and a number of pharmaceutical manufacturers and academic groups are currently conducting studies. The strengths and weaknesses of this database will become evident when these studies are completed.[70]

The Kaiser Permanente, Los Angeles, group has recently computerized an outpatient pharmacy covering 1.2 million HMO beneficiaries. Prescriptions filled through these pharmacies can be linked with Kaiser system hospital discharge diagnoses.[66]

Clinical Databases. Clinical databases that capture drugs, diagnoses, symptoms, and laboratory values are presently not disseminated widely enough to constitute an important resource for PMS studies. However, pharmacoepidemiologists have not yet taken full advantage of these databases or worked with their originators to ensure that they capture essential data on drugs, adverse reactions, and disease outcomes. Presently, these systems cover only limited segments of the population, but can provide valuable information for these groups. An excellent review of clinical databases has been published by Pryor et al.[71]

The Composite Health Care System (formerly the Tri Military Information System) of the U.S. Armed Forces provides additional evidence that the proliferation of these systems is inevitable. This comprehensive clinical information system currently is being tested in one alpha site and modules in a number of beta sites. The goal of the Defense Department is to implement the entire system in all of its 167 health installations.

Current U.S. Postmarketing Surveillance

Many components of an integrated PMS system are in place and occasionally interact in a systematic way. There have been a number of recent efforts to improve coordination by allowing for an interchange of ideas and information, to better train professionals, and to develop the new scientific tools needed to interpret large automated databases linking drugs and disease. However, a significant amount of work remains. In October 1989, the International Society for Pharmacoepidemiology (ISPE) was formed by colleagues in 20 countries to promote the development of the science of pharmacoepidemiology. ISPE will provide a multidisciplinary, multinational forum for the interchange of ideas and information.[72]

Pharmacoepidemiology has benefited from a number of independent reviews. In 1980, the Joint Commission on Prescription Drug Use and an Expert Committee under the Experimental Technology Incentives Program (ETIP) of the FDA and the Department of Agriculture met independently to make recommendations on future directions for U.S. PMS. Both of these studies concluded that PMS is feasible and must rely heavily on the epidemiologic techniques outlined in this chapter. In addition they suggest that multiple, simultaneous approaches must be employed and that the responsibility for such a system of monitoring the efficacy and safety of all drugs must be shared by universities, government, and industry communities. Further, ETIP recommendations concentrated on the problem of identifying rare UDEs occurring with newly marketed drugs and the major recommendation to resolve this monitoring problem entailed the establishment of pharmacy panels to enlist patients prescribed a new drug in prospective cohort studies. However, the recommendations of these committees have not been translated into public policy.[73-75]

A manufacturer or an independent investigator may conduct a postmarketing research study for a number of reasons. These often include a question of drug safety that arose during premarketing phases; an interest in modifying the label to include a new indication for use; a spontaneous report to the FDA, the manufacturer, or in the medical literature; and development of a disease prevention strategy or emergence of an alternative therapy.

When a question of safety or efficacy has been defined, it is reasonably straightforward to determine whether there is sufficient information within one of the existing databases (Table 2) to design a study or whether new data must be collected. The type of study conducted will depend on the incidence and prevalence of the disease, the hypothesized effectiveness of the therapy in reducing morbidity or mortality, the percentage of the market share owned by the drug, the availability of alternative therapies, and the estimated rate of UDEs from previous studies. Typically, a mixture of epidemiologic methodologies is used to test a hypothesis. Studies involve physicians, pharmacists, university researchers and administrators, industry, and voluntary sectors.

Tilson and Whisnant provide an excellent illustration of the use of a number of epidemiologic techniques and databases required to address a question of potential carcinogenicity. Azathioprine, used to treat rheumatoid arthritis, may cause lymphoma. The approach used to investigate this possible effect included monitoring spontaneous reports, reviewing cases from premarketing clinical studies, searching the medical literature, establishing a rheumatoid arthritis azathioprine registry, and monitoring the database of the province of Saskatchewan to identify the incidence of neoplasms in azathioprine users.[76]

Table 2 presents a listing of the major pharmacoepidemiologic methods and some examples of the major components of the current U.S. postmarketing system and the methodologic approaches employed. An attempt to portray how regulatory agencies and manufacturers interact, either with each other of with the academic community and nonregulatory agencies, is beyond the scope of this chapter. However, a few points about the role of the FDA, pharmaceutical manufacturers, major disease research programs, and academic institutions are important to understanding the present system.

The FDA, because of its regulatory responsibilities and management of the spontaneous reporting system, acts as one focal point in PMS. The FDA, however, does not finance the majority of postmarketing research conducted in the U.S. and lacks the scientific staff and resources to answer major postmarketing drug questions.

A much greater proportion of financial support for postmarketing research is provided by private industry, other government agencies, voluntary associations, and private foundations. Research may be initiated by either the sponsor or the investigator. The manufacturer naturally focuses on comprehensive programs of research comparing its own drugs with competing products. NIH and academic-based medical research programs have tended to concentrate on understanding specific disease etiologies and prevention of these diseases. With few exceptions, NIH-sponsored efforts have shied away from collecting adequate drug information to answer a broad array of pharmacoepidemiologic questions. Most NIH-sponsored studies seek answers to efficacy questions and are not intended to identify rare UDEs and interactions. Fortunately, compiling the medical research and literature from a number of disciplines provides broad coverage of many diseases and therapies in the absence of an integrated postmarketing strategy. This broad coverage is largely due to the effectiveness of peer review policies employed by most scientific organizations and periodicals in setting their own funding and pub-

Table 2
U.S. Postmarketing Drug Surveillance System—Major Resources

Controlled clinical trials
conducted primarily in academic research centers under National Institutes of Health or pharmaceutical manufacturer's sponsorship
Demographic studies
National Center for Health Statistics Vital Statistics Program, etc.
Bureau of Census
Canadian Public Health Association—reports on hospital discharges
Observational epidemiologic studies
cohort studies
HMO/insurance-generated
Puget Sound HMO (BCDSP)—historical cohorts
Kaiser Permanente
Medicaid
specially enrolled
hospital-based—PEDS study (SEU)
pharmacy panels—Upjohn (see Borden Phase IV)
physician panels—special studies, e.g., cimetidine
national sample—NHANES (NCHS) Epidemiologic Follow-up Survey
case-control studies
HMO/insurance-generated
Puget Sound HMO (BCDSP)
Kaiser Permanente
Mayo Clinic
hospital-based
BCDSP—enrollment now curtailed
SEU—continued enrollment of targeted conditions
population-based
cancer registries (SEER)
stroke registries (California)
cross-sectional studies
NCHS—NHANES
National Nursing Home Survey
National Ambulatory Care Survey

Drug utilization survey
IMS America—Pharmacy Bases
special surveys—Minnesota Heart Survey
NCHS
Spontaneous reports
drug experience reports (1639) to FDA
worldwide system—WHO voluntary reporting system—limited
access to data for non-FDA reasons
worldwide medical literature
PEM system—England
Automated databases
capturing disease
  Kaiser Permanente Oakland, Portland
  Mayo Clinic
  Manitoba Health Plan
capturing drugs and disease data
  Medicaid
  Group Health Cooperative (BCDSP)
  Saskatchewan Health Plan
clinical databases
  TRW
  Regenstreif
  COSTAR
  ARAMIS
  Harvard Community Health Plan
	Table 2, cont'd.
	U.S. Postmarketing
	Drug Surveillance
	System—Major
	Resources

BCDSP = Boston Collaborative Drug Surveillance Program; HMO = Health Maintenance Organization; NCHS = National Center for Health Statistics; NHANES = National Health and Nutrition Examination Survey; PEM = Prescription Event Monitoring; SEU = Slone Epidemiology Unit; WHO = World Health Organization.

lication priorities. As discussed previously, Venning dramatically documented how much we have relied on this "ad hoc" system in the recent past.[8-10]

Summary

No matter which methodology is elected in pharmacoepidemiology, good scientific technique is required to ensure valid results. This includes reviewing the scientific literature, clearly specifying study objectives, selecting study methodology, pretesting and validating data collection procedures, and careful data analyses and interpretation of the results from statistical and biological vantage points. The survival and growth of pharmacoepidemiology as a scientific discipline depends on the value society places on the questions this discipline examines. The availability of scientific techniques and high-quality data to pursue the answers, the development of high-quality training programs to prepare scientists to address pharmacoepidemiologic questions, a growing body of knowledge recognized by other disciplines, and forums for exchanging knowledge are also critical factors. Finally, successful application of this new knowledge to important problems is essential.

References

1. Blackwell B, Stolley PD, Buncher R, et al. Panel 4: phase IV investigations. *Clin Pharmacol Ther* 1975;18:653-6.

2. Borden EK, Gardner JS, Westland MM, et al. Postmarketing drug surveillance (letter). *JAMA* 1984;251:729.

3. Gross FH, Inman WHW. Drug monitoring. New York: Academic Press, 1977.

4. Slone D, Shapiro S, Miettinen OS, Finkle WD, Stolley PD. Drug evaluation after marketing. *Ann Intern Med* 1979;90:257-61.

5. Wardell WM, Tsianco MC, Anavekar SN, Davis HT. Postmarketing surveillance of new drugs. I. Review of objectives and methodology. *J Clin Pharmacol* 1979;19:85-94.

6. Feinstein AR, Sosin DM, Wells CK. The Will Rogers phenomenon: state migration and new diagnostic techniques as a source of misleading statistics for survival in cancer. *N Engl J Med* 1985;312:1604-8.

7. Venning GR. Identification of adverse reactions to new drugs. I. What have been the important adverse reactions since thalidomide? *Br Med J* 1983;286:199-202.

8. Venning GR. Identification of adverse reactions to new drugs. II. How were 18 important adverse reactions discovered and with what delays? *Br Med J* 1983;286:289-92.

9. Venning GR. Identification of adverse reactions to new drugs. II (continued). How were 18 important adverse reactions discovered and with what delays? *Br Med J* 1983; 286:365-8.

10. Venning GR. Identification of adverse reactions to new drugs. III. Alerting processes and early warning systems. *Br Med J* 1983;286:458-60.

11. Remington RD. Post-marketing drug surveillance: a comparison of methods. *Am J Pharm* 1978;150:72-80.

12. Strom BL, Miettinen OS, Melmon KL. Postmarketing studies of drug efficacy: when must they be randomized? *J Clin Pharmacol* 1983;34:1-7.

13. Strom BL, Miettinen OS, Melmon KL. Postmarketing studies of drug efficacy: how? *Am J Med* 1984;77:703-8.

14. Gehan EA, Freireich EJ. Non-randomized controls in cancer clinical trials. *N Engl J Med* 1974;290:198-203.

15. Stolley PD. Prevention of adverse effects related to drug therapy. In: Clark DW, MacMahon B, eds. Preventive and community medicine. 2nd ed. Boston: Little, Brown, 1981:141-8.

16. Rawlins MD, Thompson JW. Pathogenesis of adverse drug reaction. In: Davis DM, ed. Textbook of adverse drug reactions. Oxford: Oxford University Press, 1977:44.

17. Mausner JS, Kramer S. Epidemiology: an introductory text. Philadelphia: WB Saunders, 1985.

18. Kleinbaum DG, Kupper LL, Morgenstern H. Epidemiologic research: principles and quantitative methods. New York: Van Nostrand Reinhold Company, 1982.

19. Feinstein AR. The case-control study: valid selection of subjects. *J Chronic Dis* 1985; *38*:551-2.

20. Miettinen OS, Cook EF. Confounding: essence and detection. *Am J Epidemiol* 1981;*114*: 593-603.

21. Meinert C. Clinical trials: design, conduct, analysis. Oxford: Oxford University Press, 1986.

22. Friedman LM, Furberg CD, Demets DL. Fundamentals of clinical trials. Boston: John Wright, PSG Inc., 1984.

23. Louis TA, Shapiro SH. Critical issues in the conduct and interpretation of clinical trials. *Ann Rev Public Health* 1983;*4*:25-46.

24. Aspirin Myocardial Infarction Study Research Group. A randomized, controlled trial of aspirin in persons recovered from myocardial infarction. *JAMA* 1980;*243*:661-9.

25. Veterans Administration Cooperative Study on Antihypertensive Agents. Effects of treatment on morbidity in hypertension: I. Results of patients with diastolic blood pressure averaging 90 through 114 mm Hg. *JAMA* 1970;*213*:1143-51.

26. Smith WM. The U.S. Public Health Service Hospitals Cooperative Study Group. Treatment of mild hypertension: results of a ten-year intervention trial. *Circ Res* 1977;*40*(suppl):I-98-105.

27. Smith WM, Edlavitch SA, Krushat WM. Public Health Service Hospitals intervention trial in mild hypertension. In: Onesti G, Klimt C, eds. Hypertension determinants, complications and intervention. New York: Grune and Stratton, 1977:381-99.

28. Hypertension Detection and Follow-up Program Cooperative Group. The hypertension detection and follow-up program. *Prev Med* 1976;*5*:207-15.

29. Hypertension Detection and Follow-up Program Cooperative Group. Five-year findings of the hypertension detection and follow-up program. I. Reduction in mortality of persons with high blood pressure, including mild hypertension. *JAMA* 1979;*242*:2562-71.

30. Multiple Risk Factor Intervention Trial Research Group. Multiple risk factor intervention trial: risk factor changes and mortality results. *JAMA* 1982;*248*:1465-77.

31. Hulley S, Furber C, Gurland BJ, et al. The Systolic Hypertension in the Elderly Program (SHEP): antihypertensive efficacy of chlorthalidone. *Am J Cardiol* 1985;*56*:913-20.

32. Byar DP, Simon RM, Friedewald WT, et al. Randomized clinical trials: perspectives on some recent ideas. *N Engl J Med* 1976;*295*:74-80.

33. Feinstein AR. Should placebo-controlled trials be abolished? (editorial) *Eur J Clin Pharmacol* 1980;*17*:1-4.

34. Strom BL, Miettinen OS, Melmon KL. Postmarketing studies of drug efficacy: why? *Am J Med* 1985;*78*:475-80.

35. Guyatt GH, Sackett D, Taylor DW, et al. Determining optimal therapy—randomized trials in individual patients. *N Engl J Med* 1986;*889*:3-14.

36. Rossi AC, Knapp DE, Anello C, et al. Discovery of adverse drug reactions: a comparison of selected phase IV studies with spontaneous reporting methods. *JAMA* 1983;*249*:2226-8.

37. Edlavitch S. Practical perspectives on postmarketing surveillance—phase IV. In: Nwangwu PU, ed. Concepts and strategies in new drug development. New York: Praeger, 1983:223-42.

38. Jabbari B, Bryan GE, Marsh EE, Gunderson CH. Incidence of seizures with tricyclic and tetracyclic antidepressants. *Arch Neurol* 1985;*42*:480-1.

39. Vessey MP, Lawless M, Yeates D. Oral contraceptives and stroke: findings in a large prospective study. *Br Med J* 1984;*289*:530-1.

40. Heinonen OP, Slone D, Shapiro S. Birth defects and drugs in pregnancy. Littleton, MA: PSG, 1977.

41. Kurland LT, Molgaard CA. The patients record in epidemiology. *Sci Am* 1981;*245*:54-63.

42. Sartwell PE. Retrospective studies: a review for the clinician. *Ann Intern Med* 1974; *81*:381-6.

43. Spitzer WO. Ideas and words: two dimensions for debates on case controlling (editorial). *J Chronic Dis* 1985;*38*:541-2.

44. Miettinen OS. The "case-control" study: valid selection of subjects. *J Chronic Dis* 1985; *38*:543-8.

45. Schlesselman JJ. Valid selection of subjects in case-control studies. *J Chronic Dis* 1985; *38*:549-50.

46. Axelson O. The case-referent study: some comments on its structure, merits and limitations. *Scand J Work Environ Health* 1985;*11*(suppl 3):207-13.

47. Miettinen OS. Author's response. *J Chronic Dis* 1985;*38*:557-8.

48. Hurwitz ES, Barrett MJ, Bregman D, et al. Public health service study on Reye's syndrome and medications. *N Engl J Med* 1985;*313*:849-57.

49. Herbst AL, Ulfelder H, Poskanzer DC. Adenocarcinoma of the vagina: association of maternal stilbestrol therapy with tumor appearance in young women. *N Engl J Med* 1971; *284*:878-81.

50. Lawson DH, Jick H. Comparative drug utilization in hospitalized patients. In: Hollman M, Weber E, eds. Drug utilization studies in hospitals. Stuttgart, FRG: FK Schattauer Verlag, 1980:39-41.

51. Catalog of public use data tapes from the National Center for Health Statistics. Hyattsville, MD: U.S. Department of Health and Human Services, 1980. DHHS publication no. (PHS) 81-1213.

52. Gillum RF, Hannan PJ, Prineas RJ, et al. Coronary heart disease mortality trends in Minnesota, 1960-80: the Minnesota Heart Survey. *Am J Public Health* 1984;*74*:360-2.

53. National Center for Health Statistics. Hyattsville, MD: U.S. Department of Health and Human Services, 1983. DHHS publication no. (PHS) 83-1200.

54. Baum C, Kennedy D, Forbes M, Jones J. Drug use in the United States in 1981. *JAMA* 1984;*25*:1293-7.

55. Draft of guidelines for postmarketing reporting of adverse drug reactions. Rockville, MD: Division of Drug and Biological Products Experience, Center for Drugs and Biologics, 1985 [docket no. 85D-0249].

56. Jue SG, Clark BG, Araki MA. Inservice teaching and adverse drug reactions in a nursing home. *Drug Intell Clin Pharm* 1985;*19*:483-6.

57. Abrutyn E. Better reporting of adverse drug reactions. *Ann Intern Med* 1985;*102*:264-5.

58. Louik C, Lacouture PG, Mitchell AA, et al. A study of adverse reaction algorithms in a drug surveillance program. *Clin Pharmacol Ther* 1985;*38*:183-7.

59. Koch-Weser J, Sellers EM, Zacest R. The ambiguity of adverse drug reactions. *Eur J Clin Pharmacol* 1977;*11*:75-8.

60. Naranjo CA, Busto U, Sellers EM, et al. A method for estimating the probability of adverse drug reactions. *Clin Pharmacol Ther* 1981;30:239-45.

61. Schmidt LG, Dirschedl P, Grohmann R, Scherer J, Wunderlich O, Muller-Oerling-hausen B. Consistency of assessment of adverse drug reactions in psychiatric hospitals: a comparison of an algorithmic and an empirical approach. *Eur J Clin Pharmacol* 1986;30:199-204.

62. Inman WHW. Prescription-event monitoring. *Acta Med Scand* 1984;683(suppl):119-26.

63. Lane DA, Hutchinson TA, Jones JK, Kramer JK, Naranjo CA. A Bayesian approach to causality assessment 1: Foundations. Minneapolis: University of Minnesota technical report no. 461, 1986.

64. Lane DA, Hutchinson TA. Assessing causality assessment methods. Minneapolis: University of Minnesota technical report no. 460, 1986.

65. Jones JK, Van de Carr SW, Rosa F, Morse L, Leroy A. Medicaid drug-event data: an emerging tool for evaluation of drug risk. *Acta Med Scand* 1984;683(suppl):127-34.

66. Friedman GD, Collen MF, Harris LE, Van Brunt EE, Davis LS. Experience in monitoring drug reactions in outpatients. *JAMA* 1971;217:567-72.

67. Friedman GD. Screening criteria for drug monitoring. *J Chronic Dis* 1972;25:11-20.

68. Roos NP. Hysterectomies in one Canadian province: a new look at risks and benefits. *Am J Public Health* 1984;74:39-45.

69. Danielson DA, Douglas SW III, Herzog P, Jick H, Porter JB. Drug-induced blood disorders. *JAMA* 1984;252:3257-60.

70. Tilson HH. Getting down to bases—record linkage in Saskatchewan (editorial). *Can J Public Health* 1985;76:222-3.

71. Pryor DB, Califf RM, Harrell FE, et al. Clinical data bases: accomplishments and unrealized potential. *Med Care* 1985;23:623-47.

72. New international society is formed. *Epidemiol Monit* 1990;(Feb):5.

73. IMS America Ltd., Health Care Services Research Group. Draft report of task B: an experiment in early post-marketing surveillance of drugs. Rockville, MD: Department of Health, Education, and Welfare/Public Health Service, 1978.

74. IMS America Ltd., Health Care Services Research Group. Final report—task C: an experiment in early post-marketing surveillance of drugs. Rockville, MD: Department of Health and Human Services/Public Health Service, 1980.

75. The 1984 report of the Joint National Committee on Detection, Evaluation, and Treatment of High Blood Pressure. Bethesda, MD: U.S. Department of Health and Human Services, 1984. NIH publication no. 84-1088.

76. Tilson HH, Whisnant J. Pharmaco-epidemiology—drugs, arthritis, and neoplasms: industry contribution to the data. *Am J Med* 1985;78(suppl 1A):69-76.

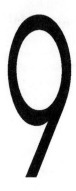

Basic Statistical Methods in Pharmacoepidemiologic Study Designs

Abraham G. Hartzema
Gary G. Koch

Abstract

This chapter reviews the major observational study methods used in pharmacoepi-demiologic studies. The importance of observational studies in pharmacoepidemiology is outlined. Observational studies are especially suited to study unintended drug effects because of the low incidence of such effects and the often long latency time for the ef-fects to occur. The emphasis in the discussion is on cohort and case-control methodolo-gy. The relationship between these two methodologies is demonstrated. Cohort meth-odology is discussed with an emphasis on handling bias due to differentiated dropouts. Relative risk calculations are discussed and illustrated with case examples. Criteria for the evaluation of cohort studies also are listed. The discussion of case-control studies is focused on the two major issues determining the validity of these studies: (1) a clear definition of the population from which cases and controls are drawn and (2) the im-portance of the matching procedure for cases and controls. The calculation of the odds ratio is demonstrated and the relationship between odds ratio and relative risk is pro-vided. Major statistical procedures are discussed, including probability assessment of the relative risk, the calculation of the confidence interval, log-linear model analysis, the calculation of attributable or excess risks, and sample size considerations.

Outline

The most common pharmacoepidemiologic study designs are observational in nature. Observational methods include case analysis, case series analysis, secular trend analysis, cross-sectional studies, cohort studies, and case-control studies. Observational studies are characterized by the data being collected without intentionally interfering with the course of the system. Drug exposure is observed in observational studies.

In clinical trials, the study protocol defines who receives the treatment and who does not. Consequently, clinical trials (experimental studies) intervene in the healthcare system by determining who receives the drug. Another difference between experimental and observational studies in pharmacoepidemiology is the character of the study outcome. In experimental studies, the focus of the study outcome is on the drugs' effectiveness, whereas for observational studies in pharmacoepidemiology, the focus is on unintended drug effects (UDEs). This chapter focuses on the analytical techniques used in pharmacoepidemiologic observational studies with an emphasis on cohort and case-control designs.

In cross-sectional, case-control, and cohort studies the assignment of drug exposure is determined by the prescriber. Thus, drug use is observed in a naturalistic environment, the customary way the drug is prescribed and used in society. Moreover, the focus of outcome in observational studies is the UDE, which has a smaller probability of occurrence than the drugs' therapeutic effects. Also, the latency time, the time between drug exposure and occurrence of the effect, may be prolonged for UDEs. Observational methods are more comprehensive and efficient in studying UDEs.

Although observational studies do not intend to interfere with the practice environment, one has to be aware that observation itself can introduce small changes in that same environment. For example, if the researchers are looking for some drug outcomes, then the accuracy of reporting may increase because the medical and nursing staff become more aware of it. Also, the individuals observed may feel supervised, and as a result become more compliant with their drug therapy. In psychology, this is called the Hawthorne effect; being observed may introduce changes in individuals' behaviors and so affect the outcome of the study.

Observational studies can be cross-sectional, retrospective, or prospective in design. A cross-sectional study measures drug exposure and any UDEs at one point in time and compares populations or geographic regions. A retrospective pharmacoepidemiologic study identifies previous drug exposure for cases and controls through pharmacy records, patient interviews, or other data sources. Thus, in retrospective studies drug exposure information is obtained in the study after the drug use has taken place. A prospective study is one in which a cohort of people exposed to the drug or not exposed to the drug is followed for the occurrence or nonoccurrence of UDEs over time. In the analysis of data from a prospective study, the occurrence of the UDEs as related to the drug exposure of the cohort usually is measured throughout or at the end of the study.

Case control and cohort studies, the two major observational designs used in pharmacoepidemiology, differ in their approach for selecting cases and controls. In case-control studies, subjects having the UDEs are identified upon hospital admittance, clinic visits, or review of medical records. Matching controls then are selected from the same population. Controls are often patients admitted to the same hospitals in which the cases are identified, or visiting the same clinics; or they are patients identified by physicians or selected from population or patient registries. These controls are matched for all factors that may influence the drug outcome except for the UDE and the drug exposure. Drug exposure is measured and compared in both the cases and controls.

The cases and controls are classified in four cells according to UDE present (cases) with or without drug exposure and UDE absent (controls) with or without drug exposure. This information can conveniently be grouped in a 2×2 contingency table.

The cohort study defines the populations on the basis of exposure. A cohort of individuals is a group of people whose membership is delineated in a clearly defined manner. Examples are all individuals visiting a particular clinic, all women between the ages of 30 and 35 who are residents in a particular city as of January 1, 1990, or all physicians practicing in the U.S. The cohort study then identifies individuals exposed and not exposed to the drug and follows these subgroups over time to count the individuals developing the UDE in the drug-exposed group and in the unexposed-drug group. As with the case-control study, the population can be classified in a 2×2 table, those exposed further classified as those with and without the UDE and those not exposed further classified as with and without the UDE present. Thus, cohort designs are appropriate if one needs accurate estimates of the incidence of the study outcome, while case-control designs are well suited for studies with a low probability of the study outcome or a long latency time for the study outcome to occur.

The major difference between case-control designs and cohort designs is how we arrive at the content of the cells in the 2×2 table. In the cohort design, one selects the population based on drug exposure; in the case-control design, one selects

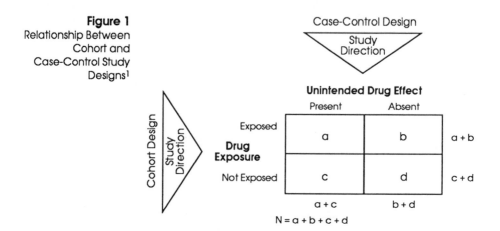

Figure 1
Relationship Between Cohort and Case-Control Study Designs[1]

the population based on the presence or absence of the outcome under study. Case-control studies usually are retrospective; cohort studies often are prospective in design. Figure 1 displays the relationship between case-control and cohort studies, where a, b, c, and d are the cell frequencies; a+b, c+d, a+c, and b+d are the row and column marginal frequencies; and N the total number of subjects.

Our approach in classifying individuals as exposed or not exposed to the drug makes the somewhat simplistic assumption of dichotomy of exposure. In clinical practice, individuals may be exposed to the drug for varying lengths of time, for different levels of exposure, or with characteristics such as intermittent use, and these factors may be important in a particular study design. Researchers often find it necessary to classify drug exposure on more than two levels. Classifying the drug exposure vector on more levels according to dosing strength, duration of drug exposure, etc., has certain advantages. It is statistically more comprehensive, allows for the examination of dose-response relationships, and provides for the estimation of risk in extreme exposure categories. The drug exposure vector is discussed in more detail in Chapter 10.

Cohort Design

BASIC ANALYSIS OF COHORT DESIGNS

The analysis of cohort designs involves the comparison of the incidence rate for the UDE in the drug-exposed population to the incidence rate of the UDE in the not-exposed control population. The not-exposed population also is often called a reference population if they are exposed to another drug or if the exposure level of this population is lower or different. The incidence of the UDE in the exposed cohort also can be compared with the incidence rate in the general population. However, in this situation, the exposed population should be similar to the general population in the distribution for variables, such as age, sex and other pertinent characteristics that may influence the rates of the UDE. Alternatively, when differences in population structure exist, then comparisons need to be based on methods that apply adjustment to a common structure.

In prospective cohort studies, fixed numbers of subjects with and without drug exposure are followed over time. Because the sample sizes for the drug exposure and nonexposure groups are determined by the researcher, the data will not allow estimates of the proportions of the population exposed. Calculations of estimates of the conditional probability of UDEs given drug exposure or nonexposure only are feasible (Figure 2).

A primary statistical measure used in cohort studies is the relative risk. The relative risk in the cohort design is the ratio of the rate of UDEs in the exposed population a/(a+b), versus the rate of the UDEs in the population not exposed c/(c+d). The ratio, which is called the relative risk,[2] then is:

$$\frac{a/a+b}{c/c+d} \qquad \text{Eq. 1}$$

In example 1, a cohort study reported by Vessey,[3] the results presented in Figure 3 are obtained:
The relative risk can be calculated for this study as:

$$\text{relative risk*} = \frac{10/(10+9538)}{3/(3+7494)} = \frac{0.0010473}{0.0004001} = 2.62 \qquad \text{Eq. 2}$$

This relative risk estimate of 2.62 implies that women exposed to oral contraceptives have a 2.62 times higher risk of cardiovascular death than women who never have used oral contraceptives. An extensive critique of pharmacoepidemiologic studies of oral contraceptive use and cardiovascular disease, including cohort and case-control designs, was presented by Realini and Goldzieher.[4]

Data for the second example are taken from a study by Guess et al. A cohort is followed in the Canadian province of Saskatchewan to measure the incidence rates of fatal upper gastrointestinal (GI) hemorrhage or perforation during use or no use of nonsteroidal antiinflammatory drugs (NSAIDs). The denominator for the no usage or not exposed group is defined as persondays of observation, the denominator for the exposed group is defined as persondays of therapy.[5] Thus, these person-time denominators play the same role in relative risk determination as the sample sizes (a+b) and (c+d) in Figure 2. This type of study is also called an incidence density study.

Persondays of therapy are calculated by counting each NSAID prescription as 30 persondays of exposure. If a refill prescription is picked up at the pharmacy too early, the overlapping days between the old and new prescription are not counted as persondays of therapy. Persondays of observation are calculated by multiplying the number of persons in the cohort by 365, the number of days in the year, and subtracting from the total number of persondays of observation the total number of persondays of therapy. Among the cohort of women aged 75 and older, 6 cases of death due to GI hemorrhage or perforation are observed for 1 171 970 persondays of therapy and 6 GI deaths for 6 211 957 persondays of observation (no use). The relative risk can then be calculated as follows:

$$\text{relative risk} = \frac{6/1\,171\,970}{6/6\,211\,957} = \frac{5.12 \cdot 10^{-6}}{9.66 \cdot 10^{-7}} = 5.30 \qquad \text{Eq. 3}$$

The relative risk estimate of 5.30 implies that women aged 75 and older exposed to NSAIDs have a 5.30 times higher risk of GI death than women in the cohort not using NSAIDs.

---

*The results of the calculations presented in all equations may be different from those published elsewhere, because of different approaches taken in handling or adjusting for confounders. This is valid for all examples presented throughout this chapter.

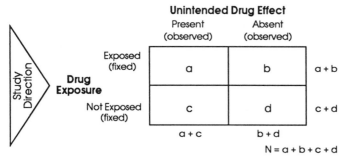

Figure 2
Schematic
Representation of
a Cohort Design
with Two Classes
of Exposure

	Cardiovascular Death		Total
	Present	Absent	
Ever Users	10 (a)	9538 (b)	9548
Oral Contraceptives			
Never Users	3 (c)	7494 (d)	7497
Total	13	17 032	N = 17 045

Figure 3
Cardiovascular
Death
and Oral
Contraceptive
Use

DROP OUTS IN COHORT STUDIES

In prospective cohort studies, certainly those examining UDEs with a long latency period in which individuals must be followed for a long time, individuals will be lost for follow-up. The number of individuals lost depends on many factors, but the following are the most important:

1. Study duration: The longer the follow-up period, the more individuals will be lost.

2. Intensity of detection of the UDE: The more intense the follow-up is or when more effort is expected from the individuals (e.g., participation in extensive medical examinations or filling out lengthy questionnaires), the more individuals will be lost for follow-up.

3. Maturation of the cohort population: In elderly populations (most drugs are used by the elderly) individuals may be lost through death by natural causes.

4. Convenience of alternate treatments over the study treatment: The difference in treatment intensity or efficacy between the drug under examination and other drugs on the market may adversely affect the drop-out rate. The perception of the severity of the UDEs may also affect the drop-out rate.

The effect of having a proportion of individuals lost is similar to having no data or incomplete data on individuals entering the cohort groups. Loss of data can take place at the drug exposure and the outcome level. At the outcome level, it is not possible to ascertain the UDE; or at the exposure level, it can not be ascertained that the person is exposed to the drug. These losses of data on drug exposure and outcomes have different impact on the calculation of relative risk ratios.

The loss of data both on drug exposure and outcome will affect the relative risk ratios for exposure categories only if it is biased in drug exposure as well as in outcome. Losses of data for drug exposure only (and with no association with outcome) should have no impact on the outcome if proper adjustment is made for the loss of data in the analysis. Losses in data on the outcome, the UDE, will impact the absolute levels of the rates of the outcome, but not the relative levels between different exposure categories (given that there is no association of such losses with exposure). If these losses are considerable, they may introduce significantly undesirable changes in the actual calculated rates, even if the ratios of relative risk for the exposure categories are not changed.

Different approaches can be taken to adjust or prevent the loss of data on drug exposure and outcome. These approaches are:

1. When the individuals are examined regularly for the UDEs or have to complete screening instruments at regular intervals, it is best to drop the individuals with missing data from the numerator and the denominator. (In calculation of person/year of exposure, exclusion would occur immediately after the last examination or contact with which they have complied.) The denominator then will be the number of individuals actually assessed for the UDE on each scheduled examination or survey date. Individuals with missing outcome data should not be included in the denominator data because we have no data about the presence or absence of the UDE for the time period encompassing the scheduled examination or interview. Thus, because of lack of numerator data on this individual, the individual should also be eliminated from the denominator.

2. Background information for the outcome or UDE sometimes allows us to record the date or time the event takes place. Some of these possiblities are: (1) If the time or date the person leaves the cohort is known as well as the status of the UDE, then it can be taken into account. A clear example is death as the UDE; death certificates contain the date that the subject left the cohort. (2) Occasionally, an adjustment is made if a subject drops out between two scheduled examinations or interviews by considering the subject as part of the cohort for half of the time expired between the two measuring points. (3) Another approach is to establish a range of the risk based on the calculation of two denominators. One denominator is based on the assumption that the individuals are lost from the study directly after their last examination or survey and the other is based on the assumption that they are lost immediately prior

to the first examination or interview that they are known to be absent. The true rate is within the range of rates calculated from the two estimated denominators.

Some difficulty arises in the analysis when the drop-out rate differs in the cohort groups, particularly if there is association with outcome. The only real solution to the problem of drop outs from a cohort study in this situation is not to have any; however, this is not always possible. Thus, the introduction of error in the calculation of relative risk due to bias both in drug exposure measurement and in ascertainment of UDEs must be handled in the analysis, although there may be limitations on how well this can be done.

In this regard, one possible approach is to establish the range within which the true rate should lie. This range can be established through two assumptions. First, one considers the assumption that none of the individuals lost to follow-up experienced the UDE, and then views all the individuals lost to follow-up as developing the UDE. This method provides an estimate of the range of rates possible in each exposure category. However, this method is useful only in cohort studies in which the proportion of individuals lost to follow-up is small and the incidence of the UDE is high.

In most cohort studies, the incidence of UDEs is smaller than the proportion of individuals lost to follow-up; consequently, the range between the estimates of outcome frequency often will be too large for meaningful interpretation. The range of relative risk estimates based on this range of true rates should not be confused with the confidence interval for the relative risk ratio, which is a measure of its reliability. The confidence interval for the relative risk is discussed later in this chapter. Sources of misclassification of drug exposure and outcome are discussed in more detail in Chapter 10 on drug exposure and outcome misclassification. Criteria for the evaluation of the quality of cohort studies as developed by Feinstein are summarized in Table 1.[6-8]

Case-Control Design

DESIGN CONSIDERATIONS

The case-control design can be very elegant and useful in pharmacoepidemiology. It is a cost-effective method for studies in which the UDE has a low incidence or a long latency time. Case-control studies are also cost-effective alternatives to cohort studies. However, an accurate definition of the population from which the cases with the UDE are identified and the procedure of matching cases with controls are two important methodological considerations in case-control designs. Both need to be executed carefully to assure the internal and external validity of any case-control study.

For case-control studies, specification of a common population from which cases and controls are selected is an important condition for the validity of the odds ratio for relative risk estimation. Most case-control studies are retrospective, where cases are selected from hospital records, death registers, or any source that records individuals' outcomes in a systematic way. The outcome, the UDE, is the criterion on which the cases are selected; however, the population that these cases represent cannot always be defined accurately nor its size determined.

In cohort studies, groups are selected according to their exposure; in general, two groups are defined in the study protocol: one group of individuals exposed to the drug and another group not exposed to the drug. The incidence of the UDEs in both groups then is examined. Consequently, the denominator in cohort studies is defined more clearly and reflects the populations under study more accurately. Accurate denominator data allow the researcher to calculate the relative risk.

Occasionally, it is possible to estimate the relative risk in case-control studies by accurately defining the population from which the cases derive. An accurate definition of this population allows one to select the controls from the same population. If we know all cases or the sample of cases included in the study and also are able to precisely define the population from which these cases are derived and the matching control group is representative of the same population, estimates of the probabilities of the UDEs in exposed and unexposed individuals can be established and used to calculate estimates of the relative risk.

More typically, the data cannot be related to a defined population. For exam-

---

Table 1
Evaluation Criteria
for Cohort Studies

1. Randomization in exposure; this will assure that exposed and not-exposed subjects have equal susceptibility for developing the UDE relative to factors other than drug exposure. However, it is not always feasible to randomize the exposure.

2. The exposed and not-exposed cohort should be comparable with respect to demographics and other background characteristics that may affect the likelihood of developing the UDE. This is assured by randomization when it is feasible.

3. The exposed and not-exposed cohort should be comparable with respect to clinical characteristics (pharmacogenetics) which may affect the likelihood of developing the UDE.

4. Drug exposure including compliance should be ascertained equally in both groups.

5. Medical surveillance for the UDE should be equal in the exposed and nonexposed cohorts.

6. The same diagnostic criteria and examination should be used in the exposed and nonexposed cohorts.

7. Dropout rates and characteristics of dropouts in the exposed and nonexposed cohorts should be similar.

8. The cohort should be representative of the population that normally uses the drug.

9. The cohort should have the characteristics of an inception cohort, the subjects are followed from the beginning of the drug exposure.

ple, this occurs when the individuals are attending selected hospitals and no attempt is made to limit the subject group to place of residency or to determine the coverage these individuals represent for all individuals in the catchment area of the hospitals. Similarly, the control group often is selected from individuals with other diseases or other complaints. One assumes that these individuals represent the same catchment areas from which the individuals with the UDEs are selected, but other aspects of structure are not known.

A hospital or clinic can have different catchment areas for different medical specialties based on regional reputation. When cases are identified in one specialty area and controls in another specialty area, the catchment areas or populations from which the cases and controls come may overlap, but they are not necessarily identical. Patients attending oncology clinics may come from a wider geographic area than the patients visiting internal medicine clinics. Since the nature of the population at risk sometimes is not known, it is impossible to derive estimates of the rates of UDEs in the exposed and the unexposed populations. However, it is possible to derive an estimate of the relative risk in case-control studies, by use of a quantity called the odds ratio.

A crucially important component of case-control studies is the matching procedure followed in selecting the controls. In case-control studies, the strength of the study design depends on the approach one takes in matching the cases with controls. The most compatible matching among human beings occurs with the case and the control being identical twins. Identical twins have the same genes and often are raised together and thus have been exposed to the same environment. Consequently, in an observational study, a strong scientific inference can be made if appropriate pairs of twins are found. If one had identical twins raised in the same environment where one of the twins smoked and the other did not, then prospective follow-up for the incidence of lung cancer, general health, and survival experience could provide quite strong scientific inferences as to the health effects of smoking.

The difficulty with twin studies is that sufficient numbers of identical twins cannot be located, where one of the twins is exposed to the drug while the other is not. There are limited numbers of identical twins and it is most likely that both are exposed or not exposed. Thus, the number of epidemiologic studies employing twins is small, and no pharmacoepidemiologic studies using twins have been reported in the literature. Although this approach is logistically not feasible, other methodological approaches can be taken. These approaches are:

1. Matched pair approach: A control or multiple controls are identified for each case on the basis of similarity (or identity) with regard to all variables pertinent to the study except for the UDE outcome. Thus, in many studies, individuals are matched with regard to age, sex, race, and some indicator of social or economic status. Still, the possibility exists that the case and control are not truly comparable because of some unrecognized variable.

2. Matched control group approach: An entire control group is selected. Through careful consideration of the study question and insight, it is assumed that the control group will in some sense mirror the case group with regard to the distribution of the pertinent variables.

3. Proximity matching approach: Cases and controls are not matched on specific variables but somewhat intuitively on the basis of proximity in the process of case selection. Procedures often used are to select the next person after a case with the same sex and in the same age range with an appointment in the clinic or admitted to the hospital. Or one might have a case designate a friend of the same age and sex. The rationale behind this approach is that by being a friend, the control will tend to have the same social and economic environment and often have similar ethnic characteristics.

4. Statistical adjustment to matching approach: In this approach, two groups are selected according to a protocol and pertinent variables are measured, such as the variables that one considers for matching. An analytical model then is used to make statistical adjustments to estimate what the comparisons would have been had the two groups been comparable. Two approaches can be taken: stratified analysis and analytical modeling. Stratified analysis is a more straightforward way to adjust for matching variables. In stratified analysis, one separates the data into a set of two or more 2×2 tables. For example, if we expect an age effect and the age distribution in the cases and controls to be different, the data are further partitioned in strata for those <55 years old and those ≥55 years. Analysis is performed on the two resulting 2×2 tables. In particular, the Mantel-Haenszel statistic is used for testing the overall association between drug exposure and UDE for the combined strata in a manner that controls for potential confounding from the stratification factor. Methods that control for confounding through analytical modeling include analysis of covariance and logistic regression. When the dependent variable is dichotomous, the logistic model is commonly used; when the dependent variable is continuous, analysis of covariance is used.

The selection of the controls in a case-control study is based to a large extent on the skills and expertise of the researcher. Critical considerations are identifying cases and controls that are comparable for all variables that may confound the study outcome and assuring that cases and controls arrive from the same defined population, even though the nature of that population may not be clearly known.

BASIC ANALYSIS OF CASE-CONTROL DESIGNS

In case-control studies, four types of individuals are identified. These four types arrive from two main groups: those who show the UDE, and the corresponding controls. These two groups are further subdivided into individuals exposed to the study drug and individuals not exposed to the study drug. Thus, four types

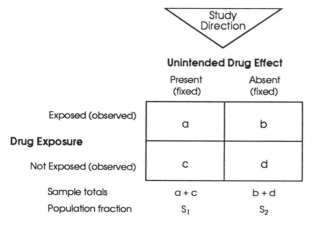

Figure 4
Schematic Representation
of a Case-Control Design
with Two Classes of Exposure

of subjects are identified: individuals with the UDE who are exposed to the drug, individuals with the UDE not exposed to the drug, and controls who were exposed or not exposed to the drug. The basic structure of a case-control study and the frequencies a, b, c, d for the four types of subjects are displayed as a 2×2 table in Figure 4.

For the case-control study in Figure 4, the column totals (a+c) and (b+d) are sample sizes for individuals with the UDE present and the controls with it absent, and so they are relevant for estimating corresponding rates of exposure. The row totals (a+b) and (c+d) for total numbers of exposed and not-exposed individuals in the study are not shown because the cases and controls represent unknown and nearly always unequal sample proportions S_1 and S_2 of the individuals with and without the UDE in the population. This aspect of the design of case-control studies usually makes (a+b) and (c+d) invalid for the estimation of rates for presence and absence of UDEs among exposed and nonexposed individuals. Consequently, the estimation of disease rates, risks, or prevalences within exposure categories usually is not feasible for case-control studies. The underlying reason for this limitation of the case-control design is that neither the size of the exposed population nor the size of the not-exposed population from which the individuals with the UDE and the controls are drawn is known. In other words, the denominator data for rates of UDEs are not known in the case-control study. Thus, rates for UDEs can not be calculated directly from a case-control study, nor can the relative risk be estimated. The measure used in case-control studies for the association of exposure status with presence versus absence of UDE is called the odds ratio.

As discussed previously, the true frequencies for presence and absence of UDEs among exposed and not-exposed individuals are not known in a case-control study. Nevertheless, for the observed frequencies, the relevant considerations are the quality of the approach taken in the identification of the cases of UDEs, the selection of controls, and the definition of the population so that cases and controls are from the same population. On this basis (a+c) and (b+d) are relevant for estimating rates (or odds) of exposure for those with and without UDEs. Accordingly, the odds or probability of being exposed or unexposed to the drug for the cases with the UDE is a/c. The odds of being exposed or unexposed for the controls is b/d. Division of these two odds provides the estimate of the odds ratio ad/bc, sometimes called the cross-product ratio. The sequence of operations to calculate the odds ratio in a 2×2 table is to multiply a×d and then b×c and then divide the products:

$$\frac{a\,d}{c\,b}$$

If the cases constitute a sample proportion S_1 of the population and the controls constitute a different sample proportion S_2, the formula can be written as:

$$\frac{a\,d}{c\,b} = \frac{aS_1\ dS_2}{cS_1\ bS_2} = \frac{(aS_2/bS_1)}{(cS_2/dS_1)} \qquad \text{Eq. 4}$$

for which the ratio $(aS_2/bS_1)=\{(a/S_1)/(b/S_2)\}$ is the odds of presence versus absence of UDEs for the entire exposed population, and $(cS_2/dS_1)=\{(c/S_1)/(d/S_2)\}$ is the corresponding odds for the entire unexposed population. Thus, without depending on the sample proportions S_1 and S_2, the odds ratio expresses the relative extent to which the risk of presence versus absence of the UDEs is larger for the exposed versus unexposed population, and for this reason is an appropriate measure of relative risk.

Moreover, it is not necessary to know the sample proportions S_1 and S_2 to calculate the odds ratio, as long as the sample of cases and controls is taken from the same population. However, because different sample proportions usually are taken for cases and controls, case-control studies do not allow for estimation of rates of UDEs within exposure categories. If S_1 and S_2 were known, these rates would be $aS_2/(aS_2+bS_1)$ for exposed and $cS_2/(cS_2+dS_1)$ for unexposed. Thus, as stated previously, unknown and unequal S_1 and S_2 make (a+b) and (c+d) invalid for estimating rates of presence and absence of UDEs among exposed and unexposed subjects.

In a third example, calculation of the odds ratio is illustrated for the data taken from the International Agranulocytosis and Aplastic Anemia Study.[9] The case-control information is displayed in Figure 5.

In this case-control study, data are collected at eight different international sites. The cases are patients admitted to the involved hospitals. Agranulocytosis is ascertained by including those patients with a granulocyte count of $<0.5\times10^9$/L, a hemoglobin concentration of >0.3, and a platelet count of $>100\times10^9$/L. Controls are enrolled without knowledge of drug exposure from patients admitted to the hospital with a diagnosis not related to pre͏ͅ us use of antithyroid drugs. Drug exposure is obtained by interview of th͏ͅ by trained interviewers. The odds ratio can be calculated as follows·

$$\text{odds ratio} = \frac{a\,d}{c\,b} = \frac{45 \times 1766}{217 \times 5} = \frac{79\,470}{1085} = 73.2 \qquad \textbf{Eq. 5}$$

Case-control studies are generally used in epidemiology to study rare diseases. Most UDEs are also rare. For this situation, there is a very close relationship between the odds ratio and the relative risk.

CALCULATION OF THE RELATIVE RISK IN CASE-CONTROL STUDIES

The relative risk often is reported in the literature for case-control studies. This can be quite appropriate, because the odds ratio approaches the relative risk when the incidence rate of the UDEs is low. Also, this condition is applicable for most of the case-control studies conducted within pharmacoepidemiology.

The relationship between the relative risk and odds ratio can be examined by looking at the ratio of these two terms:

$$\frac{\text{relative risk}}{\text{odds ratio}} = \frac{a/(a+b)}{c/(c+d)} \times \frac{c\,b}{a\,d} = \frac{b}{a+b} \times \frac{c+d}{d} \approx \frac{b}{b} \times \frac{d}{d} = 1 \qquad \textbf{Eq. 6}$$

For a UDE with a small incidence, a is small compared with b, so that b/a+b becomes approximately 1. Also, c is small compared to d, so that c+d/d becomes 1. Thus, the ratio for relative risk/odds ratio becomes 1. In other words, if the UDE has a small incidence in the population exposed to the drug and the population not exposed, the odds ratio and the relative risk are approximately the same. Accordingly, the odds ratio gives a reasonable estimate of the relative risk.

The assumptions underlying the use of relative risk for case-control studies are valid only when the following two criteria are met: (1) that the UDE incidence is relatively low, and (2) that case identification and control selection have been performed in an unbiased way. The researcher needs to review the confounders considered in their study design to address these issues. When the incidence of the UDE is higher than ten percent in either the exposed or the not-exposed subjects, then the term odds ratio should be used. When the incidence of the UDE is below ten percent in both the exposed and the unexposed individuals, the relative odds or the odds ratio approximates the relative risk so closely that it is common to use the terms interchangeably.

	Agranulocytosis	
	Present (fixed)	Absent (fixed)
Exposed	45	5
Not Exposed	217	1766
Total	262	1771

Antithyroid Drug

Figure 5
Agranulocytosis and Antithyroid Use

The second criterion is more difficult to evaluate. It requires the qualitative assessment of the procedures being used to select the cases and the definition of the population from which the cases come. Also, there must be confirmation that the selection of the controls is equivalent in all respects that may influence the distribution of the UDE or drug exposure, such as age, sex, and other potential confounding variables. Substantial insight into the circumstance of case identification, control selection, and drug exposure verification is essential here. These and other criteria to assess the quality of case-control studies are summarized in Table 2.[10]

Interpretation of the Results

THE MEANING OF THE RELATIVE RISK ESTIMATES

A relative risk of 2 implies that drug exposed individuals are twice as likely to show the UDE as not-exposed individuals. Relative risk is a summary of the relationship between counts, proportions, or probabilities in the four cells of a 2×2 table such as in Figures 1–5. Different probabilities, proportions, or counts can provide the same relative risk.

For example 4, the tables in Figure 6, in which the cell entries are represented by probabilities or counts, each has a relative risk of 2. It can be seen in Figure 6

Table 2 Evaluation Criteria for Case-Control Studies	1. Selection method for cases and controls should be defined before the study starts. 2. Level of drug exposure should be established before data analysis. 3. Data collection should be unbiased by the use of blind interviewers relative to case versus control status of subjects, and the use of structured data-collection instruments. 4. Patient drug exposure recall should be equivalent in cases and controls. 5. Exclusion criteria should be unbiased for cases or controls. 6. Equal diagnostic examination based on explicit criteria should be implemented for cases and controls. 7. Similar intensity of medical surveillance for cases and controls before enrollment in the study should be observed. 8. Equal demographic susceptibility for the use of the drug by cases and controls should be assured. 9. Equal clinical susceptibility, or pharmacogenetic attributes, by cases and controls should be assured. 10. Berkson's bias should be avoided; cases and controls should arrive from a common defined population rather than selected from patients admitted to a hospital, because patients who are both exposed and diseased often are more likely to be hospitalized than those who are unexposed and diseased or exposed and nondiseased.

Proportions of study individuals

	Unintended Drug Effect			Unintended Drug Effect	
	Present	Absent		Present	Absent
Drug Exposed **Exposure**	0.50	0.00		0.001	0.499
Not Exposed	0.25	0.25		0.0005	0.4995

Figure 6
Examples of Different
Cell Entries Resulting
in the Same Relative
Risk Estimate of 2

Counts of study individuals

	Unintended Drug Effect			Unintended Drug Effect	
	Present	Absent		Present	Absent
Drug Exposed **Exposure**	250	0*		20	9980
Not Exposed	125	125		10	9990

*A common method to deal with zero cells in odds ratio analysis is to add 0.5 to all cell entries on any 2 x 2 table containing at least one zero cell. This is called the Woolf-Haldane adjustment,[11,12] for the calculation of an odds ratio or summary odds ratio; this adjustment also can improve the statistical properties of the odds ratio when the cell entries are small, but non-zero (e.g., between 1 and 2).[13]

that many different distributions or patterns of the cells can provide the same relative risk. This is not surprising because relative risk summarizes four numbers in one. In that one summary value, separate information on drug exposure frequency and UDE incidence is contained.

To interpret the clinical significance of the relative risk, it is important to know what the underlying rates are. For UDEs with equivalent severity, one with a relative risk of two on the basis of two drug events in 10 000 individuals or one with a relative risk of two on the basis of two drug events in 100 individuals, are the same from a comparative perspective for exposed and not-exposed individuals. However, the latter may have a 100-fold greater clinical relevance in terms of rates of occurrence.

TEST OF ASSOCIATION

Both relative risk and odds ratios can be reported with p-values. The p-values indicate whether the relative risk is statistically significantly different from 1.0. In this way, whether the difference in risk between the exposed and not exposed is beyond that due to random variation can be assessed. A $p \leq 0.05$ is generally considered statistically significant. A $p < 0.05$ indicates that the probability is less than 1 in 20 for the relative risk to be at least as far from 1.0 as observed by chance when the relative risk is actually 1.0. Since $p < 0.05$ is atypical for a relative risk equal to 1.0 as a hypothesis, it indicates that relative risk is different from 1 and thereby is statistically significant.

For the statistical analysis of both the 2×2 table or contingency tables with multiple cells, the chi-square test is a reasonable method. It enables evaluation of the statistical significance of the observed differences, particularly when different exposure levels need to be managed. In this regard, it tells us about the difference in expected risk between the exposed groups (or the groups that experience different levels of exposure) and the control group of not-exposed individuals (or the group of individuals exposed to a different drug).

The most important consideration is the risk associated with the presence or absence of exposure or the level of drug exposure. Issues dealing with establishing a causal relationship between drug exposure and UDE are discussed in Chapters 5 and 6 and the issues of how to deal with confounders are discussed in Chapter 10. The question of association should be established prior to the calculation of the risk while issues of confounding can be addressed in subsequent statistical analysis.

The hypothesis of no association for 2×2 contingency tables can be tested with the Fisher's exact test for small samples and the chi-square test for larger samples.[14-17] If one or more cells in the 2×2 table include fewer than ten subjects, the Fisher's exact test is used to calculate the p-value. When all cells include at least ten subjects, evaluation of the strength of the association between drug exposure and UDE often is based on the chi-square test. The chi-square statistic provides an excellent approximation to the exact p-values from Fisher's exact test. Its result enables interpretation of whether the relative risk is different from 1.0 for a cohort study and whether the odds ratio is different from 1.0 for a case-control study. An expression for the chi-square statistic is:

$$Q = \frac{(N-1)(ad-bc)^2}{(a+c)(b+d)(a+b)(c+d)} \qquad \text{Eq. 7}$$

where N=total number of individuals in the study; a, b, c, and d are the numbers of individuals in the different cells; and a+b, c+d, b+d, and a+c are the row and column totals. See Figure 4 for the notation. As the observed relative risk or odds ratio becomes more different from 1.0, Q increases and so large values of Q are contrary to the null hypothesis of no association between exposure status and presence versus absence of UDE (i.e., true relative risk or odds ratio equals 1.0). The p-value for the test is the probability of values at least as large as Q in theoretical tabulations for the chi-square distribution with one degree of freedom; in this regard, the one degree of freedom for this test corresponds to the relative risk (or odds ratio) as its one focus.

Using the data from Example 3 (the International Agranulocytosis and Aplastic Anemia study[9]) for Equation 7, the chi-square and its p-value of the established odds ratio of 73.2 can be calculated as follows:

$$Q = \frac{(N-1)(ad-bc)^2}{(a+c)(b+d)(a+b)(c+d)} = \frac{(2033-1)\,((45\times1766)-(5\times217))^2}{(262)(1771)(50)(1983)} = 271.38 \quad \text{Eq. 8}$$

with a p-value of p<0.0001.

A "corrected for continuity" version of the chi-square statistic is suggested by Fleiss;[18] however, others do not recommend its use. The formula for the "corrected for continuity" version of the chi-square statistic is as follows:[19]

$$Q_C = \frac{(N-1)\,[\,|ab-bc|-(N/2)]^2}{(a+c)(b+d)(a+b)(c+d)} \quad \text{Eq. 9}$$

STRATIFIED ANALYSIS IN CASE-CONTROL STUDIES

Stratified analysis enables assessment of the association between drug exposure status and the presence versus absence of the UDE with adjustment for a confounding variable. Examples of potential confounders are age, gender, concurrent disease status, smoking status, and body mass. A variable is called a confounder when it is associated with exposure status and the risk of the UDE and there is an influence of these associations on the relationship between exposure status and the presence or absence of the UDE.

The two major reasons for the control of confounding variables are: (1) assurance of the internal validity of the study by adjustment for confounders that may have a different distribution in exposed and unexposed subjects and have a relationship to the distribution of the UDE; (2) improvement of the precision of the relative risk and odds ratio estimates and the power of the tests for whether they are significantly different from 1.0. One can evaluate through consideration of these factors any causal relationship between drug exposure and UDE in a more focused way, as well as obtain a deeper insight into the etiology of the UDE.

The control of confounders can take place in the design of the study through stratified selection of the sample with respect to the distribution of the confounders (e.g., separate samples for men and women) or through matching procedures in case-control studies. Alternatively, one can control for confounders in analysis by stratification adjustment or mathematical modeling. These strategies are discussed in more detail below.

In stratified analysis, all observations are categorized into separate strata after the data are collected. Three conditions are necessary for stratification to provide satisfactory control for confounders that might influence the presence or absence of the UDE in the population: (1) strata are based on the relevant confounding variable(s); (2) an appropriate categorization defining appropriate strata is established for the confounding variable(s); for example, is the age effect really controlled for by the strata age <55 and age ≥55 or are age <70 and age ≥70 more appropriate strata? Or should the strata be age <55, 55 ≤ age <70, and age >70; and (3) all strata contain sufficient numbers of subjects (i.e., each stratum has a 2×2 table like Figure 7, in which each row total exceeds 1 and each of the column totals exceeds 1).

The Mantel-Haenszel test is an appropriate method for assessing overall association in a stratified analysis. The expression for the test statistic is a direct extension of the chi-square test for a single 2×2 table. Accordingly, it is:

$$Q_{MH} = \left\{ \sum_{i=1}^{I} \frac{(a_i d_i - b_i c_i)}{N_i} \right\}^2 \Big/ \left\{ \sum_{i=1}^{I} \frac{(a_i + b_i)(a_i + c_i)(b_i + d_i)(c_i + d_i)}{N_i^2(N_i - 1)} \right\} \qquad \text{Eq. 10}$$

where $i=1, \ldots$, and I indexes the strata. The Mantel-Haenszel statistic Q_{MH} tests the association between drug exposure status and presence versus absence of the UDE for the combined strata.

When the estimates of relative risk or odds ratios within the respective strata are consistently larger (or smaller) than 1.0, then Q_{MH} tends to be large. Thus, the p-value for the Mantel-Haenszel test is the probability of values at least as large as Q_{MH}. Except for relatively small sample situations (e.g., N ≤50, or total number of cases with UDE ≤10), this p-value can be well approximated by use of the chi-square distribution with one degree of freedom.

The Mantel-Haenszel statistic Q_{MH} is applicable to both unmatched and matched data structures. Another advantage is that the accuracy of the approximation of its p-value by means of the chi-square distribution with one degree of freedom is based more on the combined sample size for the data from all strata than on the separate sample sizes within each stratum. Thus, this approximation is usually adequate as long as the total number of subjects is sufficiently large even though some strata may have a small number of subjects in them (e.g., studies where the strata correspond to matched pairs of subjects or matched sets with one case and several controls). In view of this consideration, control for more than one confounder is usually feasible provided that the resulting cell sizes do not become so small as to violate the previously stated condition (3); the reason why condition (3) is important is that there is no contribution to Q_{MH} from subjects in any stratum where either one of the row totals in the 2×2 table is zero or one of the column totals is zero. Finally, for situations with small samples, exact p-values for Q_{MH} can be obtained with methods that are extensions of Fisher's test.[20]

For example 4, the data are obtained from a case-control study conducted by Ray et al. The Michigan Medicaid database was used to identify incident cases of individuals hospitalized for proximal-femur fracture from 1980 through 1982. A stratified group of randomly selected controls with no prior diagnosis of proximal-femur fracture was selected from the same database. Controls were stratified to group matched for sex, race, age within one year, index year, and living arrangement. Five controls were randomly selected for each case from this group. The matching procedure was further designed to prevent confounding by dementia.[21]

The data in Figure 7 are constructed from the published data on the risk of proximal-femur fracture in those exposed to antipsychotics versus those not exposed to demonstrate the calculation of the chi-square statistics in stratified anal-

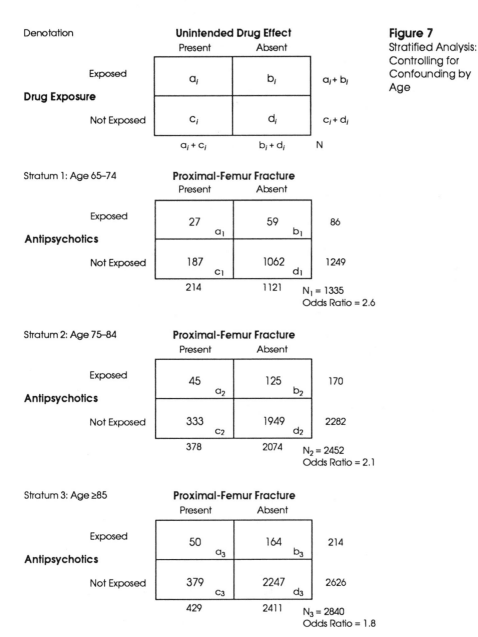

Denotation — **Unintended Drug Effect**

Figure 7
Stratified Analysis:
Controlling for
Confounding by
Age

ysis.[19] Three strata are defined to examine age as a confounder. These strata are: age 65–74, 75–84, and 85 years of age and older.

$$Q_{MH} = \left\{ \sum_{i=1}^{I} \frac{(a_i d_i - b_i c_i)}{N_i} \right\}^2 \Big/ \left\{ \sum_{i=1}^{I} \frac{(a_i + b_i)(a_i + c_i)(b_i + d_i)(c_i + d_i)}{N_i^2 (N_i - 1)} \right\}$$

Eq. 11

$$= \frac{\left\{ \dfrac{(27 \times 1062) - (59 \times 187)}{1335} + \dfrac{(45 \times 1949) - (125 \times 333)}{2452} + \dfrac{(50 \times 2247) - (164 \times 379)}{2840} \right\}^2}{\left\{ \dfrac{86 \times 214 \times 1121 \times 1249}{(1335)^2 (1335-1)} + \dfrac{170 \times 378 \times 2074 \times 2282}{(2452)^2 (2452-1)} + \dfrac{214 \times 429 \times 2411 \times 2626}{(2840)^2 (2840-1)} \right\}}$$

$$= 43.408$$

A chi-square of 43.408 with one degree of freedom has a p-value of <0.001.

STRATIFIED ANALYSIS IN COHORT STUDIES

Procedures followed in stratified analysis in cohort studies are sometimes different from those in case-control and cross-sectional studies. The control of one single confounder was emphasized for the stratified analysis of case-control designs; however, consideration of the cohort design focuses on the concept of control with multiple confounders.

An expected value for the total number $A = \sum_{i=1}^{I} a_i$ of exposed subjects with a UDE under the hypothesis of no association between exposure status and the presence or absence of the UDE is:

$$E_0(A) = \sum_{i=1}^{I} \{(a_i + b_i) c_i / (c_i + d_i)\}$$

Eq. 12

A corresponding estimate for the variance of $\{A - E(A)\}$ is:

$$V_0(A) = \sum_{i=1}^{I} \frac{N_i (a_i + b_i) c_i d_i}{(c_i + d_i)^2 (c_i + d_i - 1)}$$

Eq. 13

Given that the data from the respective strata are independent, the test statistic for the combined strata is:

$$Q_A = \{A - E_0(A)\}^2 / V_0(A)$$

Eq. 14

For situations where the sample sizes for the combined strata are moderately large, Q_A approximately has the chi-square distribution with one degree of freedom.

Example 7: Data from Guess et al., discussed in example 2, page 146, is further categorized in two classes of potential confounders.[5] These classes are age and sex. Four classes are defined for age: ≥75, 65–74, 45–64, and <45 years. For sex the data are further broken down for male and female. The following calculations are presented based on the data displayed in Figure 8 and the procedures discussed above.

$$A = 6+0+0+0+0+0+0+1=7 \qquad \text{Eq. 15}$$

$$E_0(A) = \left\{ \frac{(6+1\,171\,970)6}{(6+6\,211\,957)} + \frac{(0+605\,742)6}{(6+5\,252\,813)} + \frac{(0+1\,158\,276)1}{(1+9\,362\,715)} + \right.$$

$$\frac{(0+696\,743)2}{(2+8\,896\,999)} + \frac{(0+1\,724\,208)0}{(0+24\,850\,057)} + \frac{(0+1\,145\,069)2}{(2+25\,455\,912)} + \qquad \text{Eq. 16}$$

$$\left. \frac{(0+1\,256\,470)1}{(1+109\,272\,262)} + \frac{(1+916\,969)0}{(0+116\,129\,781)} \right\} = 2.206$$

$$V_0(A) = \frac{7\,383\,939(6+1\,171\,970)6\times6\,211\,957}{(6+6\,211\,957)^2\,(6+6\,211\,957-1)} +$$

$$\frac{5\,858\,561(0+605\,742)6\times5\,252\,813}{(6+5\,252\,813)^2\,(6+5\,252\,813-1)} +$$

$$\frac{10\,520\,992(0+1\,158\,276)1\times9\,362\,715}{(1+9\,362\,715)^2\,(1+9\,362\,715-1)} +$$

$$\frac{9\,593\,744(0+696\,743)2\times8\,896\,999}{(2+8\,896\,999)^2\,(2+8\,896\,999-1)} +$$

$$\text{Eq. 17}$$

$$\frac{26\,574\,265(0+1\,724\,208)0\times24\,850\,057}{(0+24\,850\,057)^2\,(0+24\,850\,057-1)} +$$

$$\frac{26\,600\,983(0+1\,145\,069)2\times25\,455\,912}{(2+25\,455\,912)^2\,(2+25\,455\,912-1)} +$$

$$\frac{110\,528\,733(0+1\,256\,470)1\times109\,272\,262}{(1+109\,272\,262)^2\,(1+109\,272\,262-1)} +$$

$$\frac{117\,046\,751(1+916\,969)0\times116\,129\,781}{(0+116\,129\,781)^2\,(0+116\,129\,781-1)} = 3.38$$

Since the total number of exposed subjects is relatively small, a continuity correction (0.5) is incorporated in Q_A to improve the chi-square approximation of $(7-2.206-0.5)^2/3.38=5.46$ with one degree of freedom and a p-value of $p \le 0.02$.

The statistic Q_A differs from Q_{MH} by evaluating A relative to expected values based on the experience of the unexposed subjects as opposed to all subjects in a stratum. For this reason, use of Q_A is most appealing when the number of unexposed subjects in a cohort study is very large relative to the number of exposed subjects. In this case, one approximately has:

$$V_0(A) = \sum_{i=1}^{I} \frac{(a_i + b_i)c_i \, d_i}{(c_i + d_i)^2}$$

Eq. 18

Also, Q_A and Q_{MH} are essentially identical. Thus, the Mantel-Haenszel statistic Q_{MH} is an appropriate method for testing the association between drug exposure status and the presence versus absence of UDEs in both case-control studies and cohort studies.

A direct test often is applied within each of the strata. For this purpose, Fisher's test is used for strata with small sample sizes and the chi-square test is used for strata with large sample sizes. Estimation of relative risk or odds ratios for each stratum is also important in order to enable evaluation of whether patterns of association are consistent in direction or whether opposing relationships cancel each other and thereby misleadingly give an impression of no association. When stra-

Figure 8
Stratified Analysis:
Controlling for Confounding
by Age and Sex

Crude Table: Combined for the Strata's Age and Sex

	Fatal Upper GI Hemorrhage	
	Present	Absent
NSAID Exposed	7 $\quad$ a	8 675 447 $\quad$ b
NSAID Not Exposed	18 $\quad$ c	30.542 x 10^7 $\quad$ d

Relative Risk = 13.691

Stratum 1: Age ≥75, Female

	Fatal Upper GI Hemorrhage	
	Present	Absent
NSAID Exposed	6 $\quad a_1$	1 171 970 $\quad b_1$
NSAID Not Exposed	6 $\quad c_1$	6 211 957 $\quad d_1$

Relative Risk = 5.30

Stratum 2: Age ≥75, Male

	Fatal Upper GI Hemorrhage	
	Present	Absent
NSAID Exposed	0 $\quad a_2$	605 742 $\quad b_2$
NSAID Not Exposed	6 $\quad c_2$	5 252 813 $\quad d_2$

Relative Risk = Not applicable

continued on page 165

tum specific effects are predominantly in the same direction, association is usually evident. Moreover, similarity of the magnitude of stratum specific measures of association strengthens the interpretability of corresponding summary measures for the combined strata. (Clinical importance and stability of the effects are important if published.)

SUMMARY ESTIMATES FOR THE ODDS RATIO AND RELATIVE RISK

The Mantel-Haenszel summary odds ratio (OR_S) is widely used in pharmacoepidemiology. In its computation, each stratum is weighted essentially according to sample size in the estimate of overall risk. The expression for its computation is:

$$OR_S = \left(\sum_{i=1}^{I} a_i\, d_i\, /N_i \right) \Big/ \left(\sum_{i=1}^{I} b_i\, c_i\, /N_i \right) \qquad \text{Eq. 19}$$

Stratum 3: Age 65–74, Female   **Fatal Upper GI Hemorrhage**

		Present	Absent
NSAID	Exposed	0 a_3	1 158 276 b_3
	Not Exposed	1 c_3	9 362 715 d_3

Relative Risk = Not applicable

Figure 8, cont'd.
Crude Table: Combined for the Strata's Age and Sex: Fatal Upper GI Hemorrhage and NSAID Use

Stratum 4: Age 65–74, Male   **Fatal Upper GI Hemorrhage**

		Present	Absent
NSAID	Exposed	0 a_4	696 743 b_4
	Not Exposed	2 c_4	8 896 999 d_4

Relative Risk = Not applicable

Stratum 5: Age 45–64, Female   **Fatal Upper GI Hemorrhage**

		Present	Absent
NSAID	Exposed	0 a_5	1 724 208 b_5
	Not Exposed	0 c_5	24 850 057 d_5

Relative Risk = Not applicable

continued on page 166

where n_i is the number of subjects in the i-th stratum. This statistic is also applicable when some cells in individual strata have zero entries, including those where the strata correspond to matched pairs or matched sets with one case and several controls. Another use of OR_S is to summarize results for a collection of studies as is often applied in meta-analysis. In this situation, the studies are the strata. See Chapter 13 for more details.

Taking the data from example 4, it can be seen in Figure 7 that the odds ratios for strata 1, 2, and 3 are 2.6, 2.1, and 1.8, respectively. The summary estimate for the odds ratio can now be calculated using the equation above as follows:

$$OR_S = \frac{\left\{ \left(\frac{27 \times 1062}{1335}\right) + \left(\frac{45 \times 1949}{2452}\right) + \left(\frac{50 \times 2247}{2840}\right) \right\}}{\left\{ \left(\frac{59 \times 187}{1335}\right) + \left(\frac{125 \times 333}{2452}\right) + \left(\frac{164 \times 379}{2840}\right) \right\}} = \frac{96.808}{47.126} = 2.054$$

Eq. 20

Figure 8, cont'd.   Stratum 6: Age 45–64, Male   **Fatal Upper GI Hemorrhage**

NSAID		Present	Absent
	Exposed	0 a_6	1 145 069 b_6
	Not Exposed	2 c_6	25 455 912 d_6

Relative Risk = Not applicable

Stratum 7: Age <45, Female   **Fatal Upper GI Hemorrhage**

NSAID		Present	Absent
	Exposed	0 a_7	1 256 470 b_7
	Not Exposed	1 c_7	109 272 262 d_7

Relative Risk = Not applicable

Stratum 8: Age <45, Male   **Fatal Upper GI Hemorrhage**

NSAID		Present	Absent
	Exposed	1 a_8	916 969 b_8
	Not Exposed	0 c_8	116 129 781 d_8

Relative Risk = Not applicable

Thus, the summary odds ratio estimate is 2.054 for the three strata. This is lower than the two highest odds ratios because of the large N of the stratum with the lowest odds ratio. A summary relative risk for multiple strata in a cohort study can be calculated as follows:[19]

$$RR_S = \frac{\sum_{i=1}^{I} \frac{a_i(c_i + d_i)}{N_i}}{\sum_{i=1}^{I} \frac{c_i(a_i + b_i)}{N_i}}$$

Eq. 21

For situations where the numbers a_i and c_i of subjects with the UDE are small relative to the corresponding totals $(a_i + b_i)$ and $(c_i + d_i)$ for exposed and not exposed (e.g., studies where the denominators for risks are expressed as person-time amounts), RR_S simplifies to:

$$RR_S = \frac{\sum_{i=1}^{I} \frac{a_i d_i}{(b_i + d_i)}}{\sum_{i=1}^{I} \frac{b_i c_i}{(b_i + d_i)}}$$

Eq. 22

since $(b_i + d_i) \approx n_i$, $RR_S \approx OR_S$. Thus, the Mantel-Haenszel summary odds ratio is a summary relative risk for cohort studies in which the UDE is a relatively rare event.

Example 9: The summary relative risk for example 4 can be calculated as follows:

$$RR_S = \left(\frac{6 \times 6\,211\,957}{1\,171\,970 + 6\,211\,957} + \frac{1 \times 116\,129\,781}{916\,969 + 116\,129\,781} \right) \Big/$$

$$\left(\frac{6 \times 1\,171\,970}{1\,171\,970 + 6\,211\,957} + \frac{6 \times 605\,742}{605\,742 + 5\,252\,813} + \right.$$

$$\frac{1 \times 1\,158\,276}{1\,158\,276 + 9\,362\,715} + \frac{2 \times 696\,743}{696\,743 + 8\,896\,999} +$$

Eq. 23

$$\frac{0 \times 1\,724\,208}{1\,724\,208 + 24\,850\,057} + \frac{2 \times 1\,145\,069}{1\,145\,069 + 25\,455\,912} +$$

$$\left. \frac{1 \times 1\,256\,470}{1\,256\,470 + 109\,272\,262} + \frac{0 \times 916\,969}{916\,969 + 116\,129\,781} \right) = 6.04 / 1.924 = 3.14$$

Note that the presence of many zero cells for the respective strata causes the numerator to have components for only strata 1 and 8 and the denominator to have components for only strata 1, 2, 3, 4, 6, and 7; these zeroes make the separate odds ratios for strata 2–8 undefined.

EVALUATION OF MULTIPLE LEVELS OF DRUG EXPOSURE IN THE STATISTICAL ANALYSIS

The analysis of the case-control or cohort study is concerned with the association of the presence versus absence of the UDE with the drug exposure status of subjects. Evaluation of this association in its most simple form is through a 2×2 table. Such a table is available when exposure to the drug is a simple dichotomy for exposed versus not exposed. However, often a relationship between dose and effects can be observed or hypothesized. For example, information would be lost if the data in Tables 3 and 4 would have been collapsed to the dichotomous categories exposed or unexposed. By maintaining multiple levels of exposure, relationships of UDEs to extent of exposure can be evaluated. The consideration for a broad range of exposures, as in Table 3, is statistically more comprehensive. Also, it often enables better detection of association through trends which might be less evident when exposure is collapsed to a dichotomy. Another advantage of multiple levels of exposure is that it makes possible the estimation of the risk in the more extreme exposure categories. The properties of the drug exposure vector are discussed in more depth in Chapter 10.

The association of the presence versus absence of the UDE with an ordered set of exposure levels (including no exposure) can be assessed with a chi-square statistic for linear trend.[14] This statistic can be straightforwardly expressed as $Q_{LT}=$ $(N-1)r^2$ where r is the correlation coefficient between scores of 0 and 1 for absence or presence of the UDE and scores 0, $y_1, y_2, \ldots, y_K$ for no exposure and K increasing levels of drug exposure. Often, the use of the integers 1, 2, ..., K for $y_1, y_2, \ldots, y_K$ is reasonable for assessing association with the trend test.

Example 5 employs data from a case-control study by Ray et al. examining the association between long-term use of thiazide diuretics and risk of proximal-femur fracture.[22] The database of the health insurance plan of the Canadian province of Saskatchewan is searched for individuals ≥65 years old hospitalized for proximal-femur fractures between 1984 and 1985. Nine hundred and five cases of proximal-femur fracture are identified; these cases are matched with 5137 population controls matched for age, sex, and calendar year. Thiazide use information for study subjects is obtained from computerized pharmacy records. The potential for con-

Table 3	Proximal Femur Fractures		
Trend Analysis.* Testing for an	Thiazide Exposure	Present (1)	Absent (0)	Odds Ratios
Exposure Dose-	Exposed with			
Response	Use ≥6 years (y_3)	30	384	0.413
Relationship.	Use 2–5 years (y_2)	115	795	0.764
Thiazide Use	Use <2 years (y_1)	90	420	1.132
and Proximal-	Not exposed (0)	670	3538	1.0 Reference
Femur Fractures				

*The Mantel-Haenszel test for linear trend based on the presented values is 21.29 with a p value of p<0.001.

| | Gallbladder Disease | | | Table 4 |
Estrogen Exposure	Present (1)	Absent (0)	Relative Risk	
Exposed with				
Use >50 μg (y_3)	336	11 299	1.21	
Use 50 μg (y_2)	1564	56 240	1.13	
Use <50 μg (y_1)	993	41 596	0.97	
Not exposed (0)	8403	341 478	1.0 Reference	

Table 4
Trend Analysis.*
Testing for Dose-Response Relationship.
Estrogen Use and Gallbladder Disease

*The Mantel-Haenszel test for linear trend based on the presented values is 23.28 with a p value of p<0.001.

founding is examined for the variables body mass, ambulatory status, functional status, and dementia.

Table 3 is constructed from data in the refereed article. It can be observed that the risk of proximal-femur fracture decreases significantly with increasing duration of use of thiazide. The Mantel-Haenszel extension test for linear trend is used to test for dose response relationships. The Mantel-Haenszel statistic for one degree of freedom for the values in Table 3 has the chi-square of 21.29 with a p-value of p<0.001. Based on these data a statistical significance, at the p<0.001 level dose-response relationship is present. Thiazide use reduces the risk of proximal-femur fractures in this population.

Example 6: This retrospective cohort study conducted by Strom et al. studies the association between oral contraceptive use and gallbladder disease.[23] The Computerized On-line Medicaid Pharmaceutical Analysis and Surveillance System (Compass) is used to extract gallbladder disease incidences and women exposed to oral contraceptives in the age group of 15–44 years from the Michigan and Minnesota State Medicaid files for the years 1980 and 1981.

Table 4 shows a population of users stratified according to the following usage categories: <50 μg estrogen per tablet, 50 μg per tablet and >50 μg estrogen per tablet. (This table is constructed calculating back from the published age-adjusted relative risks.)

The Mantel-Haenszel extension test for linear trend, as discussed above, is used to test for dose-response relationship between oral contraceptive dose and gallbladder disease outcomes. The Mantel-Haenszel statistic for one degree of freedom for the values in Table 4 has a chi-square of 23.28 with a p-value of <0.001. It can be concluded that a statistically significant dose-response relationship is present at the p<0.001 level.

LOG-LINEAR MODELS IN THE ANALYSIS OF COHORT AND CASE CONTROL DESIGNS

The relationship between drug exposure and UDE often is complicated with confounding variables for which control or adjustment is needed in the analysis. Moreover, there is often more than one confounder; for example, sex, age, and smoking instead of only age need to be taken into account. In dealing with more than one confounder, stratified analysis becomes more awkward and less reliable because the numbers in the strata become so small that they no longer contribute to the analysis. In this situation, log-linear modeling provides more appropriate analysis. Log-linear modeling allows the researcher to combine the adjustment for confounders as in stratified analysis, with assessment of different levels of drug exposure (trend analysis). It has this capability because the explanatory variables concerning association in this type of model can have different measurement levels. In this regard, the measurement level for exposure can be dichotomous (i.e., unexposed versus exposed) or numeric (total consumption in milligrams); among potential confounders, age can be numeric and smoking status can be categorical. Thus, log-linear regression can be a powerful method for the analysis of cohort and case-control studies.

For cohort studies, logistic regression is a log-linear modeling method for describing the relationship of the presence versus absence of UDEs with exposure status and a set of confounders. This model includes all relevant confounders and sufficient structure for multiple levels of exposure. Statistical tests can be used to assess the components of the model as well as the need to add other components to the model. The latter is sometimes done with what is called a "chunk test." When the other variables assessed by this method are found to be unnecessary, goodness of fit of the model is supported.[17]

Logistic regression analysis is based on specifying a multiplicative relationship between the odds of presence versus absence of a UDE and a set of explanatory variables:

$$\text{Odds} \left(\frac{\text{UDE presence}}{\text{UDE absence}} \right) = \exp(\beta_0 + \beta_1 x_1 + \beta_2 x_2 + \ldots + \beta_t x_t) \qquad \text{Eq. 24}$$

where $\exp(\ )$ is the exponential operator for inverting natural logarithms; x_1, x_2, $\ldots$, x_t are t explanatory variables for exposure status and confounders; β_1, β_2, $\ldots$, β_t are corresponding regression coefficients; and β_0 is a reference value which applies to subjects with $x_1 = x_2 = \ldots = x_t = 0$. The respective β_g represent odds ratios by which the presence versus absence odds are multiplied per unit change in the corresponding x_g. Through estimates for the β_g, predicted probabilities for presence of the UDE can be calculated for any set of x_1, x_2, $\ldots$, x_t by first determining the corresponding predicted odds from the model and then transforming it to the probability (UDE presence) $= \frac{\text{odds}}{(\text{odds}+1)}$. Relative risk estimates then can be calculated from the predicted probabilities, although the odds ratios $\exp(\beta_g)$ usually provide a more natural way to interpret associations of presence versus absence of UDEs with explanatory variables in logistic models.

Logistic regression models also are applicable to case-control studies. For these studies, they can be applied with respect to the presence versus absence odds for

UDEs or the exposed versus not-exposed odds. Interpretation of association pertaining to UDEs would be based on odds ratios.

CONFIDENCE INTERVAL

What is the accuracy of the relative risk estimate? This question can be addressed with a confidence interval, which is a range of values for which coverage of relative risk can be described with a probability statement. Often a 95 or 99 percent probability is selected. For example, 95 percent probability tells us that with 95 percent likelihood, a study will provide a range of values that includes the relative risk; in other words, only 5 percent of possible repetitions of a study would fail to have their confidence intervals include the relative risk. It should be noted that if the range of values includes 1, no difference in risk is found between the exposed and the not-exposed population. In this case, the group of drug-exposed individuals would be interpreted as not showing a larger tendency to develop the UDE beyond that compatible with chance.

The odds ratio confidence interval can be calculated using the following formula indicated by Breslow and Day[24] and Fleiss[18] when a, b, c, and d are large:

$$CI = (ad/bc) \exp \left[\pm Z_{(1-\alpha/2)} \sqrt{\frac{1}{a} + \frac{1}{b} + \frac{1}{c} + \frac{1}{d}} \right] \qquad \text{Eq. 25}$$

where $Z_{(1-\alpha/2)}$ is the value of the $100(1-\frac{\alpha}{2})$ percentile of a standard normal variable Z. This value is 1.96 for a 95 percent confidence interval and 2.576 for a 99 percent confidence interval. Addition of 0.5 to each of a, b, c, and d when any of them is small (e.g., <10) enhances the applicability of this approximate confidence interval. The confidence interval expression for relative risk is:

$$CI = \frac{a(c+d)}{c(a+b)} \exp \left[\pm Z_{(1-\alpha/2)} \sqrt{\left(\frac{b}{a(a+b)} + \frac{d}{c(c+d)} \right)} \right] \qquad \text{Eq. 26}$$

Using the data from Example 3, the 95 percent confidence interval for the odds ratio for the International Agranulocytosis and Aplastic Anemia case-control study can be calculated as follows:[9]

$$(ad/bc) \exp \left[\pm 1.96 \sqrt{\left(\frac{1}{a} + \frac{1}{b} + \frac{1}{c} + \frac{1}{d} \right)} \right] = 73.2 \exp \left[\pm 1.96 \sqrt{\left(\frac{1}{45} + \frac{1}{5} + \frac{1}{27} + \frac{1}{1766} \right)} \right]$$

$$= 95\% \ CI = 28.77 - 186.29 \qquad \text{Eq. 27}$$

For the 99 percent confidence interval the calculation is:

$$(ad/bc) \exp\left[\pm 2.576 \sqrt{\left(\frac{1}{a}+\frac{1}{b}+\frac{1}{c}+\frac{1}{d}\right)}\right] = 73.2 \exp\left[\pm 2.576\sqrt{\left(\frac{1}{45}+\frac{1}{5}+\frac{1}{217}+\frac{1}{1766}\right)}\right]$$

$$= 99\% \ CI = 21.45\text{--}249.68$$ Eq. 28

The 99 percent confidence has a higher probability for the odds ratio being within the confidence interval, but also is much wider.

The interpretation of a relative risk of 3 in the confidence interval (1.98, 5) is different from the interpretation of the same relative risk located in a (1.10, 20) interval. The confidence interval width expresses directly the precision of the odds ratio or relative risk estimates. A wider interval with the same probability statement indicates poor precision of the odds ratio or relative risk. The inclusion of 1 in the confidence interval indicates that no risk difference is observed between those exposed and those not exposed. The relative risk or odds ratio is considered statistically different from unity if the lower 95 percent confidence limit is >1.0 or the upper confidence limit is <1.0. Not as much information is available if a study's findings are only stated as the relative risk is 4.0 with $p \leq 0.05$.

Other approaches to calculating the confidence interval can be found in the literature.[19]

EXCESS RISK OR ATTRIBUTABLE RISK

Relative risk and excess or attributable risk, the two last terms being interchangeable, are the two most common measures of association between exposure to a drug and the risk of the UDE.[25] Relative risk is the ratio of the rate of the UDE among those exposed to the drug to the rate among those not exposed to the drug.

The data in Figure 3, discussed on page 146, display the rate of cardiovascular death among those exposed to oral contraceptives.[3] On the basis of this information, it can be seen that the risk of cardiovascular death among exposed 10/9548 or 10.5/10 000 is larger than among those not exposed 3/7497 or 4.0/10 000.

Excess risk is the part of the rate of the UDE in drug-exposed individuals that can be attributed to the exposure. The excess rate is calculated by subtracting the incidence rate of the UDE in the unexposed cohort group from the incidence rate of the UDE in the exposed cohort group. It is assumed that the causes other than the drug under investigation for potentially contributing to the same symptom pattern as the UDEs have the same distribution in the drug exposed as the not-exposed cohort group. The excess risk is then: 10.5/10 000 − 4.0/10 000 = 6.5/10 000 for this population. Thus, on the basis of this information, one can state that 6.5/10 000 of the cardiovascular deaths in the study population can be attributed to the use of oral contraceptives.

SAMPLE SIZE CONSIDERATIONS

A cohort study can be designed with sufficient sample size to have power probability (1–ß) for detecting statistical significance with two-sided $p \leq \alpha$ for relative risk (RR) when the rate of the UDE in the unexposed population is P_{NE}. A simplified expression for the appropriate sample size for each group (i.e., exposed and not exposed) is:

$$\frac{N}{2} = \frac{(Z_{(1-\alpha/2)} + Z_{(1-\beta)})^2 \, (2P_{NE}RR)(1-P_{NE}RR)}{\{P_{NE}(RR-1)\}^2}$$

Eq. 29

where $Z_{(1-\alpha/2)}$ and $Z_{(1-\beta)}$ are the $100(1-(\alpha/2))$ and $100(1-\beta)$ percentiles of a standard normal variable Z. Typically $Z_{(1-\alpha/2)} = 1.96$ for the 0.05 significance level and $Z_{(1-\beta)} = 0.84$ for 0.80 power. Also, the rates P_{NE} and $(P_{NE}RR)$ of the UDE in the unexposed and exposed populations are assumed to be between 5 and 50 percent, respectively. Somewhat better expressions for sample size determination and tables are presented by Fleiss.[18] For relatively rare events, exact methods, such as those in Haseman are sometimes useful.[26]

Sample sizes for case-control studies can be determined in a similar way. The relevant specifications are the proportion exposed among cases F_E, the odds ratio (OR), and the ratio L of the control sample size to the case sample size. Relative to this background, a simplified expression for the appropriate sample size for cases is:

$$N/(1+L) = \frac{\left\{ Z_{(1-\alpha/2)} + Z_{(1-\beta)} \right\}^2 \, F_E(1-F_E)(L+1)}{L\Delta^2}$$

Eq. 30

where $\Delta = \frac{F_E(1-F_E)(OR-1)}{\{OR(1-F_E)+F_E\}}$ and F_E is assumed to be <50 percent. Alternatively, Fleiss' methods could be used for the comparison of F_E to its counterpart $F_E/\{OR(1-F_E) + F_E\}$ for the controls.[18] Finally, for both cohort and case-control studies, consideration should be given to a range of specifications in determination of sample size so that the resulting study design is reasonably robust across them.

Discussion

Pharmacoepidemiology is a rapidly expanding field of scientific endeavor. An increase in the use of observational studies in the evaluation of UDEs can be observed in the literature. Cohort and case-control designs are the study methodologies most often employed, although the studies based on the case-control design far exceed cohort design studies.

This is not surprising, because many characteristics of the case-control design make it an attractive approach to studying these effects. In the case-control design, cases are first identified and drug exposure then is assessed. Thus, case-control studies require fewer substantial resources for data collection than those of enrollment and follow-up of large populations as in cohort studies. Moreover, because cases with the UDEs are identified, the latency time for the drug effects, which may be long, are identified. Thus, while case-control studies are most effective in pharmacoepidemiologic studies, they require strict compliance to methodological principles to ensure the clinical relevance of the statistics.

Although case-control studies have gained considerable popularity, the interpretation of their results has not always been clear. Two crucial conditions largely determine the validity of the case-control statistics. One is that the cases and controls arrive from the same population. In theory, this is a logical assumption, but in research practice it can be a relatively complex task to accomplish. A second major condition is that cases and controls are matched for all confounders, which are variables that alter the distribution of the unintended effect under consideration and/or the exposure of subjects. However, it is not always known what the confounders are and which variables may alter distribution of outcomes. An appropriate approach to selecting the important confounders rests on the clinical skills and expertise of the researcher. These considerations should be dealt with in the report for the case-control study in a forthright manner.

Study statistics published for data may differ according to the statistical method being applied. Extensive literature has been published on improvements and adjustments to the basic statistical procedures. The main purpose of these modifications is more accurate or precise estimates for the study statistics. This chapter provides a comprehensive overview of the most common statistical procedures used in pharmacoepidemiology. Although some researchers may use different statistical methods, the results often agree. For further discussion, the reader is referred to more advanced statistical methods in the biostatistical literature.

References

1. Strom BL. Medical databases in postmarketing drug surveillance. *Trends Pharm Sci* 1986;7:377-9.

2. Miettinen OS. Estimability and estimation in case-referent studies. *Am J Epidemiol* 1976; 103:226-35.

3. Vessey MP, McPerson K, Yeates D. Mortality in oral contraceptive users (letter). *Lancet* 1981;1:549-50.

4. Realini JP, Goldzieher JW. Oral contraceptives and cardiovascular disease: A critique of epidemiologic studies. *Am J Obstet Gynecol* 1985;152:729-98.

5. Guess HA, West R, Strand LM, et al. Fatal upper gastrointestinal hemorrhage or perforation among users and nonusers of nonsteroidal anti-inflammatory drugs in Saskatchewan, Canada 1983. *J Clin Epidemiol* 1988;41:35-45.

6. Feinstein AR. Clinical biostatistics X. Sources of "transition bias" in cohort statistics. *Clin Pharmacol Ther* 1971;12:704-21.

7. Feinstein AR. Clinical biostatistics XI. Sources of "chronology bias" in cohort statistics. *Clin Pharmacol Ther* 1971;12:864-79.

8. Feinstein AR. Clinical biostatistics, XLVIII. Efficacy of different research structures in preventing bias in the analysis of causation. *Clin Pharmacol Ther* 1979;26:129-41.

9. International Agranulocytosis and Aplastic Anaemia Study. Risk of agranulocytosis and aplastic anaemia in relation to use of antithyroid drugs. *Br Med J* 1988;297:262-5.

10. Horwitz RI, Feinstein AR. Methodologic standards and contradictory results in case-control research. *Am J Med* 1979;66:556-64.

11. Haldane JBS. The estimation and significance of the logarithm of a ratio of frequencies. *Ann Human Genet* 1955;20:309-14.

12. Anscombe FJ. On estimating binominal response relations. *Biometrika* 1956;43:461-4.

13. Mantel N, Fleiss JL. Minimum expected cell size requirements for the Mantel-Haenszel one-degree of freedom chi-square test and a related rapid procedure. *Am J Epidemiol* 1980;112:129-34.

14. Ostle B. Statistics in research. Ames, IA: Iowa State University Press, 1963.

15. Mantel N, Haenszel W. Statistical aspects of the analysis of data from retrospective studies of disease. *J Natl Cancer Inst* 1959;22:719-48.

16. Katz D, Baptista J, Azen SP, Pike MC. Obtaining confidence intervals for the risk ratio in cohort studies. *Biometrics* 1973;34:469-79.

17. Koch GG, Edwards SE. Clinical efficacy trials with categorical data. In: Peace KE, ed. Biopharmaceutical statistics for drug development. New York: Marcel Dekker, 1988: 403-57.

18. Fleiss JL. Statistical methods for rates and proportions. 2nd ed. New York: John Wiley & Sons, 1981.

19. Kleinbaum DG, Kupper LL, Morgenstern H. Epidemiologic research: principles and quantitative methods. Belmont, CA: Wadsworth Inc., 1982.

20. Mehta CR, Patel NR, Gray R. Computing an exact confidence interval for the common odds ratio in several 2×2 contingency tables. *J Am Stat Assoc* 1985;80:969-73.

21. Ray WA, Griffin MR, Schaffner W, Baugh DK, Melton LJ. Psychotropic drug use and the risk of hip fracture. *N Engl J Med* 1987;316:363-9.

22. Ray WA, Griffin MR, Downey W, Melton III LJ. Long-term use of thiazide diuretics and risk of hip fracture. *Lancet* 1989;1:687-90.

23. Strom BL, Tamragouri RN, Morse ML, et al. Oral contraceptives and other risk factors for gallbladder disease. *Clin Pharmacol Ther* 1986;39:335-41.

24. Breslow NE, Day NE. Statistical methods for cancer research. Volume 1. The analysis of case control studies. IARC Scientific Publications No. 32. Lyon, France: International Agency for Research on Cancer, 1980.

25. MacMahon B, Pugh TF. Epidemiology: principles and methods. Boston: Little Brown, 1970.

26. Haseman JK. Exact sample sizes for use with the Fisher-Irwin test for 2×2 tables. *Biometrics* 1978;34:106-9.

10

Sources and Effects of Drug Exposure and Unintended Effect Misclassification in Pharmacoepidemiologic Studies

Abraham G. Hartzema
Eleanor M. Perfetto

Abstract

Chapter 10 discusses the sources of misclassification of drug exposure and unintended drug effect (UDE) ascertainment. Definitions are provided for the major types of mis-classification in cohort and case-control studies. Misclassification can be nondifferential or differential and unidirectional or bidirectional. The calculation of sensitivity and specificity are presented as a measure of misclassification in cohort and case-control studies. The qualitative and quantitative dimensions of the drug exposure vector are discussed. Drug identification and description, dosage strength, and length of exposure are the major determinants of the drug exposure vector. Patient compliance is a major source of misclassification of drug exposure status. Sources of misclassification of UDEs are discussed and are related to study designs employed. Error in event ascertainment is a major source of misclassification of the UDE. Finally, the impact of misclassification of drug exposure and UDE on relative risk and odds ratio estimates are illustrated for cohort and case-control examples.

Outline

D rug exposure (DE) and unintended drug effect (UDE) misclassification have an important effect on relative risk estimation in pharmacoepidemiologic studies. Misclassification contributes to a distortion of the relative risk and odds ratio estimates because of inaccurate ascertainment of DE or UDE. This chapter defines the concept of misclassification in pharmacoepidemiologic studies, outlines potential sources of misclassification, provides a brief overview of the effect size of the misclassification introduced by these sources, and models the effect of misclassification on relative risk estimators.

Research in drug utilization and outcomes, with emphasis on safety and UDEs has made extensive use of large computerized data sources.[1,2] These large managerial or billing databases provide the advantage of increased numbers; however, many disadvantages have been described and investigated. The issues that have arisen include patient confidentiality; cost of data and/or its management; timeliness of retrieval; ability to follow a cohort of patients over time; and differences and difficulties among coding systems.[1]

These databases are predominantly designed for billing purposes. Their sources of information can include the physician's office, the pharmacy, and acute or long-term care facilities. Information also may be gathered directly from the patients. Drugs recorded as being obtained by the patient from a pharmacy may not always be used by that patient. Patient noncompliance with prescription drugs has been estimated to be as high as 90 percent.[3] Thus, many factors in pharmacoepidemiologic studies utilizing large databases, medical records, disease registries, death certificates, or specially selected study populations can introduce misclassification bias.

Previous research on the effect of misclassification in pharmacoepidemiology studies has been conducted by Graham and Smith. These researchers discussed and simulated the impact of misclassification bias on relative risk when both exposure and disease are inappropriately categorized in epidemiologic investigations using a large database. The simulations in their research assumed minimal amounts of exposure misclassification (0.1–1.0 percent) with varying levels of disease prevalence. The effects of DE misclassification on the risk ratio were large and independent of disease misclassification.[4]

The magnitude of noncompliance reported in the literature implies that DE misclassification may be higher than the data used in Graham and Smith's simulation and would result in larger effects on estimates of the relative risk. This chapter discusses the information bias that results from DE and UDE misclassification in pharmacoepidemiologic studies.

Definition of Misclassification in Pharmacoepidemiologic Studies

Misclassification is an important source of information bias and has potentially severe consequences. When selection bias occurs, the observed sample is a subset of the target population and external validity is violated. However, when misclassification occurs, a rearrangement of the target population in the 2×2 table results and internal validity is violated.[5] Figure 1 displays the rearrangement due to misclassification.

The individuals truly exposed and truly experiencing the UDE can be misclassified in each of the four cells of the table. The observed classification of a' includes a_{11}, b_{11}, c_{11}, and d_{11}; for b' it includes a_{12}, b_{12}, c_{12}, and d_{12}, and so on for c' and d'. Only a_{11}, b_{12}, c_{21}, and d_{22} are correctly classified. It can also be concluded from Figure 1 that misclassification can take place for DE, UDE, or both in the same study.

One example of rearrangement due to misclassification is a cohort study that examines the association between estrogen exposure and endometrial cancer. Women receiving estrogen therapy are more likely to have regular medical examinations, and therefore are more likely to have their cancer diagnosed. Some women who have not taken estrogen are classified as not diseased when actually their disease is undetected. This detection bias results in misclassification: some of the women (c_{22}) in d' belong in c.

Another example may be recall bias in a case-control study that examines the association between barbiturate use and neural tube defects. Patients diagnosed with neural tube defects (cases) may recall the exposure better than the controls; thus, some of the women (b_{22}) in d' belong in b. Because case-control studies are generally retrospective in design and cohort studies prospective, it is assumed that DE misclassification may be more prevalent in case-control studies and UDE ascertainment bias in cohort studies.

TYPES OF MISCLASSIFICATION

A typology of misclassification has been developed. Misclassification bias can be described as differential or nondifferential, and as unidirectional or bidirection-

Figure 1
Rearrangement Due to Misclassification

		Observed Unintended Drug Effect	
		Present	Absent
Drug Exposure	Exposed	$a' = a_{11} + b_{11} + c_{11} + d_{11}$	$b' = a_{12} + b_{12} + c_{12} + d_{12}$
	Not Exposed	$c' = a_{21} + b_{21} + c_{21} + d_{21}$	$d' = a_{22} + b_{22} + c_{22} + d_{22}$

		Correct Unintended Drug Effect	
		Present	Absent
Drug Exposure	Exposed	$a = a_{11} + a_{12} + a_{21} + a_{22}$	$b = b_{11} + b_{12} + b_{21} + b_{22}$
	Not Exposed	$c = c_{11} + c_{12} + c_{21} + c_{22}$	$d = d_{11} + d_{12} + d_{21} + d_{22}$

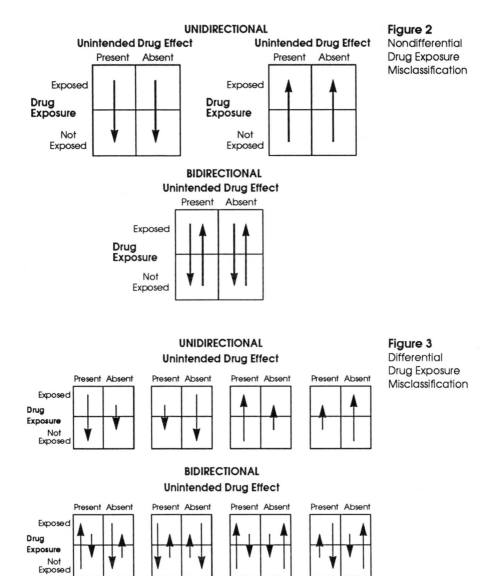

UNIDIRECTIONAL

Unintended Drug Effect

Unintended Drug Effect

Figure 2
Nondifferential
Drug Exposure
Misclassification

BIDIRECTIONAL

Unintended Drug Effect

UNIDIRECTIONAL

Unintended Drug Effect

Figure 3
Differential
Drug Exposure
Misclassification

BIDIRECTIONAL

Unintended Drug Effect

al.[4,5] This section describe these four types, and Figures 2–5 depict some of the more common rearrangements.

DE misclassification can be typed as nondifferential when the extent of error is the same for those with and without the UDE (Figure 2). Differential misclassification of exposure occurs when errors are different for those with and without the UDE (Figure 3).[5]

Similarly, nondifferential errors in classification of UDE are the same for those exposed and those not exposed (Figure 4). Misclassification of the UDE is differential when it differs among those exposed and not exposed (Figure 5).

Further, misclassification is unidirectional when only one category of a dichotomous DE or UDE variable is affected.[4] It is bidirectional when both categories are affected, equally or unequally (Figure 2).[4]

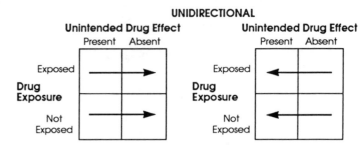

Figure 4
Nondifferential
Unintended
Drug Effect
Misclassification

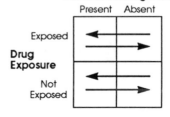

Figure 5
Differential
Unintended
Drug Effect
Misclassification

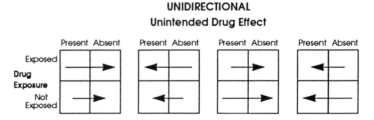
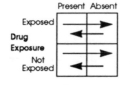

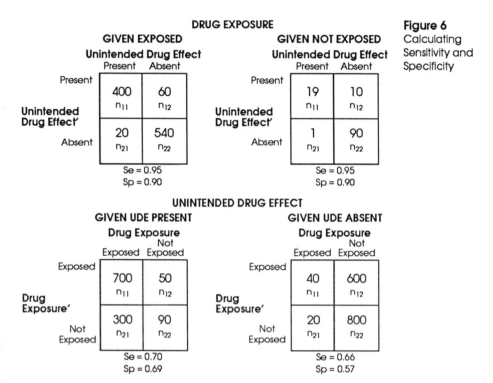

Figure 6
Calculating
Sensitivity and
Specificity

SENSITIVITY AND SPECIFICITY

Two parameters are used to provide a probability of the correct classification of the cell entries, the sensitivity (Se) and the specificity (Sp). They commonly are used in the evaluation of screening procedures or laboratory tests, and most researchers have some familiarity with them in that context.

Sensitivity and specificity can be calculated both for DE and UDE classification. Sensitivity expresses the probability that an individual with the UDE is classified as such, and specificity is defined as the probability that an individual without the UDE will be classified as such.[5] The same definitions can be stated in terms of DE.

Figure 6 shows the calculation of the sensitivity and specificity for both the DE and UDE. DE and UDE are the correct values; UDE' and DE' are the observed values. Sensitivity is calculated as $n_{11}/n_{11}+n_{21}$; specificity is calculated as $n_{22}/n_{22}+n_{12}$.

The sensitivity for UDE given exposed is $n_{11}/n_{11}+n_{21}$ or $400/400+20=0.95$. The specificity for UDE given exposed is $n_{22}/n_{22}+n_{12}$ or $540/540+60=0.90$. A sensitivity of 0.95 for UDE given DE implies that a subject who is truly exposed and who has experienced the UDE has a 95 percent probability of being classified as such. A subject who is truly not exposed and has not experienced the UDE has a 90 percent probability of being classified as such. The sensitivity for UDE given not exposed is $n_{11}/n_{11}+n_{22}$, or $19/19+1=0.95$. The specificity for UDE given not exposed is $n_{22}/n_{22}+n_{12}$ or $90/90+10=0.90$.

The sensitivity and specificity estimates can be used to calculate the impact of misclassification on odds ratio and relative risk estimates. In nondifferential misclassification the sensitivity and specificity are the same for each DE level or for each level of UDE.[6] The sensitivity (0.95) and specificity (0.90) of UDE given DE present must be equal to the sensitivity (0.95) and specificity (.90) of UDE given DE not exposed, for misclassification to be considered nondifferential.

In example 6.b (Figure 6), the misclassification of DE is differential, Se UDE present (0.70) does not equal Se UDE absent (0.66), and Sp UDE present (0.69) does not equal Sp UDE absent (0.57). The misclassification for UDE is nondifferential, and Se exposed and Sp exposed are equal to Se not exposed and Sp not exposed. In the ideal study, an assumption made in Chapter 9, sensitivity and specificity for both UDE and DE should be 1; no misclassification has occurred. The following section adresses the major sources of misclassification.

The Drug Exposure Vector

INFECTIOUS DISEASE VECTOR MODEL

The epidemiologist's earliest endeavors were mainly focussed on infectious diseases before other epidemiologic questions came to the foreground. Our knowledge of infectious diseases has increased significantly resulting in the initiation of control mechanisms based upon epidemiologic knowledge and the introduction of effective new antiinfectives. Later, the focus of the epidemiologist shifted to chronic diseases and subsequently it became clear that epidemiology is a powerful tool in making drug therapy safer.

Most infectious or communicable diseases in man are well described and categorized. Benenson has described and defined the transfer of infectious disease as: a causal agent (e.g., bacteria, virus), a reservoir, a mode of transmission, and a resulting disease outcome.[7] Elements identified in describing the vector in the infectious disease model area include: identification, occurrence, infectious agent, reservoir, mode of transmission, incubation period, period of communicability, susceptibility, and methods of control.[7]

CHRONIC DISEASE VECTOR

Chronic disease epidemiology is more complex. Most chronic diseases have multiple causal agents and many covariables or modifying variables with interactive effects. In chronic disease, environmental, genetic, lifestyle, and a multitude of other factors play a role. Chronic disease epidemiologists only recently have

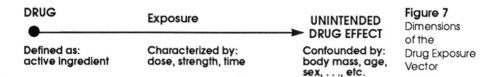

Figure 7
Dimensions of the Drug Exposure Vector

been able to establish the causes of chronic heart disease and assess their significance. For most chronic diseases epidemiologists are still sorting the contributory effects of many of these contributing causes in an effort to quantify them.

More recently, epidemiologists have become interested in the causes or distribution of the unintended effects of medications in patient populations. This is distinct from clinical trials, a powerful tool for the evaluation of the effectiveness of a drug. The DE vector is important to pharmacoepidemiology and is discussed in more detail in the following section.

DRUG EXPOSURE VECTOR DEFINED

Drug exposure can be modeled as a vector for the transmission of the UDE. The dimension of the DE vector is quite simple: the causal agent is the drug of interest, assuming that a causal association has been established. The methodology to establish a causal association between DE and UDE is discussed in Chapters 5 and 6. In Chapter 9 the statistical conditions for such an association are described (Figure 7).

In addition to causality, other dimensions of the DE vector merit attention. These include an accurate definition of the biologically active ingredient, the identification of the characteristics of the exposure, and the description of confounders. Qualifying and quantifying the DE vector are important in cohort and case-control studies to accurately classify DE.

In the most simple approach, a dichotomous exposure level (exposed versus not exposed) is assumed. In this case the exposed category is a summary of varying exposure levels. Breaking exposure down into various levels increases statistical power and allows for the testing of a dose-response relationship.[8-12]

QUALIFYING THE DRUG EXPOSURE VECTOR

The identity of the drug product under scrutiny needs to be defined in the study. The exposing agent is best defined in terms of the biologically active ingredient. Consideration of particular salts and esters can become important. The researcher is faced with the decision of inclusion or exclusion of particular compounds. The biologically active ingredient that is the focus of the research should be identified, including particular esters or salts of the drug. Although the molecular structure of a drug may be an indicator of its safety profile, the physical chemical properties of the active ingredient may not always predict its UDE profile. For example, the molecular structures of brompheniramine and zimeldine are quite similar; however, their patterns of toxicity observed postmarketing are different.[13]

Many drugs are on the market in different forms and strengths, and the strength of the product may have been changed over time. The daily dose of oral contraceptives has become lower over time, decreasing the strength of exposure. Oral contraceptives also are on the market in many dosage forms, making it difficult to obtain an exact drug identity. Approximately 30 different formulations for oral contraceptives have been or are still on the market.[14] In one study, 30 percent of the women interviewed could not recall the oral contraceptive product by brand name.[15]

Approaches taken in patient interviews to ascertain the product prescribed include the use of a prompting book with photographs of all contraceptives marketed since 1960.[14]

An extensive listing of all products (branded, branded generics, and generics), including strengths and dosage forms, that contain the active ingredient should be compiled for the study drug. Different coding systems and changes in coding schemes for historical data may be important considerations. The *USAN and the USP Dictionary of Drug Names* contains more than 5400 International Nonproprietary Names, 5800 brand names, 3906 investigational drug code designations, and 2481 official names of drug substances.[16] The usual or customary strength and recommended daily dose are also important. Properties of the pharmaceutical preparation may alter its UDE profile.[17] In retrospective studies, it may be important to know the time of market introduction for the drug and its different strengths and dosage forms. The latter can verify patient use data obtained by interview or other methods.

Changes in the formularies of health maintenance organizations (HMO) or Medicaid programs also may be an area of concern. These formularies tend to be modified over time, usually to replace more expensive drugs with less costly ones. Formularies also may limit the covered patient population from exposure to the drug.

QUANTIFYING THE DRUG EXPOSURE VECTOR

The most important dimensions of the exposure vector are dosage strength and length of exposure (Figure 7). These can become complex issues in measuring the DE vector.

Strength. Different approaches can be taken in assessing the strength of the exposure. Chapter 7 discusses units used to evaluate the strength of the DE. These units can be expressed as prescriptions, dosage, number of dosages, or defined daily doses. If different levels of DE are assessed, it is important to classify the exposure in the most common dosage levels used. Each level of exposure in the analysis represents a distinct usage pattern. When the dosing of a drug is standard, the length of exposure becomes the major dimension to be considered in the study.

Other approaches may be adapted to assess the strength of the exposure of multiple agents. Such an approach was taken when patients with leukemia were exposed to multiple alkylating agents. To quantify the patient's exposure to these agents, an alkylating agent score was developed based on the total dose/body surface area (mg/m²). A score of 0, 1, 2, and 3, for each agent was given: a 0 for no exposure to the agent and, 1, 2, and 3 for the lower, middle, and upper third of the distribution, respectively. These scores are summarized in an alkylator score of the strength of exposure.[18]

Time. Different approaches to quantifying the time dimension are available in the literature. Time can be categorized as length of exposure, time since last use, time since first use, or time in relationship to an event such as pregnancy. In pregnancy, exposure often is related to the trimester in which the exposure has taken place parallel with fetal development. The first trimester, covering early embryogenesis, is most important.[19,20]

Summary Measures. A summary measure is achieved by multiplying the time period the subject is exposed, expressed in days, weeks, months, or most commonly years by the dosing level. For example, five years of receiving 250 mg/d is equivalent to ten years of 125 mg/d. Such a summary measure of DE is the cumulative dose, as used in studies of the association between estrogen replacement therapy and breast cancer. A total milligram accumulated dose (TMD) can be calculated as the sum of the products of the dose taken in milligrams, the number of days per month it was taken, and the total months of consumption for that dose. Three categories of exposure could be defined: 0 TMD is no exposure; low exposure is <1500 TMD; and high exposure is ≥1500 TMD. For instance, 1500 TMD is equivalent to approximately three years of daily consumption of 1.25 mg of conjugated estrogens.[21]

The assumption is that the effect of the exposure is cumulative, and in both cases is the same. When the UDE is related to an individual's total exposure instead of specific blood concentrations, this approach may be quite reasonable. However, important information may be lost. Understanding the pharmacokinetic and pharmacodynamic properties of the drug assists in the appropriate classification of exposure level for trend analysis.

A measure frequently used in pharmacoepidemiologic studies is the person-time of exposure or person-time of observation. Person-time for each observation often is used in the calculation of rates for specific outcomes. The duration of time that each individual in the cohort is followed is summed. This value is used as the denominator with the incidence of the event in the numerator, resulting in the incidence density.[5] It is used when the event of interest can occur in one individual more than one time during the period of observation.

This measure also is used when all persons are not followed over the complete time period of the study. This may be due to dropouts, variation in the time periods of individual exposures, or because enrollment has taken place over an extended time period. For example, if 100 individuals were followed for two years,

200 person-years of observation would be recorded. This sum also would be obtained if 50 individuals were followed for one year and 50 individuals were followed for three years: (50×1)+(50×3)=200 person/years of observation. Cohort studies do not always use person-time of exposure in the denominator of rates of outcomes. They are not used when the observation time period is short or variation is small.

Interruption of Exposure or Erratic Dosing Intervals. Certain outcomes may occur because of interrupted or irregular use of a drug. For example, anaphylactic shock syndrome related to zomepirac sodium may have been precipitated by a patient's irregular use of the drug, producing a hypersensitivity reaction to the product.[22,23] A clear understanding of the usage pattern is necessary for the definition of appropriate exposure categories.

Sources for Misclassification of Drug Exposure and Their Relative Magnitude

Many drug use data sources are being used in pharmacoepidemiologic studies to classify subjects into those that are exposed or not exposed to a drug. Subjects can be further differentiated according to varying exposure levels. There are four primary sources of DE information. The next section of this chapter presents their inherent contributions to misclassification bias. Figure 8 diagrams the relationship between these sources and exposure misclassification, and provides an estimate of the relative magnitude of the misclassification introduced.

PHYSICIAN'S OFFICE

Subjects exposed to the drug under study can be identified in the physicians' offices. Such patients often are identified through the use of a double prescription program, in which prescriptions are written by the physician on a prescription pad with carbon copies. The researcher obtains a carbon copy of the prescription.

Other approaches to collecting prescribing and disease outcome information is through medical record abstraction or by asking physicians to record information on special forms. This information reflects the mention of drugs or prescriptions written in the physicians' offices. The National Ambulatory Care Survey and the National Disease and Therapeutic Index employ this data collection method.[24]

Although these appear to be very valid ways to identify subjects exposed to a drug, it is obvious that a drug mentioned or a prescription written does not always result in a prescription being filled at the pharmacy. It has been reported that approximately seven percent of prescriptions written by physicians are not filled.[25] In a survey conducted for the Upjohn corporation it was found that 19.4 percent of the prescriptions were not filled.[26] It also has been reported that 3–21 percent of patients admitted to not filling at least one prescription given to them by their physician.[27, 28]

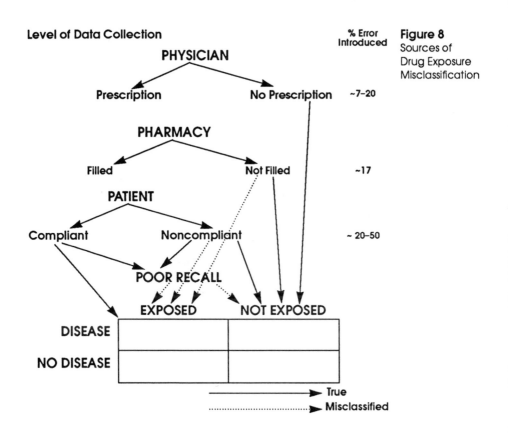

Level of Data Collection

% Error Introduced

Figure 8
Sources of Drug Exposure Misclassification

PHYSICIAN

Prescription — No Prescription ~7-20

PHARMACY

Filled — Not Filled ~17

PATIENT

Compliant — Noncompliant ~ 20-50

POOR RECALL

EXPOSED — NOT EXPOSED

DISEASE

NO DISEASE

——→ True
·········▶ Misclassified

Therefore, reliance on physician office data for DE classification can overstate the exposure rate. Establishing DE at the physician level would introduce a unidirectional misclassification bias. Seven to twenty percent of subjects are classified as exposed who actually are not exposed.

CONTROLLED ENVIRONMENTS

Hospital and nursing home drug use data also can be valuable sources of DE information (e.g., The Boston Collaborative Drug Surveillance Program).[29] These settings are controlled in the sense that medications are administered under the supervision of medically trained personnel. DE misclassification can result even in these controlled environments. It would be expected that patients receive the drug prescribed because the nursing staff is responsible for drug administration. However, the literature points out that the medication distribution systems in hospitals and nursing homes are not error free. Medication administration error rates as high as 59.1 percent have been reported in these settings.[30] Error types that may affect the misclassification of exposure are: omissions, unauthorized drugs, wrong dose, wrong route, wrong dosage form, or wrong time.

Omission, failure to give an ordered drug, is the most prevalent error that occurs in these settings. An unauthorized drug error takes place when a patient receives a drug that was not ordered. When these two error types occur together it results in bidirectional misclassification. Those subjects recorded as having received the drug, have not. Conversely, those subjects who should not have received the drug, have received it.

Omissions can occur for many reasons; medication being unavailable is fairly common. For this reason, it is more likely that omissions will occur more frequently than unauthorized drugs. Therefore, more subjects classified as exposed have not been exposed than vice versa. Misclassification errors are likely to be bidirectional, but differential.

The pharmacy dispensing recording system used in these environments also may affect exposure classification.[29] For example, a hospital emergency room may record drugs given there separately from those given after admission. Also, records may be inaccurate in that what was billed may not necessarily be what was dispensed.

PHARMACY PRESCRIPTION DATA

When a large computerized database is used, prescription billing records are largely the source of DE classification (e.g., Medicaid databases). However, it can not be assumed that a filled prescription is equivalent to exposure. The prescribed drug may not actually be the dispensed drug. Substitution, particularly therapeutic substitution, may introduce a discrepancy between the drug prescribed, the drug dispensed, and the drug recorded in a database.

In collecting prescription data in a sample of pharmacies, it was found that 4.6 percent of the prescriptions had escaped detection, resulting in underestimation of the exposure.[31]

Patient noncompliance with prescribed medications has been estimated to be 20–90 percent.[3] According to the Schering report, 15 percent of patients stop taking a drug earlier than prescribed, and 32 percent of patients do not have their prescriptions refilled.[25] In a large clinical trial, only 33.5 percent of the individuals in the control group and 32.7 percent of those in the placebo group took more than 80 percent of the doses as scheduled.[32] However, compliance may depend on the drug category studied. In examining the rate with oral contraceptives in a prospective cohort a compliance rate of 91 percent was measured.[31]

The prescribing decision can be an important modifier of the accuracy of the exposure measure. A study of the effect of multiple daily dosages found compliance rates of 67 percent for once daily, 50 percent for twice a day, 44 percent for three times a day, and 22 percent for four times a day. Other authors found a high correlation between the daily dosing schedule and compliance: 87 percent for once daily, 86 percent for twice daily, 77 percent for three times a day, and 39 percent for four times a day.[33] Simpler dosing increases compliance and consequently the accuracy of the exposure estimation.

No correlation has been found between serum concentrations and compliance. Serum concentration determination may be effective only for drugs with a long half-life. Pill counts generally overestimate compliance.[33]

Predominantly, noncompliance is manifested as under-use. This is particularly true for the elderly who report that adverse effects are occurring, that they feel over-medicated, or that the drug was not helping.[34] Those categorized as exposed based on pharmacy prescription dispensing data actually may not be exposed at all or are exposed at a much lower level than assumed. However, for drugs that are abused, the direction of the bias may be reversed; subjects may have additional drug sources and are taking more than prescribed.

PATIENT INTERVIEW

A common approach in pharmacoepidemiology studies is to obtain DE information through interviews. Patients are often a source of DE information (e.g., National Medical Care Expenditure Survey, National Medical Care Utilization and Expenditure Survey).[35,36] They routinely are questioned about drug use in the physician's office, particularly when illness or UDEs occur. Trained interviewers with a standardized questionnaire can prompt the subject for past exposure to the study drug and/or the UDE.

Patient interview information can be muddied with issues of noncompliance. Patients often report that they are more compliant than they actually are.[37,38] Thus, DE information bias can be created through inaccurate reporting of medication-taking behavior.

Norell found that, of 73 patients interviewed, only 4 percent reported two or more missed doses during a one-week period. Objective compliance assessment showed that 33 percent of the patients missed at least two doses and 16 percent missed at least six doses in that time period.[38]

Information bias may be created through selective recall if patient interview is the data source.[39] As the length of time between interview and the actual time of taking the drug is increased, the patient's ability to accurately remember declines. The occurrence of a severe UDE will prompt a patient to remember the causative agent. A patient with no UDE is more likely to forget taking the drug. These types of information bias can be bidirectional and differential and would be additional to the noncompliance misclassification.

As measure of recall bias, Werler et al. introduced recall sensitivity (Rs), the ratio of exposure reporting accuracy for cases compared with that of controls. Recall bias was recorded for a group of mothers of malformed children versus mothers of children not malformed. If the recall sensitivity estimate is >1, mothers of malformed children are more accurate in recall than mothers of children not malformed. The relative sensitivity for eight exposure factors were: nausea and vomiting, Rs=0.8; elective abortion, Rs=1.1; spotting or bleeding, Rs=1.2; antibiotic or antifungal drug use, Rs=1.2; history of infertility, Rs=1.4; urinary tract or yeast infection, Rs=2.7; and use of birth control after conception, Rs=7.6. The variation in the relative sensitivities show the recall biases for the exposure factors, and also highlight the variability in responses among the exposure factors.[40]

Other investigations have verified the validity measures of DE information from interview data in a sample of the study population.[41,42] Structured, annual (on average) interviews provided a high correlation in the data obtained between years. However, this correlation depended on the nature of the information sought. Information for medications used intermittently was poor to fair, but was good to excellent for medication used chronically. Hospitalizations and other medical factors provided good to excellent rating consistency in response.[43]

Poor quality data from interviews also may be caused by poor motivation for study participation, preconceptions about disease, or inadequately trained interviewers.[44] Patient interviews do not appear to be reliable in assessing patient exposure or compliance and can result in unidirectional or bidirectional and differential or nondifferential misclassification. Interviewers should be blinded to the outcome status of the subject to avoid exposure suspicion bias. Also, cases and controls should be interviewed the same number of times. In many instances, the interview is the only way to obtain data on DE, although it may not be as reliable as automated data sources.

In summary, these four sources of DE information can introduce misclassification bias resulting from drug information recording, medication administration errors, or patient noncompliance with the prescribed or recorded drug regimen. The errors most likely result in an overestimation of the number of exposed patients.

Some of the common considerations in the validation of DE are the use of multiple and independent data sources of drug use information in the study population or a subsample of the study populations. These should include patient interview, medical records, and pharmacy records. Interviewers and data abstracters should be blinded to the outcome status of the patient.

Chapter 20, "An Annotated Bibliography on Pharmacoepidemiologic Studies," presents the operationalization of the DE vector and its validation in pharmacoepidemiologic research.

Misclassification of the UDE

ASCERTAINMENT OF UDES

Differences in the diagnostic criteria used in identifying UDEs may introduce misclassification and make comparisons among study findings difficult. Even with defined diagnostic criteria ratings, differences may occur. In a review of the rating of 250 temporal artery biopsies, four experienced observers showed inter-observer variation that ranged from 4.3 to 13.5 percent of the cases, and intraobserver variation that ranged from 4.4 to 25.6 percent of the cases.[45]

Studies may classify histologically confirmed breast cancer as in situ or invasive. Tumor size is measured in length, width, and depth and classified accordingly, small invasive for those ≤1 cm and large invasive for those ≥1 cm.[46] Other investigators may use a detailed classification scheme to further classify tumors based on cytologic atypia.[47,48] A biopsy confirming epithelial proliferation using a pathological classification provides more information.

An accurate case definition can prevent misclassification. In a study of agranulocytosis and aplastic anemia in relation to the use of antithyroid drugs, agranulocytosis is clearly defined with the following laboratory values: granulocytes ≤0.5 × 10^9/L, hemoglobin ≥100 g/L, packed cell volume ≥0.3, and platelets ≥100 × 10^9/L.[49] Accurate case definition allows other researchers to replicate study findings.

Studies have employed survey instruments or patient self-report for case ascertainment. Formal systems for detecting new UDEs have been inadequate. The National Institute of Mental Health's Systematic Assessment For Treatment Emergent Events has described a new technique for detecting UDEs that arise during clinical trials.[50] Other authors have been successful in assessing UDEs in patient populations using structured questionnaires.[51]

Solovitz et al. found that patients were able to distinguish UDEs from other extraneous new symptoms. In 75 percent of identified symptoms, the patients deduced causality. Patient attribution was determined by personal experience, but when the patient education level was high, cognitive factors became more important. In this study patients were a good information source in the identification of UDEs.[52]

Confounding by indication may occur when a symptom such as persistent ventricular arrhythmia in postmyocardial infarction is treated with propranolol. The drug is associated with adverse outcomes such as sudden death. A UDE may be attributed to the drug when it is actually a manifestation of poor disease outcome.

Confounding by indication does not occur only in patients with poor prognosis. Patients can be selected because they are not as severely ill. In a study in which lidocaine was prescribed prophylactically to prevent death in acute myocardial infarction, it appeared that better risk patients were chosen to receive therapy.[53] To adjust for confounding by indication, the Killip scale was used to stratify the study group according to a commonly used prognostic index of infarct severity.[54] In case ascertainment the possibility of confounding by indication should be considered.

SOURCES FOR THE IDENTIFICATION OF UDEs

Medical Record Abstraction. In case-control studies, cases often are identified through medical record review and abstraction. Medical record entries are not designed for pharmacoepidemiologic research. Thus, rare UDEs may be omitted because the physician may take a watchful, waiting approach to diagnosis and treatment. A mild, reversible UDE may not be identifiable through records or survey because it was recognized and the therapy changed by the prescriber without notation.

Alternatively, information obtained through abstraction may be less biased than an interview approach. Subjects who have experienced an adverse effect are more likely to remember it. Subjects may feel that they need to please interviewers by reporting some type of UDE.

Some UDEs may be quite obvious, such as sclerosing peritonitis due to practolol, phocomelia due to thalidomide, or pulmonary hypertension due to aminorex fumarate.[55] Others may be more difficult to detect or identify. Most UDEs are not unique clinical entities, but are often similar to other conditions prevalent in the community.

An editorial in *Gastroenterology* points out the difficulties in assessing ulcer and gastrointestinal bleeding associated with drugs from the prevalence of this diagnosis in general populations. It cites the example of a 5 percent prevalence of gastrointestinal problems in the general population, with the incidence of new cases 0.2 percent per year. If associated with the drug, the incidence rises fivefold. The prevalence in a control group would be 5.2 percent and in the drug-exposed group 6 percent, a difference of only 0.8 percent.[56]

In prospective studies, incidence data collected during the length of observation should be used in the analysis instead of prevalence data. Cross-sectional identification of cases or cohort studies with long observation periods may under-report transient, fatal, minor, or latent effects. The bias that results when the evidence of exposure disappears is called Neyman's prevalence-incidence bias.[57]

A distinction needs to be made between induction and latent periods.[58] The period between causal action of the drug and the disease initiation is called the induction period. The period between disease initiation and detection is the latent period. Because it is often difficult to separate these two periods, they are called the empirical induction period when combined. Consideration of the empirical induction period is important.

In a study of malignancy following the treatment of rheumatoid arthritis with cyclophosphamide, it was found that the rate of malignancy development was greater after six years in the exposed group and that the increased rate persisted even after 13 years.[59] Other researchers found that the risk of gallbladder disease in estrogen users persisted after use of the drug was ceased.[60] Inappropriate considerations about the length of the empirical induction period in a pharmacoepidemiologic study can result in nondifferential misclassification and bias toward the null.[58]

An innocent exposure may become suspect if it causes a sign or symptom that precipitates a search for the UDE. Knowledge about a patient's prior exposure may influence both the intensity and the outcome of the diagnostic process. Media publicity may have been used to alert patients to particular dangers. For example, women exposed to estrogens are encouraged to obtain a medical examination for the detection of endometrial neoplasia. This is called diagnostic suspicion bias.[57]

DATABASES

Misclassification sources in large databases are multiple. Dick et al. reviewed 289 abstracted records for the diagnosis of non-Hodgkin's lymphoma from two databases. These databases showed a 23.4 percent disagreement in the diagnosis. The most common errors were coding and problems due to ambiguous terms in the reporting forms.[61]

A review of the Michigan Kidney Register, which collects demographic data and records the diagnosis of endstage renal disease in new cases, shows that there is variation in reporting. Some cases were characterized etiologically (e.g., lead, analgesic, diabetic nephropathy), some were characterized histologically (e.g., glomerulo- or interstitial-nephritis), and others were characterized as hypertensive nephrosclerosis with no determination of whether the kidney damage preceded or followed the hypertension.[62-64]

Other misclassification errors can be introduced because of a phenomenon called diagnosis-related group "creep." Due to Medicare's prospective payment system for reimbursement, diagnostic and procedure data may be upcoded. The provider is then reimbursed at a higher level. Controversy exists as to whether this is an increase in the accuracy of coding or intentional miscoding.[65,66]

Many sources can be used for case ascertainment. These sources include: Medicaid data bases, HMO databases, disease registries, death certificates, discharge summaries, autopsy reports, physician office and hospital inpatient records, or direct observations. The method of case ascertainment is important; however, ascertainment of controls can be difficult. Controls should have the same intensity of medical surveillance and diagnostic procedures as cases.

Direct diagnosis with pathological evaluation is more accurate than secondary data. To avoid ascertainment bias in prospective cohorts examining the association between estrogen exposure and endometrial cancer, serial endometrial biopsy in cases and controls was proposed using similar medical surveillance schedules and diagnostic procedures.[67]

CATEGORIZATION OF UDES

The diagnostic codes used in medical databases usually are obtained from the *International Classification of Diseases, Ninth Edition.*[68] Other approaches exist in the literature to classify UDEs. For example, Matthews et al. provide a method based on the following organ systems: cardiovascular, dermatologic, endocrinology, gastrointestinal, hematologic, immunologic, neurologic, ophthalmologic, otologic, pulmonary, renal, and miscellaneous. Within this classification each UDE is further defined.[69]

Many dictionaries have been developed to facilitate the coding of UDEs. These dictionaries often assign signs, symptoms, and diagnosis the same value. A thesaurus, such as FDA's COSTART (Coding Symbols for Thesaurus of Adverse Reaction Terms) may collapse terms into large categories for analysis.[70]

In summary, most UDEs have low incidence rates, particularly when the empirical induction period is long. Methods of detection become more important for rare events, including routine examination. Inaccurate diagnostic procedures, measuring devices, interview procedures, or incomplete or erroneous data sources can contribute to UDE misclassification.[57]

Inaccurate diagnostic procedures may lead to under- or over-ascertainment. Under-ascertainment may be harder to detect because it implies that all study individuals in which the UDE is not presented have to be examined. Over-ascertainment is detected more easily because it can be handled by reexamining all cases.

Sackett provides a catalog of biases to be considered in pharmacoepidemiologic research.[57] Chapter 20 provides an overview of the UDEs surveyed and the validation of the UDEs in the annotated studies.

Identification of Exposure and Outcome Confounders

Confounders are risk factors for UDEs that are distributed unequally among the exposed and the not exposed; thus, they modify the true effect of the exposure on the outcome. To estimate the true effect, the confounder needs to be controlled for. Confounders modify the DE–UDE association by altering the pharmacokinetic and pharmacodynamic parameters. Age, sex, and weight (with respect to lean body weight) are major factors to consider.

In the evaluation of the UDE, confounding by disease plays an important role. The worsening or progression of the disease for which the drug was prescribed is mistakenly identified as an unintended effect of the drug. Confounding by disease can lead to ascertainment bias in case selection. Retrospective studies using case-control design are more likely to be biased in this respect. In prospective studies with a control group, DE and symptoms that are attributed to treatment can be more easily confirmed.

The most extensive approach in controlling for confounding can be found in the oral contraceptive neoplasm literature. In a case-control study examining the relationship between diethylstilbestrol and clear cell adenocarcinoma, Herbst et al. controlled for the following confounders: use of other hormones, mother's age and pregnancy history, daughter's birth month and weight, age at menarche, use of diethylstilbestrol in pregnancy, and prior spontaneous abortions.[71] In examining the association between oral contraceptive use and breast cancer other authors have examined up to 25 potential confounders.[14]

In a retrospective cohort study of the association between the use of nonsteroidal antiinflammatory drugs (NSAIDs) and upper gastrointestinal tract bleeding, the following confounders were examined: age; sex; state; alcohol-related diagnoses at any time; anticoagulant use at any time; preexisting abdominal conditions; antacid, cimetidine, or steroid exposure; and indication for NSAID therapy.[72] A review of the literature of the UDE under survey may assist identifying risk factors that may conclusively link with the UDE.

The use of large databases can restrict the ability to control for confounding. Not all biologically or clinically relevant confounders are captured in the data available. For example, the Quetelet's body mass index (height in inches/weight in pounds^2 ×100), which is used to measure obesity, may not be easily deduced from Medicaid databases.[73] An approach taken in examining confounders not available in a database is to conduct a medical record review for pertinent information on a sample of subjects in the study.[8]

There are several other considerations of misclassification that are beyond the scope of this chapter, and therefore will be briefly mentioned. Misclassification of exposure can spuriously introduce effect modification of risk estimates by covariates or confounders.[74] When a confounder has been misclassified, stratification or modeling of a misclassified data set reintroduces confounding in the estimates.[74] The reader is referred to the literature cited for further discussion of methodological and statistical considerations in the misclassification of confounders.

Calculating the Correct Risk Estimate from the Observed Study Sample

SIZING THE EFFECT OF MISCLASSIFICATION

Two assumptions are made in further discussions of the effect of misclassification. DE and UDE are dichotomous variables (DE exposed or not exposed; UDE present or absent), and a statistically significant association is observed between DE and the UDE. This allows us to demonstrate the adjustment procedures for misclassification in the observed population.

Misclassification can be nondifferential or differential and bidirectional or unidirectional in case-control, cohort, and cross-sectional studies. Two parameters, sensitivity and specificity, indicate the misclassification. The following eight probabilities in terms of sensitivity (Se) and specificity (Sp) estimate the misclassification of DE and UDE of a 2×2 table:

Se_1 for UDE present given DE exposed
Sp_1 for UDE present given DE exposed
Se_2 for UDE present given DE not exposed
Sp_2 for UDE present given DE not exposed
Se_3 for DE exposed given UDE present
Sp_3 for DE exposed given UDE present
Se_4 for DE exposed given UDE absent
Sp_4 for DE exposed given UDE absent

Accordingly, the following conditions can be derived for the major types of misclassification ($\neq$ indicates equal or not equal to):

1. For no misclassification:
$$Se_1 = Se_2 = Se_3 = Se_4 = 1 \text{ and } Sp_1 = Sp_2 = Sp_3 = Sp_4 = 1$$

2. For UDE nondifferential, unidirectional misclassification:
$$0 \leq Se_1 = Se_2 < 1, \text{ and } Se_3 = Se_4 = 1, \text{ and } Sp_1 = Sp_2 = Sp_3 = Sp_4 = 1, \text{ or}$$
$$0 \leq Sp_1 = Sp_2 < 1, \text{ and } Sp_3 = Sp_4 = 1, \text{ and } Se_1 = Se_2 = Se_3 = Se_4 = 1$$

3. For UDE nondifferential, bidirectional misclassification:
$$0 \leq Se_1 = Se_2 < 1, \text{ and } Se_3 = Se_4 = 1, \text{ and } 0 \leq Sp_1 = Sp_2 < 1, \text{ and } Sp_3 = Sp_4 = 1$$

Here Se_1 and Se_2 or Sp_1 and Sp_2 can, but do not have to have the same values.

4. For DE nondifferential, unidirectional misclassification:
$$Se_1 = Se_2 = 1, \text{ and } 0 \leq Se_3 = Se_4 < 1, \text{ and } Sp_1 = Sp_2 = Sp_3 = Sp_4 = 1, \text{ or}$$
$$Sp_1 = Sp_2 = 1, \text{ and } 0 \leq Sp_3 = Sp_4 < 1, \text{ and } Se_1 = Se_2 = Se_3 = Se_4 = 1$$

5. For DE nondifferential, bidirectional misclassification:
$$Se_1 = Se_2 = 1, \text{ and } 0 \leq Se_3 = Se_4 < 1, \text{ and } Sp_1 = Sp_2 = 1,$$
$$\text{and } 0 \leq Sp_3 = Sp_4 < 1$$

Here Se_3 and Se_4, or Sp_3 and Sp_4 can, but do not have to have the same values.

6. For UDE differential, unidirectional misclassification:
$$0 \leq Se_1 \neq Se_2 < 1, \text{ and } Se_3 = Se_4 = 1, \text{ and } Sp_1 = Sp_2 = Sp_3 = Sp_4 = 1$$

7. For UDE differential, bidirectional misclassification:
$$0 \leq Se_1 \neq Se_2 < 1, \text{ and } Se_3 = Se_4 = 1, \text{ and } 0 \leq Sp_1 \neq Sp_2 < 1,$$
$$\text{and } Sp_3 = Sp_4 = 1$$

8. For DE differential, unidirectional misclassification:
$$Se_1 = Se_2 = 1, \text{ and } 0 \leq Se_3 \neq Se_4 < 1, \text{ and } Sp_1 = Sp_2 = 1,$$
$$\text{and } 0 \leq Sp_3 \neq Sp_4 < 1$$

9. For DE differential, bidirectional misclassification:
$$Se_1 = Se_2 = 1, \text{ and } 0 \leq Se_3 \neq Se_2 < 1, \text{ and } Sp_1 = Sp_2 = 0,$$
$$\text{and } 0 \leq Sp_3 \neq Sp_4 < 1$$

10. For misclassification both in DE and UDE any combination of 2, 3, 6, 7, and 4, 5, 8, 9 can occur.

The values of Se and Sp can be obtained through validation of the DE and UDE classification in the study population. Patient interviews can be validated by secondary and tertiary data sources such as medical and pharmacy records, by examining the true DE and UDEs in a subsample of the study population, or through use of data from other studies or information published in the literature. For example, prescribing information (DE) in a population-based cohort study is obtained from medical records in physician offices. It appears that five percent of the individuals do not have their prescriptions filled. This is a nondifferential unidirectional misclassification with $Se_3 = Se_4 = 0.95$.

Using this information the eight sensitivity and specificity probabilities can be derived. The true or correct population can be estimated from the observed population.

Given the values for Se_{1-4} and Sp_{1-4} for each category, a general mathematical solution to correct for misclassification can be used.[5] In matrix terms this solution is:

$$Y = W^{-1} \times Y'$$

where, $Y = [a,b,c,d]$, the true or correct cell entry vector; $Y' = [a',b',c',d']$, the observed cell entry vector, and

$$W = \begin{bmatrix} Se_1 \ Se_3 & (1-Sp_1)Se_4 & Se_2 \ (1-Sp_3) & (1-Sp_2) \ (1-Sp_4) \\ (1-Se_1)Se_3 & Sp_1 \ Se_4 & (1-Se_2) \ (1-Sp_3) & Sp_2 \ (1-Sp_4) \\ Sp_1(1-Sp_3) & (1-Sp_1)(Se_4) & Se_2 \ Sp_3 & (1-Sp_2) \ Sp_4 \\ (1-Se_1) \ (1-Se_3) & Sp_1(1-Se_4) & (1-Se_2) \ Sp_3 & Sp_2 \ Sp_4 \end{bmatrix}$$

Thus,

$$\begin{bmatrix} a' \\ b' \\ c' \\ d' \end{bmatrix} \times W^{-1} = \begin{bmatrix} a \\ b \\ c \\ d \end{bmatrix} \qquad \text{Eq. 1}$$

(observed)   (true or correct)

Results of the computation should be evaluated with care. Accurate and realistic probabilities for the sensitivity and specificity parameters are necessary. Negative or erroneous cell values result when the sum of Se_1 or Se_2 and Sp_1 or $Sp_2 = 1$, or when the sum of Se_3 or Se_4 and Sp_3 or $Sp_4 = 1$. This would result in zero denominators, which makes the formula indeterminate.[5]

In the following section, two examples are presented for establishing the true or correct population from the observed population using Equation 1.

Sizing the Effect of Nondifferential Classification. In a hypothetical example of a cohort study, validation of the procedures of medical surveillance and diagnostic ascertainment followed in the study design indicate that an exposed individual showing a UDE has an 80 percent probability of being classified as such and a 20 percent probability of being misclassified. An individual without DE or the UDE has a 90 percent probability of being classified as such and a 10 percent probability of being misclassified. Thus, UDE is misclassified with a sensitivity of 0.8 and a specificity of 0.9.

For the UDE the following probabilities are derived: $Se_1 = Se_2 = 0.8$ and $Sp_1 = Sp_2 = 0.9$. There is no misclassification for DE in this prospective cohort study, $Se_3 = Se_4 = 1$ and $Sp_3 = Sp_4 = 1$. The misclassification of UDE is the same for those exposed and not exposed, therefore nondifferential and bidirectional. The observed cell entries for the study are displayed in Figure 9.

The misclassification rearrangement is reflected in Figure 10. In the notation, UDE represents the true cell entries, and UDE' is the study's observed classification of the UDEs.

From Figure 10, the relationship between the observed population and the actual or correct population can be observed, as demonstrated earlier in Figure 6. The column marginals for UDE given exposed and UDE not exposed provide the cell entries for the observed population (a' = 310; b' = 690; c' = 170; and d' = 830). The row marginal show the cell entries for the actual or corrected population (a = 300, b = 700, c = 100, and d = 900). Using Equation 1 the true or correct cell values can be estimated as follows:

The observed cell value vector:

$$\begin{bmatrix} a' \\ b' \\ c' \\ d' \end{bmatrix} = \begin{bmatrix} 310 \\ 690 \\ 170 \\ 830 \end{bmatrix}$$

The derived probabilities for sensitivity and specificity:

$$Se_1 = 0.8 \qquad Se_3 = 1$$
$$Sp_1 = 0.9 \qquad Sp_3 = 1$$
$$Se_2 = 0.8 \qquad Se_4 = 1$$
$$Sp_2 = 0.9 \qquad Sp_4 = 1$$

Figure 9
The Observed
Population

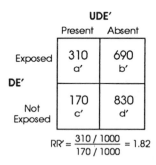

$$RR' = \frac{310 / 1000}{170 / 1000} = 1.82$$

Figure 10
Misclassification
Rearrangement

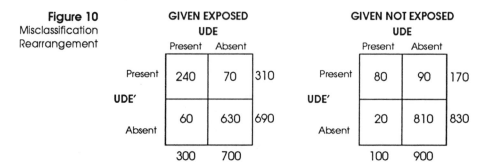

The matrix of Se and Sp probabilities:

$$W = \begin{bmatrix} 0.8 & 0.1 & 0 & 0 \\ 0.2 & 0.9 & 0 & 0 \\ 0 & 0 & 0.8 & 0.1 \\ 0 & 0 & 0.2 & 0.9 \end{bmatrix}$$

Using Equation 1, the following results are obtained:

$$\begin{bmatrix} a \\ b \\ c \\ d \end{bmatrix} = \begin{bmatrix} 1.286 & -0.143 & 0 & 0 \\ 0.286 & 1.143 & 0 & 0 \\ 0 & 0 & 1.286 & -0.143 \\ 0 & 0 & -0.286 & 1.143 \end{bmatrix} \times \begin{bmatrix} 310 \\ 690 \\ 170 \\ 830 \end{bmatrix}$$

$a = 300, b = 700, c = 100,$ and $d = 900.$

The relative risk estimate for the observed population is 1.82, while the relative risk estimate for the actual population is 3.0 (Figure 11). A bias index can be calculated as follows:

$$RR' - RR/RR = 1.82 - 3/3 = -0.39$$

The bias index should be equal to zero in the case of no misclassification; here it is negative, toward null. In nondifferential misclassification the bias is toward the null and the observed relative risk is closer to one than the true value.

Sizing the Effect of Differential Misclassification. In the following example, data are presented for a case-control study. Most case-control studies are retrospective in design, making the ascertainment of DE difficult (patient interview, etc.). Therefore, differential DE misclassification will be discussed. Three controls were selected for each case. The observed odds ratio (OR) is calculated as 2.39.

Validation studies, in which patient recall of DE is compared with documented DE data, indicate that the exposure misclassification has a sensitivity of 0.7 and a specificity of 0.9 for UDE cases and a sensitivity of 0.6 and a specificity of 0.9 for controls. No misclassification of the UDE is assumed. Thus $Se_1 = Se_2 = 1$, $Sp_1 = Sp_2 = 1$ and $Se_3 = 0.7$, $Sp_3 = 0.9$, $Se_4 = 0.6$, and $Sp_4 = 0.9.$

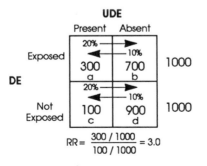

Figure 11
The Actual
Population
(Nondifferential
Bidirectional)

The sensitivity of 0.7 for UDE cases and 0.6 for controls may reflect that cases have better recall, differences in compliance, or differences in methodology to obtain exposure data. The classification of observed data is as follows:

Figure 12 demonstrates the relationship between the observed cell entries and the true entries. The row marginal shows the observed value of the cell entries (a' = 290, b' = 550, c' = 210, and d' = 950, see Figure 13). The column margins show the true cell entries (a = 400, b = 800, c = 100, and d = 700, see Figure 14). This relationship is demonstrated in Figure 6.

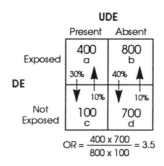

Figure 12
Misclassification
Rearrangement

GIVEN UDE PRESENT

DE

	Exposed	Not Exposed	
Exposed	280	10	290
DE' Not Exposed	120	90	210
	400	100	

GIVEN UDE ABSENT

DE

	Exposed	Not Exposed	
Exposed	480	70	550
DE' Not Exposed	320	630	950
	800	700	

Figure 13
The Observed
Population

UDE'

	Present	Absent
Exposed	290 a'	550 b'
DE' Not Exposed	210 c'	950 d'

$$OR' = \frac{290 \times 950}{550 \times 210} = 2.39$$

Figure 14
The Actual
Population
(Differential
Bidirectional)

UDE

	Present	Absent
Exposed	400 a	800 b
	30% ↑	40% ↑
	↓ 10%	↓ 10%
DE Not Exposed	100 c	700 d

$$OR = \frac{400 \times 700}{800 \times 100} = 3.5$$

Based on the identified probabilities for Se and Sp and the observed cell values in Figure 12, the true or correct cell values can be calculated from Equation 1 as follows:

The observed cell value vector:

$$\begin{bmatrix} a' \\ b' \\ c' \\ d' \end{bmatrix} = \begin{bmatrix} 290 \\ 550 \\ 210 \\ 950 \end{bmatrix}$$

The derived probabilities for sensitivity and specificity:

$$\begin{array}{ll} Se_1 = 1 & Se_3 = 0.7 \\ Sp_1 = 1 & Sp_3 = 0.9 \\ Se_2 = 1 & Se_4 = 0.6 \\ Sp_2 = 1 & Sp_4 = 0.9 \end{array}$$

The matrix of Se and Sp probabilities:

$$W = \begin{bmatrix} 0.7 & 0 & 0.1 & 0 \\ 0 & 0.6 & 0 & 0.1 \\ 0.3 & 0 & 0.9 & 0 \\ 0 & 0.4 & 0 & 0.9 \end{bmatrix}$$

Using Equation 1, the following results are obtained:

$$\begin{bmatrix} a \\ b \\ c \\ d \end{bmatrix} = \begin{bmatrix} 1.50 & 0 & -0.167 & 0 \\ 0 & 1.8 & 0 & -0.2 \\ -0.5 & 0 & 1.167 & 0 \\ 0 & -0.8 & 0 & 1.2 \end{bmatrix} \times \begin{bmatrix} 290 \\ 550 \\ 210 \\ 950 \end{bmatrix}$$

with a result of a = 400, b = 800, c = 100, and d = 700. The true 2×2 table is shown in Figure 14.

The odds ratio estimate for the observed population is 2.39, and the odds ratio estimate for the true or corrected population is 3.5. The bias index can be calculated as follows:

$$OR' - OR/OR = 2.39 - 3.5/3.5 = -0.317$$

For differential misclassification the bias index can move toward or away from the null.

Correct classification of DE and UDE so that sensitivities and specificities of 1.0 are achieved would be an ideal approach in obtaining valid study outcomes. A number of strategies and considerations in achieving correct classification have been discussed. However, if correct classification cannot be achieved, steps must be taken to adjust for the misclassification and rearrangement of cell entries. The first step in adjusting for misclassification is to obtain estimates of the sensitivity and specificity of the procedures employed in DE and UDE ascertainment.

Estimates of the sensitivities and specificities usually can be determined from previous research examining comparable populations, the same DE, and UDE associations. Other approaches include obtaining accurate ascertainment of DE and/or UDE in a subsample of the population. References from the published literature on compliance in similar populations for the same categories of study drugs may be helpful in assessing misclassification.

Misclassification that arises from differences in the selection of cases versus controls for case-control studies or selection of exposed versus unexposed subjects in cohort studies deserve particular consideration. It is advisable to correct for misclassification using sensitivity and specificity parameters derived from one's own study rather than adopting population-based parameters.[5]

Summary

Misclassification of DE and UDE ascertainment can introduce substantial bias in estimates of risk. Misclassification of DE can be introduced through inappropriate identification of drug product or class. Other errors are due to less than optimal consideration of the DE vector with regard to dosage strength and length of exposure. Faulty coding schemes or procedures, unreliable medical or pharmacy records, and patient recall bias contribute to the information bias created by DE misclassification.

Noncompliance is an important source of DE misclassification. Noncompliance is worthy of considerable notation because of its documented prevalence with regard to drug use. Epidemiologic researchers must recognize noncompliance as a considerable source of information bias. Noncompliance can overestimate the number of patients believed to be exposed. This misclassification will most likely be nondifferential, unidirectional and will bias estimates of the relative risk toward one.

The misclassification of UDEs can also result in biased risk estimates. The major sources of misclassification of UDEs are implicit and vaguely defined diagnostic criteria, prevalence-incidence bias, susceptibility bias, and empirical induction time considerations. Information bias includes medical record entry and coding errors. Most likely, these errors are differential and bidirectional.

Prospective, retrospective, case-control, or cohort study design has an effect on the type and nature of the misclassification that has to be considered in the study protocol. Prospective data are preferable to retrospective, since the latter is more subject to measurement errors that introduce misclassification. Cohort studies are often prospective in design; therefore, disease status ascertainment is the greater problem than exposure ascertainment. Detection bias may be influenced by differential surveillance in exposed and unexposed groups, exposure influence of the diagnostic investigator or exposure influenced test interpretation. Exposure ascertainment may be the greatest source of error in case-control studies, because case-control studies are retrospective in design.

Using sensitivity and specificity estimates, the true or correct cell entries can be derived for observational studies using the presented statistical equations. The shown examples use relatively low sensitivity and specificity probabilities that exaggerate the effect of misclassification on the relative risk and odds ratio estimates. These effects, even with Se and Sp probabilities closer to one, are important.

Misclassification error sources and their effects on relative risk and odds ratio estimates deserve consideration in every pharmacoepidemiological study protocol. As the extent of pharmacoepidemiologic studies grows so must the research that evaluates potential biases in DE and UDE outcomes.

References

1. Guess HA. Computer-based medical records linkage systems (lecture). Chapel Hill, North Carolina: University of North Carolina, September 1988.

2. Faich GA. Postmarketing surveillance of prescription drugs: current status. Washington, DC: Office of Epidemiology & Biostatistics, Center for Drugs and Biologics, U.S. Food and Drug Administration, October 1986.

3. Fincham JE. Patient compliance in the ambulatory elderly: a review of the literature. *J Geriatric Ther* 1988;2(4):31-52.

4. Graham DJ, Smith CR. Misclassification in epidemiologic studies of adverse drug reactions using large managerial data bases. *Am J Prev Med* 1988;4(suppl 2):15-24.

5. Kleinbaum D, Kupper L, Morgenstern H. Epidemiologic research-principles and quantitative methods. New York: Van Nostrand Reinhold Company, 1982:221-41.

6. Bross ID. Misclassification in 2×2 tables. *Biometrics* 1954;10:478-86.

7. Benenson AS. Control of communicable diseases in man. 15th ed. Washington, DC: American Public Health Association, 1990.

8. Ray WA, Griffin MR, Downey W, Melton LJ III. Long-term use of thiazide diuretics and risk of hip fracture. *Lancet* 1989;1:687-90.

9. Strom BL, Tamragouri RN, Morse ML, et al. Oral contraceptives and other risk factors for gallbladder disease. *Clin Pharmacol Ther* 1986;39:335-41.

10. Shy CM, Kleinbaum DG, Morgenstern H. The effect of misclassification of exposure status in epidemiological studies of air pollution health effects. *Bull NY Acad Med* 1978;54:1155-65.

11. Gladen B, Rogan WJ. Misclassification and the design of environmental studies. *Am J Epidemiol* 1979;109:607-16.

12. Copeland KT, Checkoway H, Holbrook RH, McMichael AJ. Bias due to misclassification in the estimate of relative risk. *Am J Epidemiol* 1977;105:488-95.

13. Agurell S. The research and development of a 5-HT selective reuptake blocker. *Acta Psychiatr Scand* 1983;308(suppl):19-24.

14. Centers for Disease Control and the National Institute of Child Health and Human Development. Oral contraceptive use and the risk of breast cancer, the cancer and steroid hormone. *N Engl J Med* 1986;315:405-11.

15. Rosenberg L, Shapiro S, Slone D. Epithelial ovarian cancer and combination oral contraceptives. *JAMA* 1982;247:3210-2.

16. Heller WH, Fleeger CA, eds. USAN and the USP dictionary of drug names. Rockville, MD: United States Pharmacopeial Convention, Inc., 1990.

17. Ellrodt AG, Murata GH, Riedinger MS, Stewart ME, Mochizuki C, Gray R. Severe neutropenia associated with sustained-release procainamide. *Ann Intern Med* 1984;100:197-201.

18. Tucker MA, Meadows AT, Boice JD. Leukemia after therapy with alkylating agents for childhood cancer. *J Natl Cancer Inst* 1987;78:459-64.

19. Mitchell AA, Rosenberg L, Shapiro S, Slone D. Birth defects related to Bendectin use in pregnancy. *JAMA* 1981;245:2311-3.

20. Resseguie LJ, Hick JF, Bruen JA, Noller KL, O'Fallon WM, Kurland LT. Cogenital malformations among offspring exposed in utero to progestins. Olmsted County, Minnesota, 1936-1979. *Fertil Steril* 1985;43:514-9.

21. Ross RK, Paganini-Hill A, Gerkins VR, et al. A case-control study of menopausal estrogen therapy and breast cancer. *JAMA* 1980;243:1635-9.

22. Strom BL, Carson JL, Morse ML, West SL, Soper KA. The effect of indication on hypersensitivity reactions associated with zomepirac sodium and other nonsteroidal antiinflammatory drugs. *Arthritis Rheum* 1987;30:1142-8.

23. Levy DB. Anaphylactic reaction due to zomepirac. *Drug Intell Clin Pharm* 1984;18: 983-4.

24. IMS America. National disease and therapeutic index. IMS America, Plymouth Meeting, PA, March 1988.

25. Schering Laboratories. The forgetful patient: the high cost of improper patient compliance. Schering Report IX, Schering Laboratories, Kenilworth, New Jersey, 1987.

26. Upjohn Company. Results of a national prescription buyer survey conducted for the Upjohn Company by Market Facts, Inc., Chicago, Il, 1988.

27. Green LW, Mullen PD, Stainbrook GL. Programs to reduce drug errors in the elderly: direct and indirect evidence from patient education. In: Improving medication compliance, Washington, DC: National Pharmaceutical Council, November 1984.

28. Burrell CD, Levy RA. Therapeutic consequences of noncompliance. In: Improving medication compliance. Washington, DC: National Pharmaceutical Council, November 1984.

29. Platt R, Stryker S, Komaroff A. Pharmacoepidemiology in hospitals using automated data systems. *Am J Prev Med* 1988;4(suppl 2):39-47.

30. Allan EL, Barker KN. Fundamentals of medication error research. *Am J Hosp Pharm* 1990;47:555-67.

31. Persson I, Adami HO, Johansson E, Lindberg B, Manell P, Westerholm B. Cohort study of estrogen treatment and the risk of endometrial cancer: evaluation of method and its applicability. *Eur J Clin Pharmacol* 1983;25:625-32.

32. The Coronary Drug Project Research Group. Influence of adherence to treatment and response of cholesterol on mortality in the coronary drug project. *N Engl J Med* 1980;303: 1037.

33. Cramer JA, Mattson RH, Prevey ML, Scheyer RD, Ouellette VL. How often is medication taken as prescribed? A novel assessment technique. *JAMA* 1989;261:3273-7.

34. Cooper JK, Love DW, Raffoul PR. Intentional prescription nonadherence (noncompliance) in the elderly. *J Am Geriatric Soc* 1982;30:329-33.

35. U.S. Department of Health and Human Services, NCHSR National Health Care Ex-

penditures Study. Prescribed medicines: use expenditures, and sources of payment. Washington, DC: U.S. Government Printing Office. April 1982;DHEW publication no. (PHS)82-3320.

36. Bonham GS. Procedures and questionnaires of the national medical care utilization and expenditure survey. Washington, DC: Public Health Service, March 1983 (Methodological Report No. 1 Series A).

37. Evans L, Spelman M. The problem of noncompliance with drug therapy. *Drugs* 1983;*25*:63-76.

38. Norell SE. Accuracy of patient interviews are estimates by clinical staff in determining medication compliance. *Soc Sci Med* 1981;*15*:57-61.

39. Austin MA, Criqui MH, Barrett-Connor E, Holdbrook MJ. The effect of response bias on the odds ratio. *Am J Epidemiol* 1981;*114*:137-43.

40. Werler MM, Pober BR, Nelson K, Holmes LB. Reporting accuracy among mothers of malformed and not malformed infants. *Am J Epidemiol* 1989;*129*:415-21.

41. Persson I, Adami HO, Bergkirst L, et al. Risk of endometrial cancer after treatment with oestrogens alone or in conjuction with progestogens: results of a prospective study. *Br Med J* 1989;*298*:147-51.

42. Goodman MT, Nomura AMY, Wilkens LR, Kolonel LN. Agreement between interview information and physician records on history of menopausal estrogen use. *Am J Epidemiol* 1990;*131*:815-25.

43. Kelly JP, Rosenberg L, Kaufman DW, Shapiro S. Reliability of personal interview data in a hospital based case-control study. *Am J Epidemiol* 1990;*131*:79-90.

44. Gordis L. Assuring the quality of questionnaire data in epidemiologic research. *Am J Epidemiol* 1979;*109*:21-4.

45. McDonnell PJ, Moore GW, Miller NR, Hutchins GM, Green WR. Temporal arteritis: a clinicopathologic study. *Ophthalmology* 1986;*93*:518-30.

46. Kleinerman RA, Brinton LA, Hoover R, Fraumeni JF. Diazepam use and progression of breast cancer. *Cancer Res* 1984;*99*:1223-5.

47. Rohan TE, Cook MG, Potter JD, McMichael AJ. A case-control study of diet and benign proliferative epithelial disorders of the breast. *Cancer Res* 1990;*50*:3176-81.

48. Rohan TE, Cook MG. Alcohol consumption and risk of benign proliferative epithelial disorders of the breast in women. *Int J Cancer* 1989;*43*:631-6.

49. International Agranulocytosis and Aplastic Anaemia Study. Risk of agranulocytosis and aplastic anaemia in relation to use of antithyroid drugs. *Br Med J* 1988;*297*:262-5.

50. Levine J, Schooler NR. SAFTEE: a technique for the systematic assessment of side effects in clinical trials. *Psychopharmacol Bull* 1986;*22*:343-81.

51. Borden EK, Lee JG. A methodologic study of post-marketing drug evaluation using a pharmacy-based approach. *J Chronic Dis* 1982;*35*:803-16.

52. Solovitz BL, Fisher S, Bryant SG, Kluge RM. How well can patients discriminate drug-related side effects from extraneous new symptoms. *Psychopharmacol Bull* 1987;*23*:189-92.

53. Horwitz RI, Feinstein AR. Improved observational method for studying therapeutic efficacy: suggestive evidence that lidocaine prophylaxis prevents death in acute myocardial infarction. *JAMA* 1981;*246*:2455-9.

54. Killip T, Kimball JT. Treatment of myocardial infarction in a coronary care unit: a two year experience with 250 patients. *Am J Cardiol* 1967;*20*:457-64.

55. Mann JI. Principles and pitfalls in drug epidemiology. In: Inman W, ed. Monitoring for drug safety. Philadelphia: JB Lippincott, 1980:401-15.

56. Kurata JH, Elashoff JD, Grossman MI. Inadequacy of the literature on the relationship between drugs, ulcers, and gastrointestinal bleeding (editorial). *Gastroenterology* 1982;82: 373-82.

57. Sackett D. Bias in analytic research. *J Chronic Dis* 1979;32:51-63.

58. Rothman KJ. Induction and latent periods. *Am J Epidemiol* 1981;114:253-9.

59. Baker GL, Kahl LE, Zee BC, Stolzer BL, Agarwal AK, Medsger TA. Malignancy following treatment of rheumatoid arthritis with cyclophosphamide. *Am J Med* 1987;83:1-2.

60. Petitti DB, Sidney S, Perlman JA. Increased risk of cholecystectomy in users of supplemental estrogen. *Gastroenterology* 1988;94:91-5.

61. Dick FR, VanLier SF, McKeen K, Everett GD, Blair A. Nonconcurrence in abstracted diagnoses of non-Hodgkin's lymphoma. *J Natl Cancer Inst* 1987;78:675-7.

62. Steenland NK, Thun MJ, Ferguson CW, Port FK. Occupational and other exposure associated with male end-stage renal disease: a case-control study. *Am J Public Health* 1990;80:153-7.

63. Weller J, Port F, Swarz R, et al. Analysis of survival of end-stage renal disease patients. *Kidney Int* 1982;21:78-83.

64. Weller J, Wu S, Ferguson W, et al. End stage renal disease in Michigan. *Am J Nephrol* 1985;5:84-95.

65. Steinwald B, Dummit LA. Hospital case-mix change: sicker patients or DRG creep? *Health Affairs* 1989;8:36-47.

66. Horn SD, Horn RA, Sharkey PD, Beall RJ, et al. Misclassification problems in diagnosis-related groups. *N Engl J Med* 1986;314:484-7.

67. Whitehead MI, McQueen J, King RJB, Campbell S. Endometrial histology and biochemistry in climacteric women during estrogen and estrogen/progestogen therapy. *J Royal Soc Med* 1979;72:322-7.

68. The International Classification of Diseases, Clinical Modification. ICD-9-CM. 9th ed. Ann Arbor, Michigan: Commission on Professional and Hospital Activities, 1978.

69. Matthews SJ, Schneiweiss F, Cersosino RJ. A clinical manual of adverse drug reactions. Norwalk, Connecticut: Appleton, Century, Crofts, 1986.

70. Food and Drug Administration. National adverse drug reaction directory "COSTART." Rockville, MD: Food and Drug Administration, 1970.

71. Herbst AL, Anderson S, Hubby MM, Haenszel WM, Kaufman RH, Noller KL. Risk factors for the development of diethylstilbestrol associated clear cell adenocarcinoma: a case control study. *Am J Obstet Gynecol* 1986;155:814-22.

72. Carson JL, Strom BL, Soper KA, West SL, Morse L. The association of nonsteroidal anti-inflammatory drugs with upper gastrointestinal tract bleeding. *Arch Intern Med* 1987; 147:85-8.

73. Machado EBV, Gabriel SE, Beard CM, Michet CJ, O'Fallon WM, Ballard DJ. A population-based case-control study of temporal arteritis: evidence for an association between temporal arteritis and degenerative vascular disease. *Int J Epidemiol* 1989;18:836-41.

74. Greenland S. The effect of misclassification in the presence of covariates. *Am J Epidemiol* 1980;112:564-9.

11

Quality of Life: Methodologies in Pharmacoepidemiologic Studies

J. Gregory Boyer
Raymond J. Townsend

Abstract

The pharmacoepidemiologist seeks to understand the effects of drug therapy on patient populations. A complete understanding cannot be achieved without information describing the full range of a drug's impact on those who take it. Clinical data are vital to this study; however, they are insufficient as the sole data source. Data reflecting a drug's impact on patients' physical, social, and emotional functioning, and sense of well-being must be evaluated in concert with the clinical findings if a complete understanding is to be achieved. Quality of life assessments offer the pharmacoepidemiologist a convenient and reliable method for documenting both the positive and negative consequences of drug therapy. Increasingly, quality of life assessments are included in clinical drug studies. The full scope of their usefulness, however, has yet to be realized. It seems certain that quality of life assessments will become data sources central to the study of pharmacoepidemiology.

Outline

Many new words and phrases have been added to the vocabulary of the pharmaceutical scientist to describe the ever-expanding field of drug research. Postmarketing surveillance, pharmaceutics, pharmacoepidemiology, and pharmacoeconomics have been included in the lexicon to describe a particular research activity that evolved into an identifiable and distinct area of study. One of the most recent additions to this list is the term "quality of life."

Quality of life has long been used in sociology, economics, public policy, and marketing, but its meaning is neither consistent across nor within disciplines.[1,2] Fayers and Jones observed that "the term 'quality of life' and various synonyms are widely used throughout the social, psychological, and medical sciences but definitions are elusive."[3] Depending on the discipline, the objective, and the perspective of the researcher, quality of life can refer to economic components such as income, housing, and working conditions; to the availability of public services; or to those components of a patient's life affected by his or her state of health.[1] Addressing the 1986 conference entitled "Measuring Quality of Life in Clinical and Epidemiology Research" (better known as "The Portugal Conference"), Spitzer commented on the nebulousness of quality of life as it pertains to health care. In reference to quality of life, he noted: "What is said, what is written, and what is done seems to be determined at times by the theme of the conference one attends or the title of the book to which one contributes a chapter."[4] Feinstein expressed similar sentiments when he described quality of life as a kind of umbrella under which is placed many different indices, each having a focus reflecting the user's particular interest.[5]

Despite the lack of a universally accepted definition of quality of life within the healthcare arena, much research effort is directed toward its study. Quality of life research generally involves the assessment of nonclinical parameters using patient self-administered questionnaires. Face-to-face interviews, telephone interviews, and patient observations are other ways quality of life data are captured. In certain situations, questionnaires completed by a parent, spouse, or significant other can provide useful information about a patient's quality of life.

Efforts to measure and quantify the subjective endpoints assessed in quality of life evaluations have given rise to an exciting new focus for drug research. Borrowing heavily from the research tools of the social and behavioral scientists, those conducting quality of life assessments are expanding the scope of many research projects. Findings from these assessments are changing the mix of attributes considered when prescribing decisions are made.

The Theoretical Framework

Schipper described the interest in studying quality of life as the result of an evolutionary process that began with the study of the basic sciences and progressed in a stepwise fashion to the study of patient-outcome measures. He observed that "at every level of development the biologic process is studied from a different perspective: the molecule, the cell, the organ, the disease, and the patient."[6] Focusing on the total patient as the unit of analysis, quality of life research is the most recent progression on this evolutionary path. The World Health Organization's (WHO) conceptualization of health is offered by many researchers as the theoretical origin for the study of quality of life as it is influenced by health and medical care.[7-9] In its 1947 constitution, WHO declared that "health is a state of complete physical, mental, and social well-being and not merely the absence of disease or infirmity."[10] By expanding the definition of health to include total well-being, traditional measures of morbidity and mortality became inadequate as the sole indicators of health status. Morbidity and mortality provide useful benchmarks for evaluating health from some perspectives; however, these aggregations are not adequate as evaluation parameters when other perspectives are taken. When focusing on the health status of one patient or a small group of patients, it is necessary to use a multidimensional approach that addresses physical, social, and emotional functioning and a sense of well-being in everyday life. Capturing data that reflect the impact of pharmacotherapy on patients' physical, social, and emotional functioning and sense of well-being in their daily lives is the crux of quality of life assessments undertaken by pharmaceutical scientists.

The WHO definition of health established a foundation from which researchers have proposed a number of models for conceptualizing quality of life as it relates to health and healthcare interventions. These models differ in complexity, but are linked by a common regard for the multidimensionality and dynamic nature of health. A simple model depicts health as a continuum anchored on one end by death, progressing through negative health to positive health, and anchored by well-being on the opposite end.[11] Ware proposed a more complex model that con-

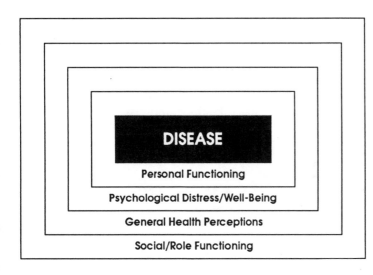

Figure 1
Framework for Discussing Disease and its Impact on Quality of Life[12]

DISEASE

Personal Functioning

Psychological Distress/Well-Being

General Health Perceptions

Social/Role Functioning

siders the impact of disease on personal, psychological, and social functioning.[12] As shown in Figure 1, this model is composed of a series of five concentric boxes, with the center and smallest box representing disease. Progressing outward, the next slightly larger box in the series represents personal functioning. Continuing outward, the three remaining boxes, each one slightly larger than the one preceding it, focus on psychological distress and well-being, general health perceptions, and social and role functioning.

Guided by these and other theoretical models depicting health as a multidimensional concept, researchers increasingly became interested in assessing the outcomes or consequences of drug therapy in terms traditionally reported anecdotally. It was a logical progression that health assessments of everyday life be included in studies evaluating alternative therapeutic agents. The use of activity of daily living (ADL) scales, originally developed to assess the level of disability in institutionalized patients and in the elderly, was expanded to include the assessment of physical activities of patients receiving alternative therapies. Used alone, however, ADL scales provide little or no information about the social, psychological, and well-being dimensions of health. A complete evaluation of patient response to treatment is obtained only when the quality of life assessment reflects the multidimensionality of health.

The term "quality of life assessment" generally has been adopted by the pharmaceutical scientist to refer to the evaluation of the various dimensions of health within a clinical research protocol designed to study patient response to specific therapies. The advances in treatment options and the clinical successes offered make the findings from quality of life evaluations important for prescribers, patients, and policy makers. Additionally, quality of life data are useful to pharmacoepidemiologists as they study the impact of drug therapies on patient populations.

Chronic Diseases and Quality of Life

It is no longer news to report that managing chronic diseases has replaced treating acute infections as the primary activity within healthcare today.[13-15] The successful treatment of life-threatening infections, the aging population, the lifestyle changes within the population, and the advances in health technology all contribute to the current domination of healthcare by activities associated with managing chronic diseases. Additionally, although advances in oncology have yielded successful treatments for Hodgkin's disease, testicular cancer, and many childhood cancers, cures remain unavailable for most metastasized solid-tumor malignancies. For many oncology patients, the treatments used make cancer a chronic condition characterized by a series of exacerbations and remissions.[16-18] Managing symptoms, restoring function, and limiting disease progression are the primary objectives of medical care received by patients with chronic maladies.[19]

Because patients with a chronic illness receive treatment for long periods, quality of life assessments can be useful in following their responses to prescribed pharmacotherapy. There is often a disjunction between what the physician can offer and what the individual patient desires. Quality of life assessments have a role to play in finding the optimal therapy. Patients are unlikely to accept a particular treatment, regardless of its scientific merit, if they perceive it to have no positive impact on their lives.[6]

In a literature review focusing on quality of life in cancer patients, DeHaes and Van Knippenberg suggest that quality of life research is meaningful in three ways. First, findings from quality of life studies may provide insight into the patients' reactions to their disease and its treatment. Second, such assessments can provide information needed in the decision process when prescribing therapy. Finally, quality of life evaluations may enhance the supportive care provided to patients by family members and medical professionals.[20] These comments are relevant to quality of life assessments of patients with other chronic diseases.

Patrick and Erickson also offer uses for quality of life findings, including monitoring and assessing patient status, selecting treatments, monitoring the effects of the treatments selected, and developing a shared view of the disease and the treatment outcomes with patients.[21] The usefulness of quality of life information in describing patients and evaluating the impact of treatment has been noted by other researchers as well.[15,22,23]

The premise underlying the application of quality of life research findings to clinical situations is that this information is important for understanding the full impact of prescribing decisions. Clinical assessment, such as a hemoglobin A1c value, a sedimentation rate, or a white blood cell count, provides invaluable insights into a patient's response to specific pharmacotherapy; however, evaluating only laboratory values cannot provide a complete response profile. By considering quality of life findings in conjunction with relevant clinical laboratory results, the clinician is better able to determine the patient's complete response to an intervention. Quality of life assessments offer a way for clinicians to capture data in objective and reproducible formats. How and what data to collect depend on the characteristics, the severity, and the prognosis of the conditions being treated.[19,22,24] Characteristics of the patients being studied also must be considered when deciding the format and the content of a quality of life assessment.

Capturing Quality of Life Data

Karnofsky and Burchenal were early proponents of assessing quality of life variables in clinical research.[25] Their 1949 paper reporting the use of the Karnofsky Performance Status Scale (KPSS), a ten-point scale for assessing the performance status of cancer patients, is regarded as a significant early contribution to the discipline.[4,8] The ten levels for assessing performance using the KPSS are detailed in

Table 1. Being observation-based, the KPSS has been criticized because it frequently does not yield scores that correlate with patients' own assessments of their situation and because it fails to address important components of health and well-being.[26] Nonetheless, the KPSS has been used extensively and has been extremely influential.[27]

From 1949 to 1990, there have been significant advances in assessing quality of life, both in terms of instruments available and assessments undertaken. An array of quality of life scales, indices, and profiles now exist for capturing data. It has been suggested that there may now be too many instruments purporting to measure health status and quality of life.[4] Among the many tools for assessing global quality of life or health status are the Sickness Impact Profile,[28,29] the Nottingham Health Profile,[30,31] the McMaster Health Index,[32,33] and the Duke-UNC Health Profile.[34] Recent reports suggest that the Medical Outcomes Study-Short Form (MOS–SF) is a global assessment tool that holds great promise for future quality of life research.[35-37] The MOS–SF contains items that measure physical functioning,

Table 1 Karnofsky Performance Status Scale[25]	Condition	Performance Status (%)	Comments
	A. Able to carry on normal activity and to work; no special care is needed.	100	Normal, no complaints. No evidence of disease.
		90	Able to carry on normal activity. Minor signs or symptoms of disease.
		80	Normal activity with effort. Some signs or symptoms of disease.
	B. Unable to work. Able to live at home, care for most personal needs. A varying degree of assistance is needed.	70	Cares for self. Unable to carry on normal activities or to do active work.
		60	Requires occasional assistance, but is able to care for most of his or her needs.
		50	Requires considerable assistance and frequent medical care.
	C. Unable to care for self. Requires equivalent of institutional or hospital care. Disease may be progressing rapidly.	40	Disabled; requires special care and assistance.
		30	Severely disabled; hospitalization is indicated although death is not imminent.
		20	Hospitalization is necessary; very sick; active supportive treatment necessary.
		10	Moribund; fatal processes progressing rapidly.
		0	Dead.

Measure	Definition
Physical functioning	extent to which health interferes with a variety of activities (e.g., sports, carrying groceries, climbing stairs, walking)
Role functioning	extent to which health interferes with usual daily activity such as work, housework, school
Social functioning	extent to which health interferes with normal social activities such as visiting with friends during past month
Mental health	general mood or affect, including depression, anxiety, and psychological well-being during the past month
Health perceptions	overall ratings of current health in general
Pain	extent of bodily pain in past four weeks

Table 2
Definitions of Health Concepts Used in the MOS–SF Instrument[35]

MOS–SF = Medical Outcomes Study–Short Form.

Reference	Name of Instrument	Disease
16	Functional Living Index—Cancer	cancer
25	Karnofsky Performance Status Scale	cancer
41	Arthritis Impact Measurement Scale	arthritis
44	Breast Cancer Chemotherapy Questionnaire	brease cancer
45	Burn Specific Health Scale	severe burn injury
46	Chronic Respiratory Disease Questionnaire	COPD
47	Health Assessment Questionnaire disability and pain scales	arthritis
48	Linear Analog Self-Assessment Scale	breast cancer
49	QL-Index	cancer
50	Quality of Life Index for Patients with Cancer	cancer

Table 3
Partial Listing of Disease-Specific Quality of Life Instruments

social functioning, role functioning, and well-being. Table 2 contains a brief definition of each of the dimensions measured by the MOS–SF.

Instruments also are available for assessing quality of life as it is influenced by a specific disease and its treatment. Among these disease-specific instruments are the Functional Living Index–Cancer[16,38] and the Arthritis Impact Measurement Scale.[39-43] A partial listing of disease-specific instruments is found in Table 3.[44-50] Assessments undertaken using a combination of disease-specific and general quality of life instruments offer the researcher greater insight into a treatment's impact on quality of life than is offered when only a disease-specific or a general quality of life tool is used.

Guyatt et al. provide a development sequence to assist the researcher in organizing the activities germane to the development of a disease-specific quality of life instrument. Although a number of disease-specific instruments are available, specific questions investigators want to address may be inadequately covered in existing scales. In these situations, the investigators must develop an instrument to capture the data necessary to answer their questions. The sequence of development steps includes: item selection, item reduction, questionnaire formatting, questionnaire pretesting, reproducibility and responsiveness determination, and validity determination. This six-step sequence also is useful to the investigator who must evaluate the appropriateness of existing quality of life questionnaires for a particular research project. Reports of instrument development that address each of these six steps assist the investigators in their quest to select well-conceived and rigorously developed assessment tools.[51]

VanDam et al. suggest that patients are the best judge of their quality of life.[52] Most recent quality of life studies use patient self-administered questionnaires to collect the data necessary to assess quality of life. Popular quality of life scales included in clinical studies use either a visual analog or a Likert format. These two approaches are most useful because they allow the detection of small changes that may occur during the clinical trial. Using a 10-cm line anchored by the extremes of the item being measured, the visual analog scales allow the respondent to record the response at any point between the two extremes. Modifications of the visual analog scale include capturing the response on a line divided into equal segments[16] and capturing the response in a 10-cm boxed area.[49] It has been suggested that the selection of either the visual analog or the Likert format is appropriate for self-administered questionnaires.[51] Figure 2 provides an illustration of a modified visual analog scale and a Likert scale.

Quality of Life in Clinical Trials

Increasingly, quality of life assessments are being included in comparative clinical trials.[8,19] As evidenced by Karnofsky's seminal work,[25] quality of life evalua-

Figure 2
Two Formats for
Capturing Patients'
Responses in
Quality-of-Life Studies

Modified Visual Analog Scale
—question from the Functional Living Index—Cancer Scale[16]

How much is pain or discomfort interfering with your daily activities?

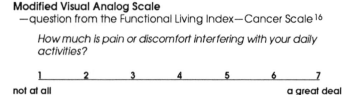

| 1 | 2 | 3 | 4 | 5 | 6 | 7 |

not at all   **a great deal**

Likert Scale
—question from the Medical Outcomes Study–Short Form[35]

How much bodily pain have you had during the past 4 weeks?
1 none
2 very mild
3 mild
4 moderate
5 severe

tions have been included in cancer research for some time. Today, they are becoming commonplace in investigations comparing treatments for coronary artery disease, hypertension, rheumatoid arthritis, and other chronic diseases. Numerous reports of such studies can be found in the medical literature.[42,53-57]

It has been suggested that quality of life assessments are not appropriate in all clinical trials. The studies in which these evaluations are most relevant include those in which the treatments under investigation are anticipated to yield only marginal differences in survival, trials in which one treatment is expected to increase survival while producing severe unintended drug effects when compared with alternative therapies, and trials comparing interventions for the lifelong treatment of a chronic disease characterized by mild symptoms.[19,58]

Reliability, Validity, and Sensitivity of Instruments

Whether selecting a single instrument or a battery of instruments to assess quality of life, a number of psychometric properties of an instrument should be considered. Unfortunately, there are no published criteria that explicitly state the minimum requirements needed to declare a quality of life instrument valid, although the need for such guidelines has been expressed.[8] Nonetheless, failure to consider an instrument's reliability, validity, and sensitivity can render the data collected suspect at best.

RELIABILITY

The reliability of a measurement refers to the proportion of observed variation that is true as opposed to random error.[59] Deyo defines reliability as the ratio of information to random error;[60] others have defined this term as the extent to which a measuring procedure is free from the effects of random error,[61] the tendency toward consistency of results upon repeated trials,[62] and the degree to which measurements are repeatable.[63] Reliability is a prerequisite for the use of a measurement for any purpose.[64]

The reliability of a quality of life instrument is determined by one or more of three possible approaches: internal consistency, test-retest, and inter-rater. Internal consistency and test-retest reliabilities are reported most often. Inter-rater reliability usually is provided for instruments designed to capture quality of life data through patient observation.

Internal consistency is an estimate of reliability based on the average correlations among items and the number of items in the scale.[65] The general approach used in determining this reliability estimate is known as the split-halves method and involves dividing the instrument into halves and then correlating the half-scale scores. If the original scale is composed of homogeneous items, the two half-scale scores will be highly correlated. A statistical formula, known as Cronbach's coefficient alpha, offers a way to determine the mean reliability coefficient for all possible ways of splitting the instrument into halves. Because it is based on data obtained from single administration of a scale, internal-consistency reliability is the least expensive and easiest method for determining an instrument's reliability.[21]

The test-retest method correlates data obtained from two administrations of the scale to the same group of respondents under the same conditions. A two-week interval generally separates these administrations.[64] Because the inherent assumptions of no recall from the first administration and of no change in conditions are weak ones, the test-retest approach is insufficient as the sole determination of an instrument's reliability.

Inter-rater reliability is an important parameter for instruments designed to capture quality of life data by direct observation of individuals. Inter-rater reliability reflects the degree of agreement among different raters using the same instrument to evaluate the same individuals at the same time.[66]

When selecting an instrument for a quality of life study, it is important to understand that reliability coefficients are based on empirical data. These estimates are properties of both the instrument used to capture the data and the population selected to provide the data; the same instrument completed by different populations may give different reliability estimates. It is necessary to consider both the demographic profile and the data collection procedure when evaluating a reported reliability coefficient. Reliability estimates above 0.9 are suggested when making comparisons between individuals. A coefficient between 0.5 and 0.7 allow comparisons between groups.[64] As a rule of thumb, Nunnally suggests that coefficients greater than 0.7 strongly support reliability.[63]

VALIDITY

Random error is not the only threat to accurate measurement. Nonrandom, or systematic, error can be problematic because of its biasing effect on measurement. The extent to which an instrument is free from nonrandom error is referred to as its validity.[61] Validity is expressed in coefficients that estimate the degree to which an instrument measures what it is intended to measure.[21] Frequent references to content, criterion, and construct validity are encountered in the quality of life literature.

Content validity refers to the representativeness of the items included in the instrument. From the domain of all questions that could be asked about a specific dimension of health, only a few make up a quality of life scale or subscale targeting that dimension. If the few selected are well representative of this domain, content validity exists. Expert opinion most often serves as the determinant of content validity. Content validity is not empirically based and does not provide sufficient evidence of an instrument's validity.

Criterion validity refers to the extent to which a measure corresponds to some other measure or observation that accurately measures the phenomenon of interest. An agreed-upon gold standard is an assumed prerequisite for determining criterion validity. Since no gold standard exists in the measurement of quality of life,[4,67] determining the criterion validity of quality of life instruments is not feasible.

When there is no gold standard, more importance is placed on construct validity, which refers to the strength of the relationship between two or more measurements purporting to measure the same construct. Instruments or subscales within instruments measuring the same construct should be strongly correlated; instruments or subscales within instruments measuring different constructs should be weakly correlated. When data from many independent studies consistently confirm these hypothesized relationships, confidence in a particular instrument's ability to capture information addressing specific constructs is justified. Nunnally suggests that construct validity is established by circumstantial evidence.[63]

Additionally, construct validity can be determined by assessing the relationship between standard clinical assessments and quality of life findings. Examples of this approach to validity assessment are found in reports describing the development of the Arthritis Impact Measure Scale (AIMS)[43] and the Chronic Respiratory Diseases Questionnaire (CRDQ).[46] In the AIMS development, correlations between the subscale scores and such standard clinical assessments as grip strength and the number of tender joints were reported. In the CRDQ development, scale scores were correlated with forced expiratory volume and slow vital capacity. For both instruments, logical relationships between scale scores and clinical findings were confirmed to support validity claims.

SENSITIVITY

The ability to detect either change over time within an individual or current differences among individuals is referred to as sensitivity.[8,60] To be useful, an instrument must be able to detect differences that are meaningful. As with reliability and validity, sensitivity must be addressed empirically. A complete profile of an instrument's reliability, validity, and sensitivity requires data analysis to be approached from both the population and patient levels. Unfortunately, an instrument's ability to detect change within an individual often is investigated inadequately. Because of this deficiency, the psychometric profiles of many quality of life instruments lack detailed reports of their sensitivity.

Summary

Quality of life assessments in which data are collected using instruments with acceptable psychometric properties can be useful in the study of pharmacoepidemiology. These evaluations document the outcomes of drug therapy from the patient's perspective. Determining the impact of a pharmaceutical product on a patient's physical, emotional, and social functioning and sense of well-being is vital to understanding a drug's effects on a patient population.

Several texts are now available that address important issues surrounding quality of life and the instruments developed to evaluate it. These works will assist the pharmaceutical scientists in their efforts to identify questionnaires appropriate and applicable to specific research questions.[65,68,69]

In Chapter 19, Tilson states that "the occurrence of harmful UDEs is an undesirable aspect of the practice of medicine, including pharmaceutical medicine." Quality of life studies offer the pharmacoepidemiologist an invaluable tool for capturing and quantifying data necessary for a total understanding of a pharmaceutical's effects—those that are beneficial as well as those that are adverse.

References

1. Friedman LM, Ferbe CD, DeMets DL. Assessment of quality of life in fundamentals of clinical trials. Littleton, MA: PSG Publishing, 1985:161-71.

2. Mosteller F. Implications of measures of quality of life for policy development. *J Chronic Dis* 1987;40:645-50.

3. Fayers PM, Jones DR. Measuring and analyzing quality of life in cancer clinical trials: a review. *Stat Med* 1983;2:429-46.

4. Spitzer WO. State of science 1986: quality of life and functional status as target variables for research. *J Chronic Dis* 1987;40:465-71.

5. Feinstein AR. Clinimetric perspectives. *J Chronic Dis* 1987;40:635-40.

6. Schipper H. Why measure quality of life. *Can Med J* 1983;128:1367-9.

7. Katz S. The science of quality of life. *J Chronic Dis* 1987;40:459-63.

8. Aaronson NK. Quantitative issues in health-related quality of life assessment. *Health Policy* 1988;10:217-30.

9. Ware JE, Brook RH, Davies-Avery A, et al. Conceptualization and measurement of health for adults in the health insurance study: Vol. 1. Model of health and methodology. R-1987/1-HEW, 1980.

10. The first ten years of the World Health Organization. Geneva: World Health Organization, 1985.

11. Patrick DL, Erickson P. What constitutes quality of life? Concepts and dimensions. *Qual Life Cardiovasc Care* 1988;4:103-27.

12. Ware JE. Conceptualizing disease impact and treatment outcomes. *Cancer* 1984;53: 2316-26.

13. Read JL. The new era of quality of life assessment. In: Walker SR, Rosser RM, eds. Quality of life: assessment and application. Lancaster, England: MTP Press Limited, 1988: 181-203.

14. Najman JM, Levine S. Evaluating the impact of medical care and technologies on the quality of life: a review and critique. *Soc Sci Med* 1981;15F:107-15.

15. Fletcher AE. Measurement of quality of life in clinical trials of therapy. *Recent Results Cancer Res* 1988;111:216-30.

16. Schipper H, Clinch J, McMurray A, Levitt M. Measuring the quality of life of cancer patients: the functional living index–cancer: development and validation. *J Clin Oncol* 1984;2:472-83.

17. Ganz PA, Rofessant J, Polinsky ML, Schag CC, Heinrich RL. A comprehensive approach to the assessment of cancer patients' rehabilitative needs: the cancer inventory of problem situations and a companion interview. *J Psychosoc Oncol* 1986; 4(3):27-42.

18. Tannock IF. Treating the patient, not just the cancer. *N Engl J Med* 1987; *317*:1534-5.

19. Wenger NK, Mattson ME, Furgerg CD, Elinson J. Overview: assessment of quality of life in clinical trials of cardiovascular therapies. In: Wenger NK, Mattson ME, Furberg CD, Elinson J, eds. Assessment of quality of life in clinical trials of cardiovascular therapies. New York: Le Jacq Publishing, 1984:1-22.

20. DeHaes JCJM, Van Knippenberg FCE. The quality of life of cancer patients: a review of the literature. *Soc Sci Med* 1985;*20*:809-17.

21. Patrick DL, Erickson P. Assessing health-related quality of life for clinical decision making. In: Walker SR, Rosser RM, eds. Quality of life: assessment and application. Lancaster, England: MTP Press Limited, 1988:9-49.

22. Siegrist J, Junge A. Conceptual and methodological problems in research on the quality of life in clinical medicine. *Soc Sci Med* 1989;*29*:463-8.

23. Tarlov AL, Ware JE, Greenfield S, Nelson EC, Perrin E, Zubkoff M. The medical outcome study, an application of methods for monitoring the results of medical care. *JAMA* 1989;*262*:925-30.

24. Fletcher AE, Bulpitt CJ. Measurement of quality of life in clinical trials of therapy. *Cardiology* 1988;*75*(suppl 1):41-52.

25. Karnofsky DA, Burchenal JH. The clinical evaluation of chemotherapeutic agents in cancer. In: Macleod CM, ed. Evaluation of chemotherapeutic agents. New York: Columbia University Press, 1949:191-205.

26. Schmale AH. Clinical trials in psychosocial medicine: methodologic and statistical considerations: Part 1. Introduction. *Cancer Treat Rep* 1980;*64*:441-3.

27. Selby P. Measuring the quality of life of patients with cancer. In: Walker SR, Rosser RM, eds. Quality of life: assessment and application. Lancaster, England: MTP Press Limited, 1988:181-203.

28. Bergner M, Bobbitt RA, Pollard WE, Martin DP, Gilson BS. The sickness impact profile: validation of a health status measure. *Med Care* 1976;*14*:57-67.

29. Bergner M, Bobbitt RA, Carter WB, Gilson BS. The sickness impact profile: development and final revision of a health status measure. *Med Care* 1981;*19*(8):787-805.

30. Hunt SM, McKenna SP, McEwen J, Williams J, Papp E. The Nottingham health profile: subjective health status and medical consultations. *Soc Sci Med* 1981; *15A*:221-9.

31. Hunt SM, McKenna SP, McEwen J, Backett EM, Williams J, Papp E. A quantitative approach to perceived health status: a validation study. *J Epidemiol Commun Health* 1980;*34*:281-6.

32. Chambers LW, Sackett DL, Goldsmith CH, Macpherson AS, McAuley RG. Development and application of an index of social function. *Health Serv Res* 1976; *11*:430-41.

33. Sackett DL, Chambers LW, Macpherson AS, Goldsmith CH, McAuley RG. The development and application of indexes of health: general methods and a summary of results. *Am J Public Health* 1977;*67*:423-8.

34. Parkerson GR, Gehlbach SH, Wagner EH, James SA, Clapp NE, Muhlbaier LH. The Duke-UNC health profile: an adult health status instrument for primary care. *Med Care* 1982; *19*:806-23.

35. Stewart AL, Hays RD, Ware JE. The MOS short-form general health survey. *Med Care* 1988;*26*:724-35.

36. Wells KB, Stewart A, Hays RD, et al. The functioning and well-being of depressed patients: results from the medical outcomes study. *JAMA* 1989;*262*:914-9.

37. Stewart AL, Greenfield S, Hays RD, et al. Functional status and well-being of patients with chronic conditions: results from the medical outcomes study. *JAMA* 1989;262:907-13.

38. Schipper H, Levitt M. Measuring quality of life: risks and benefits. *Cancer Treat Rep* 1985;69:1115-35.

39. Meenan RF, Gertman PM, Mason JH, Dunaif R. The arthritis impact measurement scales: further investigation of a health status measure. *Arthritis Rheum* 1982;25:1048-53.

40. Meenan RF, Pincus T. The status of patient status measures. *J Rheumatol* 1987;14:411-4.

41. Meenan RF, Gertman PM, Mason JH. Measuring health status in arthritis: the arthritis impact measurement scales. *Arthritis Rheum* 1980;23:146-52.

42. Mason JH, Anderson JJ, Meenan RF. A model of health status for rheumatoid arthritis: a factor analysis of the arthritis impact measurement scales. *Arthritis Rheum* 1988;31:714-20.

43. Meenan RF, Anderson JJ, Kazis LE, et al. Outcome assessment in clinical trials. *Arthritis Rheum* 1984;27:1344-52.

44. Levine MN, Guyatt GH, Gent M, et al. Quality of life in stage II breast cancer: an instrument for clinical trials. *J Clin Oncol* 1988;6:1798-810.

45. Blades B, Mellis N, Munster AM. A burn specific health scale. *J Trauma* 1982;22:872-5.

46. Guyatt GH, Berman LB, Townsend M, Pugsley SO, Chambers LW. A measure of quality of life for clinical trials in chronic lung disease. *Thorax* 1987;42:773-8.

47. Fries JF, Spitz PW, Young DY. The dimensions of health outcomes: the health assessment questionnaire, disability and pain scales. *J Rheumatol* 1982;9:789-93.

48. Priestman TJ, Baum M. Evaluation of quality of life in patients receiving treatment for advanced breast cancer. *Lancet* 1976;1:899-901.

49. Spitzer WO, Dobson AJ, Hall J, et al. Measuring the quality of life of cancer patients. *J Chronic Dis* 1981;34:585-97.

50. Padilla GV, Presant C, Grant MM, Metter G, Lipsett J, Heide F. Quality of life index for patients with cancer. *Res Nurs Health* 1983;6:117-26.

51. Guyatt GH, Bombardier C, Tugwell PX. Measuring disease-specific quality of life in clinical trials. *Can Med Assoc J* 1986;134:889-95.

52. VanDam FSAM, Somers R, Van Beck-Couzijn AL. Quality of life: some theoretical issues. *J Clin Pharmacol* 1981;21:166S-8S.

53. Croog SH, Levine S, Testa MA, et al. The effects of antihypertensive therapy on the quality of life. *N Engl J Med* 1986;314:1657-64.

54. Bombardier C, Ware J, Russell IJ, Larson M, Chalmers A, Reed JL. Auranofin therapy and quality of life in patients with rheumatoid arthritis. *Am J Med* 1986;81:565-78.

55. Williams GH, Croog SH, Testa MA, Sudilovsky A. Impact of antihypertensive therapy on quality of life: effects of hydrochlorothiazide. *J Hypertens* 1987;5(suppl):S29-35.

56. Liang MH, Cullen KE, Larson M. Measuring function and health status in rheumatic disease clinical trials. *Clin Rheum Dis* 1983;9:531-9.

57. Fletcher AE, Hunt BM, Bulpitt CJ. Evaluation of quality of life in clinical trials of cardiovascular disease. *J Chronic Dis* 1987;40:557-66.

58. Miller L, Dalton M, Vestal R, Perkins JG, Lyon G. Quality of life 1. Methodological and regulatory/scientific aspects. *J Clin Res Drug Dev* 1989;3:117-28.

59. Erickson P, Patrick DL. Guidelines for selecting quality of life assessment: methodological and practical considerations. *J Drug Ther Res* 1988;13:159-63.

60. Deyo RA. Measuring functional outcomes in therapeutic trials for chronic diseases. *Controlled Clin Trials* 1984;5:223-40.

61. Alreck PL, Settle RB. The survey research handbook. Homewood, IL: Richard C. Irwin, Inc., 1985:46, 418.

62. Carmines EG, Zeller RA. Reliability and validity assessment. 11th printing. Beverly Hills, CA: Sage Publications, 1988.

63. Nunnally JC. Psychometric theory. 2nd ed. New York: McGraw-Hill, 1978: 35-85, 225-99.

64. Ware JE. Methodological considerations in the selection of health status assessment procedures. In: Wenger NK, Mattson ME, Furberg CD, Elinson J, eds. Assessment of quality of life in clinical trials of cardiovascular therapies. New York: Le Jacq Publishing, 1984:87-117.

65. McDowell I, Newell C. Measuring health: a guide to rating scales and questionnaires. Oxford: Oxford University Press, 1987.

66. Van Knippenberg FCE, DeHaes JCJM. Measuring the quality of life of cancer patients: psychometric properties of instruments. *J Clin Epidemiol* 1988; 41:1043-53.

67. Margolese RG. The place of psychosocial studies in medicine and surgery. *J Chronic Dis* 1987;40:627-8.

68. Walker SR, Rosser RM, eds. Quality of life: assessment and application. Lancaster, England: MTP Press Limited, 1988.

69. Spilker B. Quality of life assessments in clinical trials. New York: Raven Press, 1990.

12

Evaluating the Quality of Linked Automated Databases for Use in Pharmacoepidemiology

Andy S. Stergachis

Abstract

Databases usually consist of patient-level information from two or more separate files that originally were developed primarily for nonresearch uses. Through record linkage, it is possible to create person-based longitudinal files on an ad hoc basis. Multipurpose databases should not be accepted unquestionably, for they are besieged with numerous difficulties. This chapter discusses advantages of automated linked databases (ability to study uncommon diseases and understudied defined populations, minimization of study costs, reduction in the amount of time required to complete a study, and availability of large numbers of patients). Studies based on prerecorded data, as in most record linkage studies, have all the inherent problems of the data from which they are derived. These problems relate to data completeness, patient identification, data validity, external validity, and follow-up. Examples of existing databases are provided, which show how widely they can differ in basic characteristics. Several techniques to determine the quality and validity for pharmacoepidemiologic research of automated databases are proposed.

Outline

Automated multipurpose databases are increasingly being used in postmarketing drug surveillance. These databases usually consist of patient-level information from two or more separate files, which were originally developed primarily for nonresearch applications. Through record linkage, it is possible to create person-based longitudinal files on an ad hoc basis. Multipurpose databases used in pharmacoepidemiology include databases from managed healthcare plans,[1,2] the Medicaid program,[3-5] and various other healthcare delivery programs[6,7] or defined populations.[8] In contrast to multipurpose databases, special purpose research databases are created specifically to address a research question by means of an ad hoc study.[9] Data elements contained in special purpose research databases often include information on risk factors obtained directly or indirectly from patients who are included in case-control or cohort studies. In reality, multipurpose and special purpose databases are quite complementary.[9,10]

It is important that multipurpose databases not be accepted unquestionably. Despite some long-held assumptions that record linkage approaches have wide applicability to pharmacoepidemiology, the current state of record linkage studies is besieged with numerous difficulties. A recent exchange of critiques and letters suggest some need for increased attention to the assessment of the quality of data contained in these data resources.[11-16] This chapter discusses some general characteristics of automated linked databases and proposes several techniques that should be useful in determining the quality and validity of these resources for pharmacoepidemiology. This chapter does not, however, critique the methods or findings from studies that use automated linked databases. Rather, the focus is on techniques for assessing the quality of the underlying data resources.

Multipurpose Databases and Record Linkage

Multipurpose databases or record linkage systems are resources containing longitudinal data on individual patients, which have been compiled from many sources.[9] Multipurpose databases are considered population-based if the information contained in the database is derived from a population of known size and composition. As noted by Roos et al., several characteristics of databases can facilitate their use in healthcare research:[17]

- The data must be of high quality.
- Information should be linkable across data sets.
- Individuals in the database should be traceable through time to provide longitudinal follow-up.

Generally speaking, the two principal types of files encountered in multipurpose databases are administrative records and health services files. Administrative records of programs or organizations usually include the enrollment and basic sociodemographic data of the enrolled population (e.g., age, sex). The health services databases might include information on exposures, medical events, and a limited number of potential confounding variables (e.g., preexisting or concomitant morbidities). Health services databases can be built either on the basis of each encounter with the healthcare delivery system or on the basis of claims submitted for payment. Table 1 illustrates the types of data desirable for record linkage postmarketing drug surveillance studies.

In some settings, such as the Group Health Cooperative of Puget Sound, most automated health databases originally were developed as clinical databases for both documenting the process of care and capturing clinical descriptors to facilitate running the organization in an efficient manner.[1,18] Other health services databases, such as Massachusetts General Hospital's computer-stored ambulatory record[19] and the records of the Harvard Community Health Plan, were designed to replace the traditional medical record. Many health services databases also have been developed using claims-based records. For example, the Medicaid program's claims processing files have been used extensively to provide data for pharmacoepidemiology studies.[3-5,20,21]

The use of multipurpose databases in research depends on the ability to integrate files on individuals through record linkage. Record linkage is a method for assembling information contained in two or more records and ensuring that the same individual is counted only once.[22] The concepts underlying record linkage are at least 100 years old,[23] but record linkage studies first received widespread attention when the Oxford Record Linkage Study was begun in 1962. Data on certain health events were abstracted and computerized using medical records and prescriptions from the Prescription Pricing Authority for residents of the catchment area of United Oxford Hospitals. Automated files then were linked and followed prospectively for the defined population in order to conduct ad hoc research stud-

Table 1	Variable	Database	Data Elements
Data Elements Desirable for Postmarketing Surveillance Available in Some Automated Databases	Exposure	pharmacy dispensing pharmacy billing	drug name, strength, dosage form, directions, quantity, date dispensed, patient identification
	Event	hospitalization ambulatory visit billing records disease registries vital statistics patient surveys	diagnoses (primary and secondary), procedures, reason for visit, date, provider, patient identification, disposition (alive or dead)
	Patient characteristics	membership files	patient identification (i.e., unique numeric identifier, full name, address), age, sex, tenure in plan
	Potential confounders	medical records patient surveys	age, sex, socioeconomic status, smoking, prior illnesses, family history, reproductive history

ies and health surveillance activities.[24] Another early example of record linkage is the Royal College of General Practitioners Study, designed to recruit a large group of oral contraceptive users and controls and prospectively follow their morbidity and mortality experiences.[25]

Since that time, concerns about the potential risks of marketed drugs, fueled in part by the Joint Commission on Prescription Drug Use, have led to a marked increase in the use of automated record linkage in pharmacoepidemiology. A wide variety of applications of large automated databases was developed in the 1980s, including their use in cohort studies of specific drugs,[26-28] case-control studies of events that possibly are drug-induced,[29,30] cross-sectional studies of possible drug-disease associations,[31] and studies of patterns of drug utilization.[32] Extensive other examples of the use of multipurpose databases for pharmacoepidemiology exist.

Advantages of Multipurpose Databases

In carefully designed studies of well-formed hypotheses, multipurpose databases offer a number of advantages: the ability to conduct studies of uncommon diseases or understudied defined populations (e.g., pregnant women, children, elderly), minimization of study costs, reduction in the amount of time to conduct a study, and the opportunity to study large numbers of patients. Each of these advantages will be discussed briefly.

An often-cited limitation of premarketing studies of drug effects is the exclusion of various populations of patients who ultimately use marketed drugs. Studies of the effects of drugs in children, pregnant women, and the elderly generally can be conducted only using postmarketing drug surveillance observational methodologies. Most large automated databases offer the advantage of including the health records of these relevant subpopulations. Multipurpose databases also allow the accumulation of much larger numbers of patients than those studied during premarketing drug testing. This characteristic permits the study of uncommon drug effects and the determination of more precise incidence rates than is possible through premarketing drug studies.[33]

When used properly, multipurpose databases can minimize the cost and reduce the amount of time involved in conducting pharmacoepidemiology studies. Since data already are collected and stored in a computerized format, it is possible to retrieve the data for ad hoc epidemiologic studies. As noted by Faich and Stadel, a major restriction in the conduct of most case-control and cohort studies is the time, energy, and expense necessary to assemble the case series or the series of exposed patients.[12] In acknowledging these limitations, the FDA has supported the development of automated linked databases for pharmacoepidemiology, including those for Medicaid populations and, to some degree, the Group Health Cooperative of Puget Sound (GHC).

Another advantage of most multipurpose databases is their size. Automated databases now encompass sufficiently large populations to allow the study of relatively infrequently used drugs and relatively uncommon diseases. The Medicaid files, for example, contain automated exposure information for millions of person-years of experience.[3,33] GHC's databases include outpatient pharmacy, hospitalization, and enrollment information on over 340 000 current enrollees. Moreover, it also is possible to track the health history of former GHC enrollees.[18] Collectively, the Kaiser Permanente Medical Care Program serves more than 5 million people.[34] Saskatchewan's health databases include a record of a wide range of health services provided to a province of about 1.1 million people.[35] However, more numbers are not better if a study can be done either using more traditional epidemiologic approaches, or if the data from a multisource database are irrevocably confounded or lack validity.

Another advantage is that databases containing information on prescription drugs are not subject to the limitations of incomplete recall or information bias, which are problematic for exposures remote from the index event.[33] Additionally, drug use data also can be obtained regarding deceased or impaired individuals, as well as infants and children. By examining the dates dispensed and any refill patterns, it is possible to efficiently determine dose-response and induction period relationships and the effects of in utero or periconception drug exposures.

Table 2
Illustration of Data Completeness Studies Using Data from Group Health Cooperative of Puget Sound

Methods: GHC enrollees aged 18 years and older interviewed by telephone and asked number of prescriptions written, filled at GHC, and filled at non-GHC pharmacies during previous 12 months.

Study One (1984): n = 475 random sample of GHC enrollees aged 18+ years
  2077 number of prescriptions written or authorized
   2064 (99%) prescriptions filled at GHC pharmacies
    10 (< 1%) prescriptions filled at non-GHC pharmacies
    3 (< 1%) prescriptions not filled

Study Two (1986) Sample A: n = 271 random sample of GHC enrollees (all ages) who had drug copayments ($3) and office visit copayments ($5)
  3.16 mean number of prescriptions per person/year written or authorized
   2.82 (89%) prescriptions filled at GHC pharmacies
   0.24 (8%) prescriptions filled at non-GHC pharmacies
   0.10 (3%) prescriptions not filled

Study Two (1986) Sample B: n = 206 random sample of GHC enrollees of similar age and sex as Sample A who did not have $3 drug copayments or any office visit copayments*
  3.77 mean number of prescriptions per person/year written or authorized
   3.51 (93%) prescriptions filled at GHC pharmacies
   0.18 (5%) prescriptions filled at non-GHC pharmacies
   0.08 (2%) prescriptions not filled

*This group was chosen as a random-sample comparison group to Sample A and may have included a small number of people who had a drug copayment.

Problems in Multipurpose Databases

Pharmacoepidemiology studies based on multipurpose databases are affected by a combination of conceptual and logistical impediments. These include potential limitations in the quality and completeness of the data from which they are derived; the lack of automated information on important potential confounders; and inherent limitations in the scope of exposures captured in the databases, such as the use of drug formularies or other drug restrictions implemented by managed healthcare plans or Medicaid. In some instances, investigators using large multipurpose databases have had difficulties accessing primary medical records on more than just a sample basis, thereby posing yet another potential limitation. When used alone, multipurpose databases rarely provide a sufficient basis for good epidemiologic research. Virtually all studies require at least some original data collection from either the patients' medical records or patient interviews.

The usual principles for documenting scientifically valid epidemiologic research should apply to record linkage studies;[3] however, at least five additional considerations can determine the usefulness of multipurpose databases: completeness of data, quality of patient identifiers, internal validity, external validity, and follow-up, or the ability to follow the records of individuals longitudinally. The remainder of this chapter highlights these factors that determine the utility of multipurpose databases.

DATA COMPLETENESS

Completeness of data is defined as the proportion of all exposures (e.g., prescriptions) or events (e.g., hospitalizations) in the target population that appear in a given database. For instance, if a database is population-based, all exposures and events for a defined population should appear in it. For medical events, completeness may vary considerably depending on the database. At one extreme, registration generally is estimated to be virtually complete for birth and death certificates. In contrast, registration of non-life-threatening diseases, such as minor upper respiratory infections, would be expected to be much less complete in most multipurpose databases.

The use of pharmacy databases to determine drug exposures requires that all prescriptions obtained by the population served be included in the database. At GHC, a 1984 survey of 475 randomly selected adult enrollees found that nearly all prescriptions written in the previous 12-month period were filled and obtained from GHC pharmacies.[18,36] Table 2 gives the breakdown of findings from this and a more recent study of the completeness of the GHC pharmacy database. It is interesting to note a slight decrease in the completeness of the outpatient pharmacy database over time.

As noted in the previous example, the completeness of a database can be measured by comparing information found in the database with that ascertained independently (e.g., through personal interviews). Comparisons with death vital statistics have been used to assess the completeness of cancer registries[37] and special registries for cardiovascular disease.[38] As part of an evaluation of the Illinois Trauma Registry, Goldberg et al. determined the completeness of case reporting by comparing hospital records with the trauma registry database. The completeness of case reporting was defined as the proportion of cases in the hospital records sample that also were found in the trauma registry. The authors reported a decrease in the completeness of reporting to the registry as severity of injury decreased that would have led to misleading conclusions from the uncritical use of the trauma registry.[39] The completeness of pharmacy-based surveillance by Upjohn was studied by comparing registry patients with a list of potentially eligible patients identified as receiving prescriptions for targeted drugs from a participating pharmacy.[40]

Completeness also can be determined by comparing the observed number of events (or exposures) with the number expected. The expected number is determined by applying a known incidence or prevalence rate derived from a population that is demographically similar to the study population.[39] This approach was used by Saxen et al. on a registry of congenital malformations.[41] Another approach to determining completeness is taking the database and simulating patterns of incomplete reporting to examine the possible effects on a specific variable.[39] Patterns of underreporting of burn mortality were studied in this manner by Schork et al.[42]

Because completeness rarely can be guaranteed, it is necessary to identify factors that pose systematic bias and other threats to validity. If, for example, a pharmacy database is found to be 75 percent complete and the missing data concern people with specific characteristics that could influence study findings (e.g., less affluent people, the elderly, people on certain drugs), analyses of drug effects would be misleading. This would be a potential consequence of using records from a managed care plan if the provisions of the drug benefit (e.g., deductibles, copayments) influenced certain patients to obtain some or all prescriptions from out-of-plan pharmacies. The lack of patient (particularly new enrollees) familiarity with the health plan also may result in incomplete files. There also may be differences in data completeness on the type of drugs. For example, the following types of drugs may be obtained from pharmacies whose data are not included in a given database: over-the-counter or nonlegend drugs, and nonformulary drugs.

Problems also may arise if the completeness of information varies among different types of databases for a given population. For example, the incidence of hospital unintended drug effects would be underestimated if a database included all drug acquisitions by a defined population who then sought some or all of their inpatient care from a site not included in a hospitalization database. One approach to this problem used in a retrospective cohort study of the long-term effects of tubal sterilizations is to restrict the study to those at risk for obtaining care from the hospitals included in a given database.[18] A similar problem could arise if certain specialty services were referred to a clinic or tertiary care center not contributing information to the automated database included in a study.

PATIENT IDENTIFICATION

Individuals must be identified correctly for databases to be useful for record linkage studies; otherwise, information will be linked erroneously. Individual identifiers may consist of a social security number, a unique identifying number assigned by a health plan, or some combination of other types of patient information (e.g., name, birth date, sex, address). Linkage in the Medicaid databases depends on the use of the enrollee's Medicaid identification number. Prepaid health plans, such as GHC, assign a unique medical history number to each enrollee. Once assigned, the medical history number remains with the enrollee, even if the individual leaves the program and rejoins GHC at a later date.

The linkage of databases requires each person to have a unique identifier common to the data sets that are matched. Errors in correctly identifying individuals within and across databases relate to the accuracy and precision of unique patient identifiers as well as the quality of the record linkage methodology. Having a single, unique, and permanent identification number greatly facilitates linkage; however, phonetically based methodologies such as Soundex also have been used successfully to bring together records using various combinations of name, sex, and birth date.[43] The lack of a unique identifying number in the Manitoba Health Services Commission database has been overcome through the use of a combination of family registration number, sex, and birth year.[44]

Regarding the identifiers, Acheson suggested that an ideal identification system would fulfill several criteria: uniqueness, universality, permanence, availability, and low cost. A personal identifier should be unique to the person concerned so that each individual can be distinguished from all others in a population. The identifier also should be universal, that is, all members of the defined population have unique identifiers of similar formats. Finally, personal identifiers should be permanent—from birth to death. Acheson added that, at that time (1967), no system of identification satisfying all of these criteria had been devised.[45]

DATA VALIDITY

Analysis of a database's validity is essential. Most methods used to assess the validity of automated databases involve tests of internal validity, that is, the degree that an assessment measures what it purports to measure. With automated databases, validity refers to the percentage of individuals in the database with a given characteristic (e.g., drug exposure, event, potential confounding factor) that truly has that attribute.[22] Even though multipurpose databases may contain data on drug prescriptions, hospitalizations, and limited sociodemographic factors, it usually is necessary to go to primary data sources to, at a minimum, validate the presence of medical events.

Establishing the validity of a database often involves comparisons with an external data set, preferably one collected using a different methodology. For example, if automated dispensing or billing records are used for a pharmacoepidemiologic study, then a test of validity could involve the degree of agreement between automated pharmacy records and data obtained through patient interviews. In contrast to the evaluation of data completeness, the analysis of data validity would be the concordance of specific database variables with patient responses.

Examples of data validity studies involving drug exposures can be found in several methodologic studies of the quality of both manual records and information obtained through patient interviews. Stolly et al. found high levels of agreement between prescriber records and patient-reported oral contraceptive histories on the name of the most recently used product. However, patient reports about previous oral contraceptive use were less accurate.[46] Paganini-Hill and Ross compared health-related information from multiple sources and found that agreement between data sources for ever/never drug use varied considerably, from a low of 69 percent for the use of barbiturates and related drugs to a high of 87 percent for the use of antihypertensives. Better correspondence was observed between medical records and interviews than between either medical and pharmacy records or interview and pharmacy records.[47] However, using data from the Diethylstilbesterol-Adenosis Project, Tilley et al. reported poor agreement between the mothers' recall and medical records.[48]

Similarly, assessments of the validity of data on medical events or procedures contained in automated databases usually involve comparisons with manually maintained medical records. Problems may occur in the reliability of both diagnosis and procedure codes over time because disease classifications, such as the International Classification of Diseases (ICD), periodically change. One type of check examines the actual versus the expected rates of specific diagnoses or procedures over time. For example, Sorlie and Gold reported that the ninth revision of the ICD produced an artifactual drop in ischemic heart disease mortality trends.[49]

Certain diagnoses and procedures may not be suitable for record linkage studies because they are subject to a considerable amount of physician variability in recording. Studies have shown that physicians frequently fail to list diagnoses, and sometimes list diagnoses and procedures in a way that leads to inaccurate coding onto patient discharge abstract systems. The problem of data quality in medical records[50] and hospital discharge data systems has been the subject of previous investigations.[51,52] Claims-based data systems that capture information on diagnoses and procedures have the added disadvantage of the possible influence of reimbursement policies on recording practices.

Techniques used to assess the validity of diagnostic and procedures data include the diagnostic criteria method, reabstracted record method, and the internal consistency method. In the diagnostic criteria approach, stringent criteria are applied to determine if a case is diagnosed correctly. The reabstracted record method involves reabstracting records at the ascertainment source (i.e., manual medical record). The extent of agreement between the reabstracted records and the automated database is the assessment of validity. In the internal consistency approach the database is examined, usually through cross-tabulations, for illogical combinations of data in various fields. For example, men should not be identified as having received a prescription for an oral contraceptive.

EXTERNAL VALIDITY

A study is externally valid or generalizable if it can produce unbiased inferences regarding a target population beyond the subjects in the study or an external target population.[22] For example, the results of a study conducted using a health maintenance organization population of employed people might be generalizable to employed people in the U.S., but not generalizable to low-income individuals. The evaluation of generalizability usually involves much more subject-matter judgment than does internal validity.

The sociodemographic characteristics of Medicaid enrollees not only differ from the general U.S. population, but also vary from state to state due to differences in eligibility requirements.[33] Thus, results obtained with these databases may not be generalizable to non-Medicaid populations.[53] Results from studies of members of some managed care organizations may be skewed toward middle-class, employed populations and may underrepresent the surrounding community in the extremes (e.g., very old, poor, wealthy).

The geographic location of a particular data resource also may limit the generalizability of results if the sociodemographic profile or standards of medical practice vary considerably from an external target population. Assessment of the generalizability of a particular population served by an automated database involves, at a minimum, comparisons of distributions of age, sex, race/ethnicity, and marital status.

FOLLOW-UP

Individuals in a given database should be traceable through time to permit longitudinal follow-up. Maintaining the loss to follow-up as low as possible and obtaining information on those not participating are important for high-quality research.

As noted by Cook and Ware, there are statistical benefits to lengthy follow-up.[54] Some populations represented in automated databases are fairly stable. For example, GHC membership turnover is estimated to be approximately 15 percent per year, but after two years of enrollment, turnover drops to 5 percent or less.[55] In contrast, the Tennessee and Michigan Medicaid populations experience a one-year turnover of over 20 percent and a two-year turnover of about 40 percent, with follow-up losses greatest in children and young adults.[33] Two strategies for dealing with people lost to follow-up are restriction of subjects to those having a specified minimum period of follow-up, or using person-time at risk analytic approaches (e.g., Cox regression).

Summary

The growth of interest in the use of large automated databases for postmarketing drug surveillance makes data quality and validity an appropriate topic of consideration. The development of new data resources for etiologic studies should be accompanied by methodologic assessments of the quality of the databases. The types of evaluations suggested here and elsewhere could go a long way in documenting the quality of automated linked databases.[39,44,56] In doing so, record linkage of automated databases can be used more confidently in studies of the effects of marketed drugs.

References

1. Jick H, Madsen S, Nudelman PM, Perera DR, Stergachis A. Postmarketing follow-up at Group Health Cooperative of Puget Sound. *Pharmacotherapy* 1984;4:99-100.

2. Friedman GD, Collen MF, Harris LE, et al. Experience in monitoring drug reactions in outpatients: the Kaiser-Permanente Drug Monitoring System. *JAMA* 1971;217:567.

3. Ray WA, Griffin MR. The use of Medicaid data for pharmacoepidemiology. *Am J Epidemiol* 1989;129:837-49.

4. Strom BL, Carson JL, Morse ML, et al. The Computerized On-Line Medicaid Pharmaceutical Analysis and Surveillance System: a new resource for postmarketing drug surveillance. *Clin Pharmacol Ther* 1985;38:359-64.

5. Avorn J, Everitt DE, Bright RA, Gurwitz J, Chown M. AIDS-related diagnoses and drug use among AZT users in New Jersey Medicaid (abstract). *J Clin Res Drug Dev* 1989;3:203.

6. Resseguie LJ, Hick JF, Bruen JA, et al. Congenital malformations among offspring exposed in utero to progestins, Olmsted County, Minnesota, 1936-1974. *Fertil Steril* 1985;43:514-9.

7. Guess HA, West R, Strand LM, et al. Fatal upper gastrointestinal hemorrhage of perforation among users and nonusers of nonsteroidal anti-inflammatory drugs in Saskatchewan, Canada, 1983. *J Clin Epidemiol* 1988;41:35-45.

8. Crombie IK, Brown SV, Hamley JG. Postmarketing drug surveillance by record linkage in Tayside. *J Epidemiol Commun Health* 1984;38:226-31.

9. Bortnichak EA. Coexistence of specialized and multipurpose databases. *J Clin Res Drug Dev* 1989;3:167-9.

10. Weiss NS. Complementary role of specialized and multipurpose databases in assessing the safety of prescription drugs. *J Clin Res Drug Dev* 1989;3:185-90.

11. Shapiro S. The role of automated record linkage in the postmarketing surveillance of drug safety: a critique. *Clin Pharmacol Ther* 1989;46:371-86.

12. Faich GA, Stadel BV. The future of automated record linkage for postmarketing drug surveillance: a response to Shapiro. *Clin Pharmacol Ther* 1989;46:387-8.

13. Strom BL, Carson JL. Automated data bases used for pharmacoepidemiology research. *Clin Pharmacol Ther* 1989;46:390-4.

14. Jick H, Walker AM. Uninformed criticism of automated record linkage (letter). *Clin Pharmacol Ther* 1989;46:478.

15. Tilson HH. Pharmacoepidemiology: the lessons learned; the challenges ahead (letter). *Clin Pharmacol Ther* 1989;46:479.

16. Shapiro S. Automated record linkage: a response to the commentary and letters to the editor. *Clin Pharmacol Ther* 1989;46:395-8.

17. Roos LL, Nicol JP, Cageorge SM. Using administrative data for longitudinal research: comparisons with primary data collection. *J Chronic Dis* 1987;40:41-9.

18. Stergachis A. Group Health Cooperative. In: Strom BL, ed. Pharmacoepidemiology. New York: Churchill Livingstone, 1989.

19. Barnett GO. The application of computer-based medical record systems in ambulatory practice. *N Engl J Med* 1984;310:1643-50.

20. Carson JL, Strom BL, Soper KA, et al. The association of nonsteroidal anti-inflammatory drugs with upper gastrointestinal bleeding. *Arch Intern Med* 1987;147:1054.

21. Ray WA, Griffin MR, Schaffner W, et al. Psychotropic drug use and the risk of hip fracture. *N Engl J Med* 1987;316:363-9.

22. Last JM. A dictionary of epidemiology. New York: Oxford University Press, 1988.

23. Farr W. In: Lord Herbert, Tulloch A, Farr W. Report on army medical statistics. Parliamentary paper no 366. London, 1861.

24. Acheson ED. Record linkage in medicine. Proceedings of the International Symposium, Oxford, July 1967, Baltimore: Williams and Wilkins, 1968.

25. Royal College of General Practitioners. Oral contraceptives and health. London: Pitman Medical, 1974.

26. Griffin MR, Ray WA, Fought RL, et al. Monitoring the safety of childhood immunizations: methods of linking and augmenting computerized data bases for epidemiologic studies. *Am J Prev Med* 1988;4(suppl):5-13.

27. Jick H, Watkins RN, Hunter JR, et al. Replacement estrogens and endometrial cancer. *N Engl J Med* 1979;300:218-22.

28. Friedman GD, Ury HK. Initial screening for carcinogenicity of commonly used drugs. *J Natl Cancer Inst* 1980;65:723-33.

29. Kakar F, Weiss NS, Strite SA. Thiazide use and the risk of cholecystectomy in women. *Am J Epidemiol* 1986;124:428-33.

30. Strom BL, Carson JL, Morse ML, et al. Hypersensitivity reactions associated with zomepirac sodium and other nonsteroidal anti-inflammatory drugs. *Arthritis Rheum* 1987;30:1142-8.

31. Avorn J, Everitt DE, Weiss S. Increased antidepressant use in patients prescribed beta-blockers. *JAMA* 1986;255:357-60.

32. Baum C, Kennedy DL, Forbes MB, et al. Drug use and expenditures in 1982. *JAMA* 1985;253:382-6.

33. Ray WA, Griffin MR. Use of Medicaid for pharmacoepidemiology. *Am J Epidemiol* 1989;129:837-49.

34. Friedman GD. Kaiser Permanente Medical Care Program: Northern California and other regions. In: Strom BL, ed. Pharmacoepidemiology. New York: Churchill Livingstone, 1989:161-72.

35. Strand LM, West R. Health data bases in Saskatchewan. In: Strom BL, ed. Pharmacoepidemiology. New York: Churchill Livingstone, 1989:189-200.

36. Jick H, Walker AM, Watkins RN, et al. Oral contraceptives and breast cancer. *Am J Epidemiol* 1980;*112*:577-85.

37. Freeman LS. Variations in the level of reporting by hospitals to a regional cancer registry. *Br J Cancer* 1978;*37*:861-5.

38. Elmfeldt D, Wilhelmsen L, Tibblin G, et al. Registration of myocardial infarction in the city of Gotenborg, Sweden. *J Chronic Dis* 1975;*28*:173-86.

39. Goldberg J, Gelfand HM, Levy PS. Registry evaluation methods: a review and case study. *Epidemiol Rev* 1980;*2*:210-20.

40. Borden EK, Lee LG. A methodologic study of post-marketing drug evaluation using a pharmacy-based approach. *J Chronic Dis* 1982;*35*:803-16.

41. Saxen L, Klemmetti A, Haro AS. A matched-pair register for studies of selected congenital defects. *Am J Epidemiol* 1974;*100*:297-306.

42. Schork MA, Davis DK, Roi LD. Possible effects of case selection on analyses of institutional differences in a registry—illustrated by the National Burn Information Exchange. In: Cornell RG, Feller I, eds. EMS system evaluation utilizing a national burn registry. Final grant report HS 01906, Washington, DC: Department of Health, Education, and Welfare, 1979.

43. Smith ME, Newcombe HB. Automated follow-up facilities in Canada for monitoring delayed health effects. *Am J Public Health* 1980;*70*:1261-8.

44. Roos LL, Nicol JP. Building individual histories with registries: a case study. *Med Care* 1983;*21*:955-69.

45. Acheson ED. Medical record linkage. New York: Oxford University Press, 1967.

46. Stolly PD, Tonascia JA, Sartwell PE, et al. Agreement rates between oral contraceptive users and prescribers in relation to drug use histories. *Am J Epidemiol* 1978;*107*:226-35.

47. Paganini-Hill A, Ross RK. Reliability of recall of drug usage and other health-related information. *Am J Epidemiol* 1982;*116*:114-22.

48. Tilley BC, Barnes AB, Bergstralh E, et al. A comparison of pregnancy recall and medical records: implications for retrospective studies. *Am J Epidemiol* 1985;*121*:269-81.

49. Sorlie PD, Gold EB. The effect of physician terminology preference on coronary heart disease mortality: an artifact uncovered by the 9th revision ICD. *Am J Public Health* 1987;*77*:148-52.

50. Burnum JF. The misinformation era: the fall of the medical record. *Ann Intern Med* 1989;*110*:482-4.

51. Institute of Medicine. Reliability of Medicare hospital discharge records. Washington, DC: National Academy of Sciences, 1977.

52. Lloyd SS, Rissing JP. Physician and coding errors in patient records. *JAMA* 1985;*254*:1330-6.

53. Carson JL, Strom BL, Morse ML. Medicaid data bases. In: Strom BL, ed. Pharmacoepidemiology. New York: Churchill Livingstone, 1989:173-88.

54. Cook NR, Ware JH. Design and analysis methods for longitudinal research. *Ann Rev Public Health* 1983;*4*:1-23.

55. Thompson RS, Michnich ME, Friedlander L, et al. Effectiveness of smoking cessation interventions integrated into primary care practice. *Med Care* 1988;*26*:62-76.

56. Strom BL, Carson JL. Use of automated databases for pharmacoepidemiology research. *Epidemiol Rev* (in press).

III The Application

Meta-Analysis of the Pharmacotherapy Literature

Thomas R. Einarson

Abstract

Meta-analysis is a statistical approach to the aggregation of independent research studies. Its contribution is the creation of new knowledge synthesized from existing studies. This chapter is intended as an introduction to meta-analysis for health practitioners and students. It provides a stepwise approach to planning and conducting meta-analyses by using two examples, one on fetal abnormalities and Bendectin, and the second on the impact of pharmacy services on appropriateness of drug therapy.

The literature explosion has resulted in a massive amount of information that must be analyzed and summarized in order to be useful to practitioners and their patients. Because drug information lies within the domain of pharmacy, it is the responsibility of the pharmacist to evaluate and summarize the literature for use in patient care. It therefore behooves all pharmacists, particularly those specializing in drug information, to be familiar with and utilize the various techniques of literature analysis. Conflicting results often are produced in different studies of the same topic.[1] Such differences in research outcomes need to be reconciled in order to provide quality patient care. Resolving such conflict traditionally has been done through narrative review. However, that method has many limitations [2-4] and probably has outlived its usefulness.[5] Quantitative methods of integration of research results have been used for many years, but only recently have received a great deal of attention.[6] The quantitative approach to the integration of independent research results has been termed "meta-analysis" by Glass.[3]

Definition

Leviton and Cook defined meta-analysis as "any systematic method that uses statistical analyses for combining data from independent studies to obtain a numerical estimate of the overall effect of a particular procedure or variable on a defined outcome."[7] Sacks et al. described it as a discipline that "critically reviews and statistically combines results of previous research."[8] Glass introduced the term to describe quantitative aggregation of results.[3] In this case, "meta" refers to the secondary analysis of findings since the data are derived from previously published (if not published, completed) research.

It should be noted that meta-analysis is not a single method, but an approach to summarizing findings. It is an umbrella term encompassing a great variety of methods and techniques. What these methods have in common is that they are thorough, systematic, and quantitative (i.e., produce a single overall statistic to summarize findings).

At present, meta-analysis is the preferred approach to integration of results from different studies because it incorporates all of the strengths of traditional reviews and further provides (relatively) unbiased quantitative summary estimates. Einarson et al. recommended that it become the standard approach for drug reviews.[9]

Meta-analysis is a legitimate form of research with its own methodology. Its contribution is the creation of new knowledge synthesized from existing studies. Lee has suggested that it be considered as an alternative form of research experience for nurses.[10] This suggestion is equally valid for pharmacy.

Purpose of Meta-Analysis

Sacks et al. listed four major purposes of meta-analysis of randomized controlled trials: (1) to increase power for primary endpoints and for subgroups (i.e., where sample sizes in original studies were too small to demonstrate statistical significance), (2) to resolve uncertainty when reports disagree, (3) to improve estimates of effect size, and (4) to answer questions not posed in the original trials.[8]

Other meta-analyses may be concerned with planning new studies, combining results from multicenter trials, or comparing the effectiveness of different types of services or programs. Thus, this approach to aggregation of findings can be a very useful tool to clinical practitioners, service managers, researchers, and educators.

Meta-Analysis and Drug Studies

There are two different types of drug studies: clinical (i.e., randomized controlled trials) and epidemiologic. The former are performed to determine the effectiveness of a drug or to compare drugs on the basis of effectiveness (or, occasionally, unintended drug effects [UDEs]). To be used in a meta-analysis, there must be a treatment group and a comparison group. The comparison group normally receives placebo or standard therapy, depending on the nature of the problem being treated. Patients occasionally may serve as their own controls, with outcomes compared before and after the patient has been given the drug.

Epidemiologic studies seek to quantify the relationship between a drug and a given outcome (beneficial or adverse) or to compare two drugs or events with respect to a given outcome. The two main types of epidemiologic studies are cohort and case control. Cohort studies begin with a group of patients exposed to a drug and a comparison group who are not exposed to the drug, and then compare outcome rates. Case control studies begin with a group of patients having the outcome of interest (e.g., UDE) and a group of patients who do not have the outcome (e.g., normals). Records then are examined to determine how many of each group had been exposed to the drug, and the rates are compared. Figure 1 presents a graphic presentation of a 2×2 table for epidemiologic studies.

Comparisons of the effectiveness of services or programs, such as that of Ried et al.,[11] generally have used an approach similar to that of randomized controlled trials. Usually, a comparison is made either of evaluations before and after implementation of an intervention, or of serviced versus nonserviced patient groups.

Whatever the method used, meta-analysis requires results from both a treatment and comparison group. Such studies form the raw data with which one can produce a statistical summation.

Figure 1 2×2 Table for Epidemiologic Studies		OUTCOME		
	FACTOR STATUS	DISEASE	NO DISEASE	TOTAL
	Exposure	A	B	n_1
	No exposure	C	D	n_0
	Total	m_1	m_0	N

A Brief Overview

Meta-analysis is a statistical approach to the integration and summarization of results from independent studies. It is systematic, thorough, objective, and quantitative. A variety of analytical methods can be used, including determination of effect sizes and combination of probabilities. Excellent discussions of statistical methods have been presented by Rosenthal[6] and Hedges and Olkin.[12]

Regardless of the method employed, all meta-analyses involve three major phases—the three "Ps": preparation, performance, and presentation. This sequence is the same as for any other type of research. The project must be planned in advance, then systematically carried out, followed by the reporting of results.

Phase I: Preparation

This is the planning phase of the project. During this phase, the research design is defined explicitly. It should be noted that the planning takes place *before* any data are collected. It is a serious mistake to collect studies first, and then try to analyze. Such a method introduces bias that makes interpretation of results difficult and may be misleading.

The preparation phase involves four stages: (1) statement of purpose, (2) data definition, (3) data retrieval procedure, and (4) statistical analysis. The first two steps comprise a series of definitions that clarify the research issues, and the last two steps describe the analytical procedures to be used. The aim is to answer the research question by finding all possible studies, then methodically analyzing and combining them. Adhering to an established critical protocol serves to enhance the validity of the results.

Table 1 presents a detailed listing of the steps involved in setting up the research protocol, which are discussed below. Examples are provided to illustrate meta-analyses for two different types of pharmacotherapy-related studies.

A STEPWISE APPROACH TO PLANNING META-ANALYSES

This section discusses each of the steps involved in defining the protocol for a meta-analysis.Two examples are used to illustrate these steps. The first illustrates a procedure for meta-analysis of epidemiologic studies and has been published elsewhere.[2] Results for this example are labeled "Study A." The second example illustrates a procedure for clinical studies or analyses of the impact of pharmacy services. It represents new information and is a genuine meta-analysis. Results for that example are labeled "Study B."

Step 1. Statement of Purpose: The Research Question

Every research project is undertaken to address a specific problem. It is absolutely essential that the purpose of a meta-analysis be stated explicitly and unambiguously. Without an explicit statement, it is impossible to judge whether the project accomplished its mission. Consequently, the results could be meaningless.

The statement of purpose must capture the essence of the project but does not need to include every detail. Subsequent sections define and delimit the problem by supplying operational definitions. Thus, the purpose may be stated in broad terms to allow the reader to understand what problem is being addressed.

EXAMPLE A: The purpose of Study A was to determine whether a relationship exists between maternal consumption of Bendectin during pregnancy and subsequent fetal abnormality.

EXAMPLE B: The purpose of Study B was to determine the impact of drug utilization review (DUR) programs in Canada on appropriateness of drug therapy. There is no reason that DUR studies from Canada would be any different

Table 1
Steps in Establishing the Protocol for a Meta-Analysis

Statement of purpose: the research question	Data analysis
Data definition	Analysis of individual studies
Defining acceptable studies	*Individual effect size*
Inclusion criteria	*Confidence interval or significance*
Exclusion criteria	Combinability of data
Defining acceptable patients	*Statistical analysis*
Inclusion criteria	*Graphical analysis*
Exclusion criteria	*Identification of moderator variables*
Defining acceptable diagnoses	Quality analysis of studies
Inclusion criteria	Summary statistics
Exclusion criteria	*Overall effect size*
Defining acceptable treatments	*Confidence interval or significance*
Inclusion criteria	Primary method
Exclusion criteria	Confirmatory method
Defining acceptable comparison groups	*Power considerations*
Inclusion criteria	Sample size
Exclusion criteria	Publication bias
Defining outcomes	Subgroup analyses
Inclusion criteria	*Study types*
Exclusion criteria	*Patient types*
Data extraction procedure	*Treatment levels*
Defining search procedure	*Other moderator variables*
Defining databases	**Interpretation of results**
Defining search terms	Analysis of accepted studies
Identification of acceptable articles	Analysis of rejected studies
Article retrieval	Support of studies
Blinding procedure	Other evidence
Judgment of acceptability	*Animal evidence*
Agreement of judges	*Incidental findings*
Data extraction procedure	Overall conclusions
Blinding procedure	Caveats
Data to be extracted	Implications of findings
Extractor agreement	Economic impact

from those from the U.S., Britain, or Australia, but there are differences in healthcare systems. All DUR articles from Canada had already been collected for another project; therefore, they were available and could easily be adapted as an example for this meta-analysis. In real life, studies from the U.S. and Canada would no doubt be combined, as purposes and procedures for DURs are the same and all Canadian PharmDs are trained in the U.S.

Step 2. Data Definition

As stated above, data definition occurs *before* data collection. The purpose of this section is to define variables in order to clarify the nature of data to be collected and analyzed. It provides operational definitions for the variables under study. These variables include the independent and dependent variables, the sample of studies to be analyzed, and the procedure for finding, verifying, and analyzing the studies.

Like any other form of research, we must carefully and completely define the independent and dependent variables (or their equivalents). Independent variables include the drugs, forms, doses, etc., under study. Dependent variables are outcomes that are measured, such as decreases in blood pressure, incidences of UDEs, or success rates.

It is essential to identify factors related to the outcome of interest so that only pertinent variables are included in the analysis. Three options are available when mixed results are included in a report: (1) eliminate studies that do not conform to your preestablished protocol, (2) control for factors that influence outcomes, or (3) extract data that conform. For example, if the interest is in pediatric use of a drug and a study dealing with a mixture of children and adults was found, the researcher could eliminate the study as nonconforming, stratify results by age or control for age statistically, or isolate and extract only cases that apply to the research at hand. If data can be extracted, then they should be used.

Defining Acceptable Studies

In this section, the researcher must define the aspects of the study that would be acceptable, such as its research design type, literary presentation, location, and language. As mentioned above, epidemiologic studies may be case control or cohort types and may be done either prospectively or retrospectively. Some researchers will accept all types, but some may prefer to include only data gathered prospectively, which they consider less biased. Intervention studies may be single-blind, double-blind, or open. Patients may or may not be randomized between treatment and control groups. For example, Sacks et al. analyzed the quality of meta-analyses of randomized controlled trials.[8] The researcher must decide beforehand which of the available types of research designs are acceptable for meta-analysis.

Literary presentation refers to the type of articles and publications accepted. Consideration must be given to the medium (e.g., Will studies published in books be combined with those from journals?), review status (Are nonreviewed articles equivalent to peer-reviewed articles?), prestige of the publication (Are equal weights given to articles in *New England Journal of Medicine*, which has a panel of biostatisticians on staff, and *Drug Store News*?), article type (Are letters to the editor as valid as full articles if they contain sufficient data for analysis?), and time of publication (Is it valid to combine articles published in 1960 with those from 1990?).

Another publication consideration is the language in which the original report is published. Some foreign language journals publish abstracts in English. If the abstract contains adequate information, the data may be usable. However, if a question should arise, there could be a problem with interpretation. Unless you are proficient in other languages and can guarantee a perfect scientific translation, it is preferable to limit your search to studies published in English.

The location of the research study may be important. The analyst must decide in what institutions conditions are sufficiently similar to provide comparable results. For example, differing types of hospitals may affect the results, and other times the setting may be irrelevant. Teaching hospitals may differ from general, long-term care, specialty hospitals, clinics, and community or outpatient practice. The country in which the research is done also may have an impact on the results. Pharmacy, nursing, or medical practice may differ in other countries, which could affect interpretation of results. However, effectiveness of a drug should not vary unless there are genetic differences to consider, such as differing rates of rapid acetylators in Oriental countries.

Inclusion Criteria

Inclusion criteria should list all the requirements for entry into the analysis. All studies should be primary research reports. Subsequent sections below help pinpoint those that eventually will form the source of the data to be analyzed.

STUDY A: This study accepted all research studies published in English that examined the relationship between first-trimester Bendectin administration in humans and the presence of malformations in the children. Both case-control and cohort studies were accepted, as were prospective and retrospective studies.

STUDY B: This study accepted all Canadian drug utilization reviews published in English that included an educational intervention providing feedback and/or information directly to the prescriber. Studies could be prospective or retrospective and could be in any institution with a full-time pharmacist on staff.

Exclusion criteria

Exclusion criteria should not repeat the inclusion criteria (only negative). They should present reasons for studies that met inclusion criteria to be disqualified. The most common criterion is failure to provide adequate data or data that are meaningful to the study.

They may define variables more precisely than the inclusion criteria. For example, if the inclusion criteria accepted randomized controlled trials of triazolam in geriatric patients, exclusion criteria could eliminate patients younger than 70 years of age or those over 90. Thus, "geriatric" has been defined more precisely for the purposes of that particular analysis.

Exclusion criteria also specify confounding variables and how they must be controlled (see the example under Study A below).

STUDY A: Excluded were studies that did not match or control for confounding factors, including maternal age, parity, diet, smoking, alcohol consumption, concurrent drug use (both prescription and nonprescription), drug abuse, or socioeconomic status, all of which have been shown to be related to adverse fetal outcomes.

STUDY B: Excluded were studies where the intervention was not a planned program, such as enactment of new legislation or policy change.

Defining Acceptable Patients

When comparing drug studies, there is usually an acceptable range allowable for patients. For example, studies on geriatric patients may include persons over the age of 60, 65, or even 70. Sometimes, the "old old" (i.e., >80, or even >90) are excluded because of pharmacologic differences in drug effect and disposition. Similar problems occur with pediatrics, where it may or may not be permissible to combine results from studies using different ranges of age.

Age is but one consideration. Any patient characteristic or factor that could cause a systematic difference in results needs to be identified. Methods for dealing with systematic differences (e.g., blocking) must be addressed, or such studies may have to be excluded from the analysis. It is therefore necessary for the meta-analyst to decide a priori what types of patients are acceptable for each particular research.

Inclusion criteria

STUDY A: All adult women aged 18–40 were accepted.

STUDY B: This study accepted DURs for any age of patient.

Exclusion criteria

STUDY A: Excluded were women taking drugs known to have a risk for malformation, such as anticonvulsants. Also excluded were women who had conditions that could cause fetal problems, such as uncontrolled epilepsy.

STUDY B: Excluded were patients in critical care units.

Defining Acceptable Diagnoses

It is necessary to define precisely the diagnosis. For example, when studying hypertensive patients, the researcher must define what is meant by hypertension (e.g., diastolic >90, or 100?) and how diagnosis will be determined. It is preferable to have objective measurements to verify the diagnosis (e.g., supine diastolic blood pressure >90 mm Hg).

Inclusion criteria

STUDY A: For this study, pregnancy was the diagnosis, which is rather straightforward. However, there could be a difference between first, second, or later pregnancies. If so, this must be specified. Twins or multiple births also were accepted.

STUDY B: For this study, any medical diagnosis made by a physician was considered acceptable if it involved drug therapy.

Exclusion criteria

STUDY A: Excluded were women who previously had been entered into the study. Note that epidemiologic studies often carry on for years; hence, a woman could reenter several times, if allowed.

STUDY B: Excluded were diagnoses of drug abuse or dependence, as they are special cases in which appropriateness cannot be precisely defined.

Defining Acceptable Treatments

The researcher must define the drug used and specify equivalent forms (e.g., tablets, capsules, injectables, suppositories) or products (e.g., brands, generics) that would be accepted as equivalents. The dose and route of administration should be specified (if pertinent) as well as acceptable regimens. If different doses, regimens, and so on, alter results, data may have to be stratified and analyzed separately.

In any primary study, there is a need to verify exposure to the drug, especially in epidemiologic studies or unsupervised settings. There must be a guarantee of exposure to the treatment and patient compliance must be verified.

Inclusion criteria

STUDY A: The study accepted all mother/child pairs with ingestion/exposure in utero to any amount of Bendectin during the first trimester. Studies that dealt with first-trimester exposure plus other exposures also were included. Bendectin originally was formulated with three ingredients (doxylamine, dicyclomine, and pyridoxine). However, the antinauseant effect was due to the pyridoxine and in 1976, the antispasmodic dicyclomine was removed. Thus, studies were considered acceptable if they reported on either the combination of doxylamine and pyridoxine or doxylamine, dicyclomine, and pyridoxine. Any brand was accepted (e.g., Bendectin, Diclectin, Lenotan, Debendox).

STUDY B: Any drug could serve as the focus of a utilization review for this analysis, providing criteria for appropriateness were established and accepted by the institution.

Exclusion criteria

STUDY A: Study A excluded papers that examined first-trimester exposure, but combined the data with nonfirst-trimester exposure only. That is, studies were excluded if first-trimester exposure data could not be extracted.

STUDY B: Not applicable.

Defining Acceptable Comparison Groups

Most research studies compare a treated group of subjects with a second group. Persons in the second group may receive placebo, standard therapy, or another comparable drug. Other studies may use historical controls, population comparisons, or each subject may serve as his own control (i.e., a pre- and posttest). A valid meta-analysis requires that the comparison groups be either identical or very similar. Otherwise, differences could be due to the differences in comparison groups and not due to the drug under investigation. The analyst must decide what constitutes acceptable comparisons. If different types are used, there is the option of performing sub-analyses to verify comparability.

Inclusion criteria

STUDY A: Study A accepted only patients who were not exposed to Bendectin during pregnancy. Other antinauseants could be used, providing they did not have a known association with malformations.

STUDY B: Study B accepted studies that compared data before and after implementation of a DUR in the same location.

Exclusion criteria

STUDY A: Not applicable.

STUDY B: Studies were excluded if the baseline data for comparison were more than one year old.

Defining Outcomes

For each analysis, the acceptable outcomes must be specified. It is not always necessary to have exactly the same method of measuring the outcome or even the same measurement units, as long as the different methods evaluate the same construct. It is important that measurements be objective and replicable.

Where there are categorical outcomes, each must be defined explicitly. For example, categorical outcomes for an antibiotic may be either "cured" or "not cured." Acceptable definitions must be presented for each category.

Inclusion criteria

STUDY A: For Study A, there were two possible outcomes: malformed and normal infants. Malformed included the presence of one or more major malformations or more than one minor malformation as defined by Heinonen et al.[13] Normals were defined as infants not having such malformations.

STUDY B: Appropriateness had to be defined for the drug in terms of at least one of the following parameters: indication or administration (dose, duration, route, regimen). Such appropriateness must have been defined for the study and approved for use in the institution.

Exclusion criteria

STUDY A: This study excluded case control comparisons between different types of malformations.

STUDY B: Studies that dealt only with cost were excluded.

Step 3. Data Extraction Procedure

The protocol should specify all procedures involved in data extraction, including the databases to be used, search words employed, and methods of extraction. If more than one person is involved, the tasks of each person should be specified, as well as methods for assuring inter-judge agreement.

Defining the Search Procedure

A very important requisite for meta-analysis is a thorough literature review. Glass advocates an exhaustive search through published and unpublished sources until all possible articles have been found.[3,14] The reason is that there may be some articles with differing points of view or different results published in different types of journals. It is essential that all points of view be included and all possible articles obtained.

Sources included for a literature search are computerized and printed abstracting services such as MEDLINE, *Index Medicus*, *Current Contents*, and *International Pharmaceutical Abstracts*. Dissertations and theses are available from university libraries either bound as books or on microfiche and may be located through "Dissertation Abstracts," a computerized service. Current textbooks and handbooks are often sources of original data as well as summaries of studies. Finally, the references of all retrieved articles should be investigated for further information. Additional (unpublished) data may be procured from experts in the field.

Unpublished manuscripts and theses are important. Despite being of high research quality, they may not have been published because they represented unpopular topics, or the results may have disagreed with those of others. Researchers often intend to publish material from their theses, but never find the time. Consequently, "Dissertation Abstracts" may be the only place to locate many studies.

Another overlooked source of information is the poster or podium session of scientific meetings. Abstracts often are published, such as for the annual meetings of the American Society of Hospital Pharmacists, the American College of Clinical Pharmacy, or the American Association of Colleges of Pharmacy. Finally, many pharmacy residents or Pharm.D. students perform research projects as part of their program. Those reports often are abstracted or may be located in the libraries of teaching hospitals. As stated above, it is essential that all possible articles be located, so that bias is reduced.

Defining Databases

STUDY A: In this study, the computerized database of "Bibliographic Retrieval Services" was searched using key words (see below). All references from abstracted papers and case reports were investigated. Standard textbooks containing summaries of teratogenicity data, such as those by Schardein,[15] Shepard,[16] and Briggs et al.[17] were consulted for further undetected references.

STUDY B: This study used a computerized MEDLINE search and *International Pharmaceutical Abstracts* to locate articles. All references from retrieved articles were investigated, as was the book by Carruthers et al.[18] In addition, the index edition of the *Canadian Journal of Hospital Pharmacy* was searched from 1970 to date, as were pharmacy residency projects from the University of Toronto Pharmacy Library and the abstracts of all Canadian residency projects published annually by the Upjohn Company.

Defining Search Terms

Search words are used when trying to locate articles in databases, whether manual or computerized. It is important to search for both independent (i.e., name of drug or service) and dependent (i.e., outcome) variables. Search words should include pertinent key words that are listed in *Index Medicus*. If a drug is being investigated, all tradenames and alternative generics should be used. Generic names may differ in different countries. For example, what most of the world calls salbutamol is referred to as albuterol in the U.S., and what is meperidine in the U.S. and Canada is called pethidine in Britain. Alternative names may be located in *Martindale's Extra Pharmacopoeia* or from drug information centers. Searches may be limited if the alternative names are not used.

STUDY A: Search words used included the generic names doxylamine and dicyclomine and the tradenames Bendectin, Debendox, Lenotan, and Diclectin. Also included were the terms antinauseant, birth defect, fetal abnormality, teratogenicity, malformation, and adverse outcome.

STUDY B: Search words included drug utilization review and DUR.

Identification of Acceptable Articles

The procedure should be specified here. For example, all articles may be located in the library and photocopied by a research assistant. If more than one person performs the task, it is essential that they all follow the same procedure.

Article Retrieval

STUDY A: All articles were photocopied by an assistant and assembled for analysis. Selection was done by two blinded data extractors (see below).

STUDY B: All articles were photocopied by the researcher, which possibly introduced bias at this step.

Blinding Procedure

Blinding is done to remove bias due to the perceived importance or prestige of the journal in which the report appeared, of the authors, or of sponsoring agencies. As a result, all identifying marks should be removed and articles judged solely on their own merit. Sacks et al. recommend that articles be judged on their methods—not the results. They suggest copying only the methods section and evaluating suitability based on methods only.[8] Blinding should be done by a person not involved in data analysis in any other way.

STUDY A: Methods sections were photocopied by a third person and two raters evaluated the methods based on inclusion and exclusion criteria recorded on a sheet of paper. The two judges evaluated independently.

STUDY B: Blinding was not done in this study, which imposes a further limitation on interpretation of the results.

Judgment of Acceptability

As stated above, acceptability should be based on explicit criteria that are replicable. Other researchers must be able to follow the method and arrive at similar conclusions.

Agreement of Judges

If more than one person evaluates the articles, there should be a test to ensure inter-judge agreement. It is essential that different people evaluate in the same fashion, or the results could vary substantially. Fleiss presents statistical methods for calculating kappa, the coefficient of agreement for categorical data.[19] Rosenthal discusses the calculation of effective reliability for >1 judge when dealing with continuous data (i.e., data that are measured at interval or ratio level).[6]

STUDY A: In this study, there was agreement on all cases, except one. That case involved animals, and therefore was excluded after the judges discussed the case. The result was complete agreement on case selection. (Note: another meta-analyst independently performed the same analysis and arrived at an identical list of studies, thus verifying our results).

STUDY B: Not applicable.

Table 2[13,20-35] lists the studies that were included in the analysis of Study A and Table 3 lists those rejected.[36-43] Tables 4[44-47] and 5[48-59] provide comparable data for Study B.

Data Extraction Procedure

Data extraction refers to the numbers extracted from the individual studies being analyzed. Included should be the number of observations in each group, and summaries of the outcomes. If the outcome of interest is a categorical variable (e.g., improved/not improved, success/failure), then frequencies are required for each group. If the variable is continuous, such as blood pressure, then means and standard deviations for each group should be noted. Data describing the patients may be collected, if pertinent.

STUDY A: For this study, data were entered for each article into a separate 2×2 table. In each table, rows presented data for exposed and nonexposed infants and columns separated data on malformed infants from normals.

STUDY B: In this study, data were entered into 2×2 tables with before/after in rows and appropriate/inappropriate in columns.

Reference	Study Type	Data Collection	Malformation Described
13	CH	P	any major
20	CC	R	any major
21	CH	P	any major
22	CH	P*	any major
23	CH	P	severe
24	CH	P	1 major or ≥ 3 minor
25	CC	R	cardiac
26	CC	R	cardiac
27	CH	R	any major
28	CH	P	any major
29	CH	R	any major
30	CH	P	any major
31	CC	R*	cleft lip/palate
32	CC	R*	any major
33	CH	R*	any major
34	CH	R	any major
35	CH	R*	any major

Table 2
Studies of the Teratogenicity of Bendectin Meeting the Criteria for Meta-Analysis

*Matched control group
CC = case-control; CH = cohort; P = prospective; R = retrospective.

Reference	Reason for Rejection
36	Inadequate selection of groups and poor definition of treatment
37	Reported on dicyclomine only
38	Compared specific malformations with other malfor-mations
39	
40	
41	Bendectin not separated from other antinauseants
42	
43	Used animals only

Table 3
Studies of the Teratogenicity of Bendectin Rejected from the Meta-Analysis

Blinding Procedure

Similar to the procedure in acceptance of studies, data extraction may be done by photocopying the results sections and tables, and extracting data. This serves to reduce bias and to verify numbers.

Data to be Extracted

A list of data to be extracted should be prepared. In Study A and Study B, 2×2 tables were prepared for each study to facilitate extraction. The criteria for inclusion and exclusion were kept nearby to assist in selection or to clarify points of confusion.

Extractor Agreement

When discrepancies arise, extractors must reevaluate their findings. It is essential that data be extracted accurately; as a result, there must be agreement. In both Study A and B, two extractors compared data and rechecked any discrepancies. In the end, there was total agreement.

Table 6 lists the data for accepted papers in Study A and Table 7 for those in Study B.

Step 4. Data Analysis

Once studies have been retrieved and data extracted, the focus shifts to analysis. One must consider the combinability of studies, statistics for individual studies, overall summary statistics, confidence intervals, and subanalyses.

Table 4
Studies Included in
Meta-Analysis of
Drug Utilization
Review Studies

Reference	Year	Drug
44	1977	Antibiotics
45	1983	Cimetidine iv
46	1986	Cimetidine iv
47	1978	Hypnotics

Table 5
Studies Rejected
from Meta-Analysis
of Drug Utilization
Review Studies

Reference	Year	Reason for Rejection
48	1978	Inadequate data for analysis
49	1982	
50	1981	
51	1974	
52	1987	
53	1983	
54, 55	1978, 1982	Appropriateness not verified
56	1981	
57	1973	Cost only addressed
58	1983	Intervention incidental
59	1978	

Ref.	Exposure	Congenital Defect			Chi-Square	p
		Yes	**No**	**Total**		
13	yes	79	1090	1169	0.13	0.718
	no	3169	45944	49113		
	total	3248	47034	50282		
20	yes	44	78	122	2.67	0.102
	no	659	1634	2293		
	total	703	1712	2415		
21	yes	31	589	620	0.12	0.728
	no	1208	21149	22357		
	total	1239	21738	22977		
22	yes	18	856	874	0.00	1.000
	no	19	855	874		
	total	37	1711	1748		
23	yes	14	614	628	2.80	0.094
	no	343	9234	9577		
	total	357	9848	10205		
24	yes	31	344	375	0.45	0.503
	no	93	1222	1315		
	total	124	1566	1690		
25	yes	24	46	70	3.92	0.048
	no	366	1208	1574		
	total	390	1254	1644		
26	yes	52	121	173	0.13	0.716
	no	240	607	847		
	total	292	728	1020		
27	yes	2	1362	1364	0.00	0.957
	no	4	3886	3890		
	total	6	5248	5254		
28	yes	78	1607	1685	0.38	0.538
	no	245	5526	5771		
	total	323	7133	7456		
29	yes	24	2231	2255	0.20	0.652
	no	56	4526	4582		
	total	80	6757	6837		
30	yes	2	70	72	0.05	0.815
	no	18	571	589		
	total	20	641	661		
31	yes	12	9	21	4.91	0.027
	no	184	398	582		
	total	196	407	603		
32	yes	76	88	164	0.82	0.365
	no	760	748	1508		
	total	836	836	1672		
33	yes	6	1186	1192	2.52	0.113
	no	70	6671	6741		
	total	76	7857	7933		
34	yes	28	1685	1713	0.07	0.793
	no	31	1682	1713		
	total	59	3367	3426		
35	yes	11	2207	2218	2.55	0.110
	no	21	2197	2218		
	total	32	4404	4436		
TOTAL	yes	532	14183	14715	184.79	
	no	7486	108058	115544		
	total	8018	122241	130259		

Table 6

Results of Studies Comparing Outcomes of Fetuses Exposed to Bendectin

There are many different ways to analyze data. Rosenthal[60,61] and Hedges and Olkin[12] have presented several statistical methods for combining results from independent studies. It should be noted that all methods are estimates or approximations based on various assumptions; therefore, there will be variations in the results depending on the methods used. Perhaps the best approach is to use two methods and compare the results.

Analysis of Individual Studies

In order to prepare studies for analysis, a table should be constructed listing all accepted studies. Individual statistics should be calculated for each study, including the statistical test, test value, significance, sample size, and effect size.

Individual Effect Size

For epidemiologic studies, the odds ratio is commonly used to express the risk of occurrence of a given outcome following exposure to a drug. Mathematically, it may be stated as:

$$OR = AD/BC \qquad \text{Eq. 1}$$

where A, B, C, and D are defined in Figure 1. The odds ratio is an estimate of the relative risk of an outcome when exposed to a drug. An odds ratio of unity (i.e., 1) means that the risks for exposed and nonexposed people are identical. Ratios higher than unity imply a positive association; ratios less than unity imply a negative association. Thus, an odds ratio of 2 means a person is twice as likely to experience the outcome than is a person not exposed.

For other studies, the common outcome is called an effect size. There are many different effect sizes that can be used, including Cohen's *d*, Hedges's *g*, and Glass's Δ. Another possibility is the correlation coefficient *r*, which is preferred by Rosenthal.[6] All of these coefficients are related mathematically, and all have advantages and disadvantages.

For this analysis, Cohen's *d* will be used.[62] This coefficient may be considered similar to a Student's *t* statistic except that the effect of the sample size has been removed. It should be noted that any difference between groups may be made statistically significant merely by increasing the sample size. The effect size remains constant for all sample sizes. Mathematically, it is:

$$d = 2t/\sqrt{df} \qquad \text{Eq. 2}$$

Table 7 Summary of Effect of Canadian DUR Intervention Studies on Drug Appropriateness

Reference	Before	After	χ^2	p	d	z
44	83/219	56/240	10.83	0.001	0.31	3.29
45	47/169	34/169	2.34	0.126	0.17	1.53
46	31/85	43/162	2.17	0.141	0.19	1.47
47	34/50	22/50	4.91	0.027	0.45	2.22

$d = 2t/\sqrt{df}$	**Table 8**
$d = [4\chi^2/(N-\chi^2)]^{1/2}$	Formulas for Conversion
$d = 2r/\sqrt{(1-r^2)}$	of Common Statistics to Cohen's d

Note that d represents the total difference between groups (i.e., one-tailed), whereas most t-tests are two-tailed. Table 8 presents formulas for converting various statistics to Cohen's d.

The problem with d is that there is no statistical test to qualify its magnitude. Cohen has suggested that 0.2 be considered small, 0.5 as medium, and 0.8 as large.[62] However, these descriptors are arbitrary and may not signify clinical significance. Rosenthal has shown that an effect size < 0.1 may be considered very significant clinically.[6]

As well as having a summary statistic, all individual studies should be tested for significance. Normally, such tests are reported in the original publications. However, they may not always present the exact data required for the meta-analysis. Because data will be needed for further analysis, such tests should be done.

STUDY A: This study will use the odds ratio to summarize the risk of teratogenicity from exposure to Bendectin. A ratio statistically >1 indicates a positive association and <1 indicates no association. Table 6 presents the data for all of the studies accepted for Study A.

STUDY B: This study will use Cohen's d to summarize the study effects. The significance of individual studies will be tested using chi-square analyses for 2×2 tables. Table 7 lists data for Study B.

Confidence Interval or Significance

Statistical significance of individual tests should be reported. Alternatively, the corresponding confidence interval should be reported (or both). The latter often are preferred because they provide a better estimate of the true value than do tests of significance.

STUDY A: Individual significance will be calculated for each study using the Mantel-Haenszel chi-square.[63] Along with the odds ratio, the 95 percent confidence interval will be calculated.[64] The Mantel-Haenszel chi-square is:

$$\chi^2 = \frac{(N-1)[\,|\,AD-BC\,|\,-N/2]^2}{n_1 \cdot n_0 \cdot m_1 \cdot m_0} \qquad \text{Eq. 3}$$

where N is the total number of subjects in the individual study and A, B, C, D, m, and n are defined in Figure 1.

STUDY B: Each 2×2 table will be analyzed using chi-square, and Cohen's d will be calculated from that result for each study.

Combinability of Data

Glass has espoused the theory that all studies on a given topic should be included in a meta-analysis, regardless of flaws (except grossly misleading studies), because there is a kernel of truth in every study.[3,14] This position is tantamount to stating that all of the variation between studies may be considered to be random error that cancels out in the long run. That position has not been supported by all analysts.

The other extreme, supported by many authors, is that the quality of all articles should be scrutinized and only the very best accepted for analysis. They contend that differences are due mostly to systematic error and will not cancel out, causing erroneous conclusions when varying studies are aggregated.

Perhaps the real truth lies somewhere in between. Rosenthal recommends testing studies for homogeneity of effect using statistical tests. If there is a difference, he suggests searching for moderator variables that could be responsible for systematic differences. Otherwise, combined results could be erroneous. He presents several formulas that may be used, depending on the data.[6]

Statistical Analysis

Breslow and Day presented a chi-square formula for analyzing homogeneity of epidemiologic studies. The formula is as follows:[64]

$$\chi^2 = \sum (w \bullet \ln^2 OR) - [\sum (w \bullet \ln OR)]^2 / \sum w \qquad \text{Eq. 4}$$

where OR is the odds ratio from an individual study and w is the weight:

$$w = [1/A + 1/B + 1/C + 1/D]^{-1} \qquad \text{Eq. 5}$$

This is a chi-square test with $k-1$ degrees of freedom, k being the number of individual studies analyzed.

Rosenthal presents methods for detecting heterogeneity of other study types; these methods are also chi-square tests.[6]

STUDY A: This study used the formula of Breslow and Day to detect heterogeneity.[64] The resultant chi-square was 25.19, df=16, and p=0.067, indicating no significant differences among studies.

STUDY B: This study used the method of Rosenthal and Rubin. It is a chi-square method having $k-1$ degrees of freedom and has the formula:[61]

$$\chi^2 = \sum w(d-\bar{d})^2 \qquad \text{Eq. 6}$$

where d is the effect size from each study, $\bar{d}$ is the average of all effect sizes, and w is the weight of each study. The weight is the reciprocal of the estimated variance of each d and may be approximated by the formula:

$$w = 2N/(8 + d^2) \qquad \text{Eq. 7}$$

This analysis produced a chi-square of 2.32 (df=3, p=0.956). Therefore, the studies were not heterogeneous.

Graphical Analysis

L'Abbé et al. recommended creating a graphical display to detect heterogeneity and ensure combinability.[65] Outcomes of control and treatment groups are plotted on the X and Y axes of a graph, respectively. A regression line can be calculated and tests done to identify outliers.

STUDY A: Figure 2 presents the data display for this study. Two points were identified as outliers. However, no systematic difference with other studies could be found and, since the statistical test was not significant, the decision was made to include both studies in the final analysis.

STUDY B: Due to the small number of studies and the lack of significance of statistical testing, a graph was not prepared for these data.

Identification of Moderator Variables

If heterogeneity is found on either statistical or graphical tests, a search should be made for moderator variables. Ried et al. detected such a problem and provided an analysis and discussion of how they dealt with the situation.[11]

Quality Analysis of Studies

Chalmers et al. developed a method for assessing the quality of clinical trials based on aspects of research design. Such a method may be used to assess the quality of studies and then weight results accordingly.[66] Several authors advocate such a procedure. However, quality was not assessed in the two analyses being presented here.

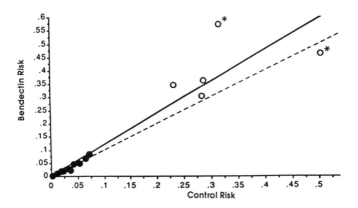

Figure 2
Plot of Bendectin Risk
Versus Control Risk
for Congenital
Anomaly
Reported[13,20-35]

Cohort studies are represented by solid circles and the case-control studies by open circles. The regressed line (solid) has an intercept of 0.002 and a slope of 1.184 which was not significantly different from unity ($t = 1.69$, $df = 16$, $p = 0.111$). The dotted line has a slope of 1 representing a relative risk of 1 for Bendectin, and the asterisks denote two studies that were identified as outliers.

Summary Statistics

The summary statistic provides the overall effect of all studies combined. This statistic answers the research question posed; in other words, this number is the reason for the meta-analysis. This is perhaps one of the easiest steps in the analysis since all of the numbers have been extracted and analyzed.

Overall Effect Size

The Mantel-Haenszel summary odds ratio (OR_s) is used widely in epidemiology. It weights each study according to sample size and provides a reasonable estimation of the overall risk. The formula is:

$$OR_s = (\Sigma\, AD/N)/(\Sigma\, BC/N) \qquad \text{Eq. 8}$$

where N is the number of subjects in the individual study.

STUDY A: For the 17 studies in this analysis, OR_s was 1.01, which was essentially unity (i.e., no relationship).

STUDY B: Average d was 0.28 for the four studies, which would be considered small, but of practical importance.

Confidence Interval or Significance

The confidence interval provides a statistical test for the significance of results. If unity (i.e., 1) is in the interval for an odds ratio, then the risk of the outcome in question is not significantly greater than for controls. If the lower limit is >1, then there is a statistically significant risk.

For studies outside of epidemiology, the matter is less clear. The effect size cannot really be tested for significance. Some authors advocate constructing a 95 percent confidence interval around the effect size based on the standard deviation of the effect sizes. The problem is in using the between-study standard deviation when we really want a (pooled) within-study standard deviation.

One option is to combine p values, which has been described by Rosenthal.[6,60] Summary statistics are converted to normal curve equivalents (Z scores), and then tested. Table 9 lists Z equivalents for various values of Cohen's *d*. Values may be calculated using the formula:

$$Z = [(N \bullet d^2)/(d^2+4)]^{1/2} \qquad \text{Eq. 9}$$

where N is the number of subjects in the study and d is the effect size. Friedman presents a table for conversion of r values to Z scores.[67]

Table 9 Conversion of Statistics into Z Values	
	$Z = r \bullet \sqrt{n}$
	$Z = \sqrt{\chi^2}$
	$Z = \sqrt{F}$
	$Z = t(1 - t^2/4df)$
	$Z = [d^2 \bullet N/(d^2 + 4)]^{1/2}$

p	One-tailed	Two-tailed
0.10	1.2816	1.6449
0.05	1.6449	1.9600
0.01	2.3263	2.5758

Table 10
Significance Values
for Z

To test the significance of the overall effect, one may use the formula:

$$Z = (\textstyle\sum Z)/ \sqrt{k} \qquad \text{Eq. 10}$$

where k is the number of studies. The sum of the individual Z scores divided by the square root of the number of studies is distributed as Z. Table 10 presents values of Z which, if exceeded, indicate significance. Note that d values in a meta-analysis represent one-tailed values.

Primary Method

STUDY A: Overall significance was tested using the formula of Mantel and Haenszel:

$$\chi^2 = [\,|\textstyle\sum A_i - \sum E(A_i)\,| - 0.5]^2 / \textstyle\sum V(A_i) \qquad \text{Eq. 11}$$

where $E(A_i) = n_i m_i / N_i$ and $V(A_i) = n_1 \bullet m_1 \bullet n_0 \bullet m_0 / [N_i^2(N_i - 1)]$. The chi-square has one degree of freedom, which provides a two-tailed result that may be halved for a one-tailed test. The chi-square value was 0.05 which had a two-tailed $p = 0.815$. Since it was not significant, no association was indicated.

STUDY B: Study B added the Zs presented above because that method can be used with any number of studies and other methods cannot be used when there are fewer than five.

For the four studies, Z was 4.25 ($p < 0.0005$). Thus, the overall result was statistically significant.

Confirmatory Method

STUDY A: Rosenthal described the widely used method of Fisher for adding logs.[6] The natural logarithm of the p value for each study is calculated and summed and this total is multiplied by -2 to arrive at an overall chi-square value that has 2k degrees of freedom (k = the number of studies). Thus, the natural log for the p values in Table 6 was determined. The chi-square value was 39.78 (df = 34, p = 0.228). This result confirmed that of the primary analysis.

STUDY B: The method for adding p values described by Rosenthal was used as a confirmatory method because it has good power and can be used with a small number of studies when p values sum to ≤ 1.[6] The formula is $p = (\textstyle\sum p)^k / k!$, where k is the number of studies and $\sum p$ is the sum of p values for individual studies. In this case, overall $p = 0.0003$, which agrees well with the original analysis.

Power Considerations

It is desirable to determine the power or robustness of results. When there are small numbers of studies, results are less conclusive than when there are large numbers. This is analogous to the finding of no difference between groups in a clinical trial of two drugs. There may be no difference between groups, or there may have been too few subjects in the study to detect the difference. With a meta-analysis, the same may be true.

Sample Size

The size of the samples in each study could have an impact on the results. Some authors suggest weighting studies by their sample size or their variance to give more weight to larger studies. That suggestion is based on the premise that studies with larger numbers of subjects are likely to provide a better estimate of the true effect than would small studies.

STUDY A: Because study A used the Mantel-Haenszel method for combining data, it in fact did weight each effect size (i.e., odds ratio) by its sample size.

STUDY B: Each study was weighted by sample size and an overall weighted d was calculated using the formula: $d_w = \sum d_i \bullet n_i / N$, where N is the sum of all subjects in all studies. The weighted d was 0.25, because the largest effect size had the smallest sample size. Thus, the value of d decreased slightly. However, results are essentially identical. Therefore, we may conclude that the effect was not an artifact of sample size.

Publication Bias

Rosenthal identified a tendency in the literature to publish only significant findings. He termed this the "file drawer problem" because it results in the accumulation of unpublished studies in the file drawers of researchers.[68] There is also the issue of bias and popularity of topics. For example, Koren et al. have shown that drug studies indicating a teratogenic effect of cocaine were much more likely to be published than those showing no UDE, despite their superior methodological quality.[69] Therefore, it is recommended that meta-analysts attempt to calculate the impact of potential unpublished reports.

Orwin has published the following formula, which may be used to determine how many studies would be needed to nullify a given outcome (i.e., effect size) from a meta-analysis:[70]

$$N_{fs} = N_0(d_0 - d_c)/(d_c - d_{fs}) \qquad \text{Eq. 12}$$

where N_{fs} is failsafe N, the number of studies required to raise (or lower, as the case may be) an effect size to any given value. N_0 is the number of studies in the meta-analysis, d_0 is the calculated effect size d, d_c is the desired effect size, and d_{fs} is the effect size of studies "to be added."

STUDY A: In this analysis, Cohen's d was calculated for each study from its chi-square value and using the formula from Table 6. The overall d was 0.013. In order to raise this effect to 0.2, which Cohen would call small, would require:

$$N_{fs} = 17(0.013-0.2)/(0.2-0.5) = 10.59 \text{ or } 11 \text{ studies}$$

Eq. 13

having an effect size of 0.5.

Since none of the published studies produced an effect size as large as 0.5 (the largest being 0.007), it would be highly unlikely that one could find 11 unpublished reports (of similar size to those in this meta-analysis) with effect sizes of that magnitude. Similarly, 33 studies having effect sizes of 0.3 would be required. It seems highly improbable that so many studies would have been overlooked on such a contentious issue.

STUDY B: For this study:

$$N_{fs} = 4(0.28-0.2)/(0.2-0) = 1.6$$

Eq. 14

That means that only two studies having a zero effect size would be needed to bring the overall d to 0.2, and eight would be needed to arrive at 0.1. It is very possible that small numbers of studies exist to disprove such findings. This is especially so since there is a tendency for pharmacy journals to publish articles that show a positive effect of clinical programs. We must conclude that more studies are required to establish the value of DUR programs.

Subgroup Analyses

Subgroups can be divided according to any moderator variables that may influence results. Moderator variables are simply names of groups to which subjects could belong. Examples may be age (e.g., pediatric, geriatric), severity of illness (e.g., mild, moderate, severe), dose of drug given (e.g., high vs. low), route (e.g., iv vs. im or po), gender, or any other factor possibly related to outcomes.

STUDY A: Since Bendectin was marketed in two forms (two and three components), a question naturally arose as to whether the three-component product could have been problematic, but the two-component product was not. Therefore, cohort studies containing only the three-component product were isolated and analyzed. The resultant OR_s was 0.87 (95% CI = 0.55–1.37), indicating no relationship.

STUDY B: Not applicable.

Study Types

If different types of studies are included, they may provide results that are dissimilar due to the data collection method. For example, case-control studies tend to have very high rates of prevalence of adverse outcomes compared with cohort studies that have low rates but comparable ratios of risk. Thus, it may be wise to separate study types to detect possible discrepancies.

STUDY A: The OR_s for cohort studies was 0.95 (95% CI 0.62–1.45), indicating no relationship. For case-control studies, OR_s was 1.17 (95% CI = 0.83–1.94), again showing no effect. Tables 11 and 12 display the data from these study types.

STUDY B: Because all studies were similar, no sub-analyses were performed.

Patient Types

The type of patient could influence outcomes. Age, gender, severity of illness, and many more factors could influence outcomes. Therefore, one should determine which factors could be important and analyze the data accordingly.

Table 11
Risk Ratios and Confidence Intervals for Cohort Studies Comparing Malformation Risk in Fetuses Exposed and Not Exposed to Bendectin

Reference	Malformation Risk		Risk Ratio	95 Percent Confidence Interval*
	Bendectin	Control		
13	0.068	0.065	1.05	0.84–1.30
21	0.050	0.054	0.93	0.65–1.31
22	0.021	0.022	0.95	0.50–1.79
23	0.022	0.036	0.62	0.37–1.06
24	0.083	0.071	1.17	0.79–1.73
27	0.001	0.001	1.43	0.26–7.78
28	0.046	0.042	1.09	0.85–1.40
29	0.011	0.012	0.87	0.54–1.40
30	0.028	0.031	0.91	0.22–3.84
33	0.005	0.010	0.48	0.21–1.11
34	0.016	0.018	0.89	0.54–1.51
35	0.005	0.009	0.52	0.25–1.08
Average	0.030	0.031	0.91	
SD	0.025	0.022		
Summary odds ratio			0.95	0.62–1.45

*$CI_i = RR_i \cdot \exp\{\pm 1.96 \cdot [(1-A_i/n_i)/A_i + (1-C_i/n_{01})/C_i]^{1/2}\}$ where $RR_i =$ the risk ratio $(A_i/n_{1i})/(C_i/n_{0i})$

Table 12
Mantel-Haenszel Estimates of Odds Ratios and Confidence Intervals for Case-Control Studies of Fetuses Exposed or Not Exposed to Bendectin

Reference	AD/N	BC/N	Odds Ratio (AD/BC)	95 Percent Confidence Interval*
20	29.77	21.28	1.40	0.96–2.05
25	17.64	10.24	1.72	1.04–2.86
26	30.95	28.47	1.09	0.76–1.55
31	7.92	2.75	2.88	1.19–6.96
32	34.00	40.00	0.85	0.62–1.17
Total	120.28	102.74	7.94	
Average odds ratio			1.58	
Summary odds ratio			1.17	0.83–1.94

*$CI_i = (A_iD_i/B_iC_i \cdot \exp[\pm 1.96 \cdot (1/A_i + 1/B_i + 1/C_i + 1/D_i)^{1/2}]$
A = number of malformed infants that had been exposed to Bendectin; B = number of nonmalformed infants that had been exposed to Bendectin; C = number of malformed infants that had not been exposed to Bendectin; D = number of nonmalformed infants that had not been exposed to Bendectin; N = total number of subjects in the study.

STUDY A: In this study, many factors could influence teratogenic outcomes. The age of the mother, alcohol ingestion, smoking, socioeconomic status, and so forth, have all been linked with adverse outcomes. However, in all of the studies involved, the investigators either matched patients or statistically controlled for all of those factors. Therefore, a sub-analysis by patient type was not needed.

STUDY B: Due to the small number of studies, sub-analyses were not performed.

Treatment Levels

The amount of drug ingested could affect the outcomes. Where possible, data should be separated to determine whether a relationship exists between drug dose and outcome.

STUDY A: A few studies documented the exact number of doses taken, but exact data were difficult to extract. As a result, differences between high and low exposure were not examined.

STUDY B: Not applicable.

Other Moderator Variables

STUDY A: Not done.

STUDY B: None was performed. With a large number of studies, one could separate specific types of services, such as pharmacokinetic monitoring, therapeutic monitoring, or anticoagulant clinics. Similarly, hospitals could be analyzed by type (e.g., teaching, community).

Step 5. Interpretation of Results

It is necessary to interpret results in the light of the data collected, size of the studies, similarity of findings, and study types. The analyst should investigate all aspects of the studies and discuss the findings while addressing all the concerns. This is especially true if controversy exists in the literature.

Analysis of Accepted Studies

STUDY A: Of the 17 studies accepted, only 2 showed a statistically significant relationship between Bendectin exposure and teratogenicity. The odds ratios were 1.72 and 2.88 and were calculated on 1644 and 603 subjects, respectively. Thus, sample sizes were smaller than the average in those studies. The study by Rothman et al. was questioned due to recall bias that resulted from the method of questioning the mothers.[25] Subsequent analysis showed no relationship.[26] Since the overall odds ratio was not significant, the conclusion is that no relationship exists.

STUDY B: Two of the four studies were significant (at the 0.05 level) and two were not. Effect sizes were not large, with an average of 0.28. The combined probability was significant. These calculations lead us to conclude that there was a small effect of those programs, but the data are not conclusive.

Analysis of Rejected Studies

STUDY A: Rejected studies could not be analyzed as they did not provide adequate data. Harron et al. did not show exposure to the drug; they merely guessed at the possible number of exposures by dividing the number of tablets dispensed in the country by the estimated number of pregnant women.[36] Results, therefore, are difficult to interpret. Three papers dealt with antinauseants in general, but data for Bendectin could not be separated. Significant problems were not reported in those studies.

Study A also did not consider studies that compared specific malformations with other malformations. Three such studies sought to establish whether Bendectin could have been responsible for a specific syndrome of malformations.[38-40] None of those studies found a relationship.

STUDY B: Inoue showed a significant pharmacist impact on drug prescribing,[54,55] as did Studnicki-Gizbert and Segal[53] and Rosser et al.[56] However, none of those authors used criteria for determining inappropriateness. Therefore, if those studies had been added, results of this meta-analysis would have been even stronger.

Support of Studies

It has been suggested that support of research could influence the results. For example, a report financed by a drug company may produce results favorable to the company.

STUDY A: In this analysis, eight (47 percent) were supported by government grants, three (18 percent) were reports from research institutions with support not stated, five (29 percent) were from physicians affiliated with a university (support not stated), and only one (6 percent) was supported solely by a pharmaceutical manufacturer. Therefore, there was little evidence of bias due to support.

STUDY B: None of the studies received support, and all reports came from teaching institutions; hence, bias was not considered to be a problem.

Other Evidence

Any other evidence, pro or con, should be presented and discussed so that all information may be analyzed. Neither study in this analysis encountered further evidence of value.

Animal Evidence

Animal studies often provide evidence that confirms or refutes human findings. The information from laboratories may help to confirm theories of malformation or drug action that can never be performed on humans. Sometimes, caution must be used in interpretation of such data or extrapolation to humans. It must be remembered that thalidomide was not teratogenic to rats or mice but, tragically, it is to humans.

STUDY A: None of the animal studies demonstrated a relationship between Bendectin administration and birth defects. This supported our findings in humans.

STUDY B: Not applicable.

Incidental Findings

If any other evidence has been discovered that may be significant to the question under investigation, it should be mentioned. However, it should be noted that those findings were incidental, not planned. Hence, their interpretation may not be straightforward. None were found in either study.

Overall Conclusions

STUDY A: Bendectin was found not to be associated with teratogenicity.

STUDY B: Canadian pharmacy DUR studies were found to have had a small, but statistically significant impact on improving the appropriateness of drug therapy.

Caveats

Caveats include limitations of the meta-analysis due to method, inclusion and exclusion criteria, or problems encountered. It helps to focus the results by stating limitations. For example, the analyst should state whether a new treatment is more effective than a former one, but perhaps must compare costs. Conclusions may only be suggestions for further research.

STUDY A: Bendectin was not associated with birth defects. However, the product has been removed from the North American market.

STUDY B: Conclusions were based on a very small number of studies; therefore, caution is recommended when interpreting the results. More studies are definitely required before solid conclusions may be made.

Implications of Findings

There should be a discussion of the meaning of the results when extrapolated to the population. Implications may be made in such areas as healthcare, patient status, and time saved for professionals.

STUDY A: Because Bendectin is not teratogenic, cases of litigation have no foundation; as a result, they should cease. Also, the only effective treatment for nausea and vomiting associated with pregnancy has been removed from the market needlessly. A cost-benefit analysis should be done to determine the economic impact of the drug's removal from the market.

STUDY B: If DURs are as effective as shown, more should be performed. Support should be obtained for adequate performance of DUR programs. The net result should be an increase in the quality of patient care.

Economic Impact

Sacks et al. have recommended discussion of the impact of new drugs or services, due to the climate of cost constraint in healthcare today.[8]

STUDY A: The impact of not using an antinauseant in pregnancy could affect hospital admissions due to nausea and vomiting of pregnancy since there is no longer a suitable alternative drug. One study has shown that this is the case: hospital admissions have increased for that indication, but cases of teratogenicity have not decreased.

STUDY B: The economic impact of DUR programs can have a substantial impact on the budget of a hospital pharmacy department. Financial savings can accrue through the appropriate use of drugs. If personnel were devoted to this task, one would expect a much greater impact. However, since these results are based on a few studies, more research is required before making recommendations.

Phase II: Performing The Analysis

In performing this phase of the research, the definitions developed in the preparation phase are applied to the available studies. This part of the analysis is straightforward and can be done relatively quickly, especially when using a spreadsheet for calculations. A well-planned meta-analysis, like other types of research, is almost done when the planning has been completed. Data collection and analysis are quite simple.

Phase III: Presentation of Results

As all researchers are aware, no project is complete until the results have been presented. For most of us, it means publication in a peer-reviewed journal that reaches the intended audience. However, other suitable means of disseminating such information are available, including books, symposia, or meetings of scientific or professional organizations.

When presenting effect size data, several techniques have been used to explain the impact of an intervention. Glass converted the effect size into a normal curve equivalent (Z score) and presented two overlapping normal curves. The effect size was displayed as the difference between the means (i.e., the peaks of the two curves).[3,14] Einarson et al. determined that patients treated with chymopapain for herniated discs had an effect size of 0.81 over placebo. The area under the curve for Z = 0.81 was 0.791, which meant that the average person in the treatment group

d	Percentile	r	BESD From	To
0.1	54.0	0.05	0.475	0.525
0.2	57.9	0.10	0.450	0.550
0.3	61.8	0.15	0.436	0.574
0.4	65.5	0.20	0.412	0.598
0.5	69.1	0.24	0.389	0.621
0.6	72.6	0.29	0.356	0.644
0.7	75.8	0.33	0.335	0.665
0.8	78.8	0.37	0.314	0.686
0.9	81.6	0.41	0.295	0.705
1.0	84.1	0.45	0.276	0.724
1.5	93.3	0.60	0.200	0.800
2.0	97.7	0.71	0.146	0.854
3.0	99.9	0.83	0.084	0.916

Table 13
Normal Curve
Equivalent Percentile
Values and BESD for
Selected Values of
Cohen's *d*

BESD = binomial effect size displays.

was better off than 79.1 percent of those in the control group.[9] Clinical results may be presented in this fashion. Rosenthal presented a method for visualizing the effect which he called the binary effect size display (BESD). He converted effect sizes to the correlation coefficient r (which is an accepted effect size itself). The experimental group success rate is calculated as 0.50 + r/2 and the control group success rate is 0.50−r/2.[6] Table 13 presents BESD for various values of *d* and r.

Summary

Meta-analysis is a statistical approach to the aggregation of independent research studies. It is an invaluable tool in evaluating the literature to arrive at an overall estimate of effect or risk. Because it provides a thorough and systematic approach to analysis, meta-analysis is to be preferred over previous methods. Drug information specialists are urged to adopt this approach to summarizing the literature. It may well become the standard method for drug evaluation in the future. Students are urged to undertake meta-analyses as research projects, and practitioners are encouraged to become familiar with the concepts involved in meta-analysis to understand and apply results to practice. Meta-analysis provides an effective tool for handling drug information.

References

1. Frieman JA, Chalmers TC, Smith H, et al. The importance of beta, the type II error, and sample size in the design and interpretation of the randomized control trial. *N Engl J Med* 1978;299:690-4.

2. Einarson TR, Leeder JS, Koren G. A method for meta-analysis of epidemiologic studies. *Drug Intell Clin Pharm* 1988;22:813-24.

3. Glass GV. Primary, secondary, and meta-analysis of research. *Educ Res* 1976;5:3-8.

4. Gerbarg ZB, Horwitz RI. Resolving conflicting clinical trials: guidelines for meta-analysis. *J Clin Epidemiol* 1988;41:503-9.

5. Teagarden JR. Meta-analysis: whither narrative review? *Pharmacotherapy* 1989;9:274-84.

6. Rosenthal R. Meta-analytic procedures for social research. Beverly Hills, CA: Sage Publications, 1984.

7. Leviton LC, Cook TD. What differentiates meta-analysis from other forms of review? *J Pers* 1981;49:231-6.

8. Sacks HS, Berrier J, Reitman D, Ancona-Berk VA. Meta-analyses of randomized controlled trials. *N Engl J Med* 1987;316:450-5.

Appendix I
Suggested
Reading List

Books

Glass GV, McGaw B, Smith ML. Meta-analysis in social research. Beverly Hills, CA: Sage Publications, 1981.

Hedges LV, Olkin I. Statistical methods for meta-analysis. Orlando, FL: Academic Press, 1985.

Hunter JE, Schmidt FL, Jackson GB. Meta-analysis: cumulating research findings across studies. Beverly Hills, CA: Sage Publications, 1982.

Light RJ, Pillemer DB. Summing up: the science of reviewing research. Cambridge, MA: Harvard University Press, 1984.

Rosenthal R. Meta-analytic procedures for social research. Beverly Hills, CA: Sage Publications, 1984.

Wolf FM. Meta-analysis: quantitative methods for research synthesis. Beverly Hills, CA: Sage Publications, 1986.

Methodologic Articles

Einarson TR, McGhan WF, Bootman JL, Sabers DL. Meta-analysis: quantitative integration of independent research results. *Am J Hosp Pharm* 1985;42:1957-64.

Einarson TR, Leeder JS, Koren G. A method for meta-analysis of epidemiologic articles. *Drug Intell Clin Pharm* 1988;22:813-24.

Gerbarg ZB, Horwitz RI. Resolving conflicting clinical trials: guidelines for meta-analysis. *J Clin Epidemiol* 1988;41:503-9.

Glass GV. Primary, secondary, and meta-analysis of research. *Educ Res* 1976;5:3-8.

Glass GV. Integrating findings: the meta-analysis of research. *Rev Res Educ* 1978; 5:351-79.

L'Abbe KA, Detsky AS, O'Rourke K. Meta-analysis in clinical research. *Ann Intern Med* 1987;107:224-33.

Rosenthal R. Combining results of independent studies. *Psychol Bull* 1978;85:185-93.

Sacks HS, Berrier J, Reitman D, Ancona-Berk VA. Meta-analyses of randomized controlled trials. *N Engl J Med* 1987;316:450-5.

Teagarden JR. Meta-analysis: whither narrative review? *Pharmacotherapy* 1989;9: 274-84.

Thacker SB. Meta-analysis: a quantitative approach to research integration. *JAMA* 1988;259:1685-9.

Walker AM, Martin-Moreno JM, Artalejo FR. Odd man out: a graphical approach to meta-analysis. *Am J Public Health* 1988;78:961-6.

9. Einarson TR, McGhan WF, Bootman JL, Sabers DL. Meta-analysis: quantitative integration of independent research results. *Am J Hosp Pharm* 1985;42:1957-64.

10. Lee KA. Meta-analysis: a third alternative for student research experience. *Nurse Educ* 1988;13(4):30-3.

11. Ried LD, McKenna DA, Horn JR. Effect of therapeutic monitoring services on the number of serum drug assays ordered for patients: a meta-analysis. *Ther Drug Monit* 1989;11:253-63.

12. Hedges LV, Olkin I. Statistical methods for meta-analysis. Orlando, FL: Academic Press, 1985.

13. Heinonen OP, Slone D, Shapiro S. Birth defects and drugs in pregnancy. Littleton, MA: PSG Publishing, 1977.

14. Glass GV. Integrating findings: the meta-analysis of research. *Rev Res Educ* 1978;5:351-79.

15. Schardein JL. Chemically induced drug defects. New York: Marcel Dekker, 1985.

16. Shepard TH. Catalog of teratogenic agents. 5th ed. Baltimore: Johns Hopkins University Press, 1986.

17. Briggs GG, Freeman RK, Yaffe SJ. Drugs in pregnancy and lactation. 2nd ed. Baltimore: Williams and Wilkins, 1986.

18. Carruthers G, Goldberg T, Segal H, Sellers E. Drug utilization: a comprehensive literature review. Toronto: Ontario Ministry of Health, 1987.

19. Fleiss JL. Statistical methods for rates and proportions. 2nd ed. New York: John Wiley and Sons, 1981.

20. Eskenazi B, Bracken M. Bendectin (Debendox) as a risk factor for pyloric stenosis. *Am J Obstet Gynecol* 1982;144:919-24.

21. Fleming DM, Knox JDE, Crombie DL. Debendox in early pregnancy and fetal malformation. *Br Med J* 1981;283:99-101.

22. Michaelis J, Michaelis H, Gluck E, Koller S. Prospective study of suspected associations between certain drugs administered during early pregnancy and congenital malformations. *Teratology* 1983;27:57-64.

23. Milkovich L, Van den Berg BJ. An evaluation of the teratogenicity of certain antinauseant drugs. *Am J Obstet Gynecol* 1976;125:244-8.

24. Morelock S, Hingson R, Kayne H, et al. Bendectin and fetal development: a study at Boston City Hospital. *Am J Obstet Gynecol* 1982;142:209-13.

25. Rothman J, Fyler DC, Goldblatt A, Kreidberg MB. Exogenous hormones and other drug exposures of children with congenital heart disease. *Am J Epidemiol* 1979;109:433-9.

26. Zierler S, Rothman KJ. Congenital heart disease in relation to maternal use of Bendectin and other drugs in early pregnancy. *N Engl J Med* 1985;313:347-52.

27. Aselton PJ, Jick H. Additional followup of congenital limb disorders in relation to Bendectin use. *JAMA* 1983;250:33-4.

28. Gibson GT, Colley DP, McMichael AJ, Hartshorn JM. Congenital anomolies in relation to the use of doxylamine/dicyclomine and other antenatal factors. *Med J Aust* 1981;1:410-4.

29. Jick H, Holmes LB, Hunter JR, Madsen S, Stergachis A. First trimester drug use and congenital disorders. *JAMA* 1981;246:343-6.

30. General Practitioner Clinical Trials. Drugs in pregnancy survey. *Practitioner* 1963; 191:775-80.

31. Golding J, Vivian S, Baldwin JA. Maternal anti-nauseants and clefts of lip and palate. *Hum Toxicol* 1983;2: 63-73.

32. Greenberg G, Inman WHW, Weatherall JAC, Adalstein AM, Haskey JC. Maternal drug histories and congenital abnormalities. *Br Med J* 1977;2:853-6.

33. Newman NM, Correy JF, Dudgeon GI. A survey of congenital abnormalities and drugs in private practice. *Aust N Z J Gynaecol* 1977;17:156-9.

34. Smithells RW, Shepard S. Teratogenicity testing in humans: a method of demonstrating safety of Bendectin. *Teratology* 1978;17:31-6.

35. Bunde CA, Bowles DM. A technique for controlled survey of case records. *Curr Ther Res* 1963;5:245-8.

36. Harron DWG, Griffiths K, Shanks RG. Debendox and congenital malformations in Northern Ireland. *Br Med J* 1980;281:1379-81.

37. Nelson MM, Forfar JO. Associations between drugs administered during pregnancy and congenital abnormalities of the fetus. *Br Med J* 1971;1:523-7.

38. Cordero JF, Oakley GP, Greenberg F, James LM. Is Bendectin a teratogen? *JAMA* 1981; 245:2307-10.

39. Mitchell AA, Rosenberg L, Shapiro S, Slone D. Birth defects related to Bendectin use in pregnancy. I. Oral clefts and cardiac defects. *JAMA* 1981;245:2311-4.

40. Mitchell AA, Schwingl PJ, Rosenberg L, Louik C, Shapiro S. Birth defects in relation to Bendectin use in pregnancy. II. Pyloric stenosis. *Am J Obstet Gynecol* 1983;147:737-42.

41. Kullander S, Kallen B. A prospective study of drugs and pregnancy. II. Anti-emetic drugs. *Acta Obstet Gynecol Scand* 1976;55:105-11.

42. Yerushalmy J, Milkovich L. Valuation of the teratogenic effect of meclizine in man. *Am J Obstet Gynecol* 1965;93:553-62.

43. Gibson JP, Staples RE, Larson EJ, Kuhn WL, Holtkamp DE, Newberne JW. Teratology and reproduction studies with an antinauseant. *Toxicol Appl Pharmacol* 1968;13:439-47.

44. Achong MR, Wood J, Theal HK, Goldberg R, Thompson DA. Changes in hospital antibiotic therapy after a quality-of-use study. *Lancet* 1977;2:1118-21.

45. Beardsell A. IV cimetidine: assessment of initial dosing regimens. Pharmacy Residency Project, St. Paul's Hospital, Vancouver, BC, 1983.

46. Ensom RJ, Jewesson PJ, Hlynka JN, Ruedy J, Kennedy JR. Effect of pharmacist intervention on appropriateness of parenteral cimetidine use. *Can J Hosp Pharm* 1986;39:6-8.

47. Tait P, Hall D. Pharmacy involvement on a psychiatric unit at St. Paul's Hospital. *Can J Hosp Pharm* 1978;31:201-4.

48. Dancey JW. Drug utilization review at Lion's Gate Hospital. *Can J Hosp Pharm* 1978; 31:55-8.

49. Danforth DH, Hlynka JN, Soon JA. Drug usage review. Part 3: implementing the long term care program. *Can Pharm J* 1982;115:9-12, 33.

50. Hlynka JH, Danforth DH, Kerr SE. Drug usage review. Part 2: implementing the ambulatory program. *Can Pharm J* 1981;114:467-70.

51. Letourneau KN. Drug utilization review in an extended care facility. *Drug Intell Clin Pharm* 1974;8:108-14.

52. Pfeifer N, Lynd L. Vancomycin cost containment through a therapeutic drug monitoring service. Pharmacy Residency Project, St. Paul's Hospital, Vancouver, BC, 1987.

53. Studnicki-Gizbert D, Segal H. Effectiveness of selected pharmacy services in long term care facilities. *J Soc Admin Pharm* 1983;1:187-93.

54. Inoue F. Implementation of clinical pharmacy services. *Hosp Formul* 1978;13:278-84.

55. Inoue F. A clinical pharmacy service to reduce psychotropic drug use in an institution for mentally handicapped persons. *Ment Retard* 1982;20:70-4.

56. Rosser WW, Sims JG, Patten DW, Forster J. Improving benzodiazepine prescribing in a family practice through review and education. *Can Med Assoc J* 1981;124:147-52.

57. Vance PH. The effect of a pharmacist drug surveillance program in an acute ward. *Can J Hosp Pharm* 1973;26:71-4.

58. Enriquez S. The effect of hospitalization on hypnotic drug use in patients admitted to an acute care unit. Pharmacy Residency Project, UBC Health Sciences Centre Hospital, Vancouver, BC, 1983.

59. Tangjerd N. Effect of a drug plan on physicians' prescribing behaviour. *Can Fam Physician* 1978;24:33-6.

60. Rosenthal R. Combining results of independent studies. *Psychol Bull* 1978;85:185-93.

61. Rosenthal R, Rubin D. Comparing effect sizes of independent studies. *Psychol Bull* 1982;92:500-4.

62. Cohen J. Power analysis for the social sciences. New York: Academic Press, 1977.

63. Mantel N, Haenszel W. Statistical aspects of the analysis of data from retrospective studies of disease. *J Natl Cancer Inst* 1959;22:719-48.

64. Breslow NE, Day NE. Statistical methods for cancer research. Volume 1. The analysis of case-control studies. IARC Scientific Publications No. 32. Lyon, France: International Agency for Research on Cancer, 1980.

65. L'Abbe KA, Detsky AS, O'Rourke K. Meta-analysis in clinical research. *Ann Intern Med* 1987;107:224-33.

66. Chalmers TC, Smith H, Blackburn B, et al. A method for assessing the quality of a randomized control trial. *Controlled Clin Trials* 1981;2:31-49.

67. Friedman H. Magnitude of experimental effect and a table for its rapid estimation. *Psychol Bull* 1968;70:245-51.

68. Rosenthal R. The file drawer problem and tolerance for null results. *Psychol Bull* 1979; 86:638-41.

69. Koren G, Graham K, Shear H, Einarson T. Against the null hypothesis: the reproductive hazards of cocaine. *Lancet* 1989;2:1440-2.

70. Orwin RG. A fail-safe N for effect size in meta-analysis. *J Educ Stat* 1983;8:157-9.

14

Pharmacoepidemiology of Psychiatric Disorders

Julie Magno Zito
Thomas J. Craig

Abstract

The pharmacoepidemiology of neuropharmacologic drugs for psychiatric disorders is the subject of this chapter. The possibilities and limitations of the existing methods of determining neuropharmacologic drug efficacy and safety in psychiatric patients are discussed. Pharmacoepidemiologic methods can improve both the scientific evaluation and clinical practice aspects of our knowledge of these drugs by providing: (1) incidence rates of drug usage and unintended drug effect rates from computerized information on large populations; (2) quantitative methods for risk-to-benefit assessments that incorporate multiple outcome measures, provide long-term effectiveness and safety data, and use statistical methods to distinguish drug-induced from illness-based behaviors; and (3) systematic epidemiologic approaches to resolve dilemmas that involve the political and social context in which drugs for psychiatric disorders are used. Collectively, these approaches seek an empirical basis for the development of clinical theory in psychiatric drug treatment.

Outline

P harmacoepidemiology is defined by Porta and Hartzema in Chapter 1 as "the application of epidemiologic knowledge, methods, and reasoning to the study of the effects (beneficial and adverse) and uses of drugs in human populations." It was also defined by Rector as "the study of the relationships of various factors to the frequency and distribution of pharmaceutical outcomes in a population."[1] Pharmaceutical outcomes consisted of three domains of measurable clinical phenomena, namely, the physiological, psychological, and socioeconomic consequences of drug use. Because pharmacoepidemiologic methods can be used to address scientific questions on all three levels of drug use impact, they can add to the existing methods of determining drug efficacy[2] and safety.[3] These methods can be directed to the special needs of drug assessment in psychopharmacology, behavioral medicine, and behavioral pharmacology. This chapter reviews pharmacoepidemiologic methods currently used to extend our knowledge of the relationship of neuropharmacologic drug usage to human behavior.

Neuropharmacologic Drugs and Behavioral Disorders

For the purpose of this discussion, neuropharmacologic drugs are defined as drugs that pass the blood-brain barrier and have intended or unintended behavioral effects. The major drug class in this category is the psychotropics, but the term neuroactive[4] has been suggested to emphasize the role of additional pharmacologic classes of agents that exhibit behavioral effects, many of which are used in the treatment of psychiatric disorders. For example, anticholinergic agents and diphenhydramine are used to treat drug-induced parkinsonism in about 50 percent of antipsychotic inpatient exposures.[5] Antiepileptic drugs also are included in this category because of the relatively high prevalence of seizure disorders in psychiatric patients[6] as well as the increasing use of carbamazepine, valproic acid, and clonazepam to treat patients with affective disorders resistant to standard drug treatment.[7] The most frequently used psychotropic drug classes are the antipsychotics (neuroleptics), antidepressants, anxiolytics-sedatives-hypnotics, and lithium. Each class produces neuropharmacologic drug responses of both an intended (positive clinical response) and unintended type (negative or adverse event). The term behavioral toxicity has been used to describe the adverse effects of drugs on behavioral or psychological functioning[8] and is receiving renewed interest in the psychiatric literature.[9-11]

In addition to the psychiatric indications mentioned above, there is separate medical literature describing the relationship between behavioral symptoms and drugs that produce neuropharmacologic effects secondary to the treatment of nonpsychiatric medical disorders. Consultation liaison psychiatrists are becoming aware of the frequency with which patients treated with digoxin at[12] and above[13] therapeutic serum concentrations initially presented as having a psychiatric disorder such as depression or dementia. Other examples include reports of depression associated with nifedipine,[14] ranitidine,[15] reserpine,[16] and beta-blockers.[17-19]

In addition, physical disorders (e.g., peptic ulcer) are being treated with psychotropics, such as the antidepressant trimipramine[20] in patients who are not well controlled by changes in lifestyle, antacids, or cimetidine. Psychobiology,[21] behavioral medicine, and behavioral pharmacology[22] are terms variously used to identify this area of specialization, although the latter term includes experimental psychological interventions such as operant conditioning, which uses drugs in a stimulus-response paradigm to alter behavior. Interest in the psychobiological aspects of drug use is growing as experts in areas such as cardiovascular medicine, oncology, rheumatology, and neurology are increasingly concerned with the role of personality and socioeconomic factors in a patient's response to long-term drug therapy. Both psychopharmacology and psychobiology would benefit from a greater coordination of terminology and methodology regarding drug use and human behavior. This would be a useful initial step in defining an area of specialization for the psychiatric pharmacoepidemiologist. The development of consultation liaison psychiatry as one of the newer specialties[23] suggests the importance of behavioral symptoms in medical patients, especially those receiving complex multidrug regimens. Curricula in this area should emphasize behavioral toxicity (i.e., drug-induced psychiatric symptoms) and the loss of effectiveness of previously stabilized psychotropics by the addition of neuroactive drugs.

The focus of this chapter is limited to the specific ways psychopharmacology can use quantitative epidemiologic methods, which are described in four sections:

1. Denominator data methods from the longitudinal monitoring of large patient populations. Subsections address problems in optimal dosing and the evaluation of clinical appropriateness.
2. Efficacy methods including limitations of the randomized, double-blind, controlled clinical trial model, and the gap between the outcome of research studies and clinical practice in large patient populations.
3. Safety methods from postmarketing surveillance programs to provide unintended drug effect (UDE) rates and to test hypotheses of possible drug-induced events.
4. Statistical methods for drug decision-making in individual patients and specific patient subgroups.

Finally, several examples are given of policy questions in which epidemiologic methods can be used to aid the benefit-to-risk assessment of psychopharmacologic drug use for controversial indications.

Denominator Data Methods

Developments in computer applications for psychiatry include office records, diagnostic tools, and specialized treatment modalities such as psychotherapy and family therapy.[24] However, more comprehensive applications related to inferences about effectiveness and safety of medications are exceptional.

Feinstein described the limitations of causal inferencing of drug effects from the standard clinical practice situation.[25] To improve upon the logic of this process, therapeutic drug monitoring, using a computerized longitudinal record of specific drug and response variables, is suggested. This method involves the use of quantitative methods derived from pharmacokinetics, pharmacodynamics, and psychometric theory for patients receiving neuropharmacologic drugs. Specifically, the drug serum concentration, pertinent laboratory or other test values, target response measures (e.g., structured scales for symptom reduction, occupational and social rehabilitation, and hospital days), and UDEs are determined at regular intervals and longitudinally entered into a computerized database. Selected variables then are arranged in bivariate displays over time (the y-axis is the positive or negative response variable and the x-axis is clinic visit or assessment time). For example, the bivariate graphing of the phenytoin plasma concentration, daily dose, and seizure frequency versus time in the antiepileptic therapy of a pregnant seizure patient during the perinatal period illustrates the inferencing process related to drug clearance, bioavailability, and dosing of phenytoin in a patient-specific situation.[26]

An alternative system that uses ward-based microcomputer entry of clinical data was developed for public psychiatric hospitals in Texas. The data collection system is intended to justify psychiatrists' choice of treatment and requires systemized drug evaluation at scheduled intervals.[27]

Linkage of the longitudinally recorded drug variables with other computerized components of the medical record permits more elaborate epidemiologic evaluations of treatment and outcome. Hypothesis-generating studies about mental health issues, such as self-reported compliance among the deinstitutionalized mentally ill, are available where national systems like Sweden have this capability.[28] In American hospitalized psychiatric populations, one example is the Mental Health Package of the Veterans Administration (VA), which uses the MUMPS program language. It is being used in more than 170 hospitals to store variables on medication, demographics, and previous treatments but, to our knowledge, large-scale drug epidemiology has been limited.[24]

Numerous epidemiologic studies were published on a pioneer system called the Multistate Information System (MSIS). When merged with computerized patient characteristics, MSIS linked diagnostic, selected clinical, and sociodemographic factors to medication usage.[29] For more than a decade, the system provided psychopharmacologic drug monitoring consisting of retrospective review of orders in exception to guidelines developed by a committee of experts.[30] The positive effect of computerized drug exception reporting on prescribing behavior was demonstrated empirically.[31] Based on users' suggestions, a revision is being implemented so that prospective review of both medical and psychotropic orders will occur. In addition, the system data can be linked to computerized outcome measures such as discharge status and length of hospitalization. Retrieval and aggregation of these data and enhancement with specific ad hoc measures (e.g., symptom severity, research diagnosis) in random subsets of patients will enable large-scale epidemiologic evaluations of drug effectiveness and safety to occur.

Using data retrieved from the MSIS database, the relationship between length of hospitalization and antipsychotic medication exposure was examined in newly admitted schizophrenic patients.[5] The univariate measure of outcome, length of hospitalization, was not related to the dose (low, moderate, high) of antipsychotics. Similarly, computerized data showed the pattern of multiple psychotropic drug usage in relation to the clinical course and outcome of the schizophrenic episodes for young adult males.[32]

Future studies in large database systems need to focus on treatment evaluation in specific patient populations using multiple outcome measures, such as symptom reduction, functional capacity, relapse rate, and patient satisfaction.[33] Multivariate analyses of treatment outcomes might specify employment history and social functioning as covariates because these variables have been identified as predictors of outcome from previous studies.[34] To the extent that the multivariate analytic approach accurately reflects the underlying nexus of patient-treatment variables, it should produce clinically meaningful, statistically significant results. Computerized and quantitative medical records will make these studies more feasible and less costly.

OPTIMAL DOSE DETERMINATION

The development of an acceptable dose range for a specific psychopharmacologic agent (e.g., a neuroleptic) is related to many factors in animal and human pharmacology. The mechanism of action of neuroleptics involves blockade of dopaminergic receptors. Despite the well-accepted role of neuroleptics in managing psychosis, research leaders now question whether antidopaminergic activity (i.e., pharmacologic effect) is a necessary and sufficient basis for antipsychotic efficacy (i.e., clinical effect) and whether antipsychotic efficacy is confounded by neurological UDEs in our studies of dose-response relationships.[35] These questions highlight the current debate on dose-response effects[36] and, more broadly, on the balance of efficacy to safety for this widely used class of psychotropics.

Because the dose-response relationship of antipsychotics is so variable (due to large interpatient variability), systematic methods to determine optimal dosing might consider empirical standards based on data from population studies.[37,38] For example, in the study of antipsychotic therapy in newly admitted schizophrenic patients, the average daily dose (chlorpromazine-equivalents) of high-potency agents was 2.7-fold greater than the dose of low-potency agents.[5] Since the excess exposure was not statistically associated with better treatment outcome, the dosing could be considered suboptimal due to the increased risk of tardive dyskinesia.[39] In addition, the excess drug exposure was translated into $1273, or 16.3 percent of the overall neuropharmacologic drug costs. This approach permits an empirically based clinical dosage and cost analysis. If the favorable outcome is the criterion, the optimal dose is defined as the dosage used in a cohort of patients with the best treatment outcome. To be a valid technique, a large population with similar baseline characteristics must be assessed. In another illustration, a stepwise multiple regression model was applied by Hargreaves et al. to analyze neuroleptic dosing trends from computerized drug data on 1490 admissions. The 50 percent decline in maximum and average daily doses over a ten-year period was not explained by fewer days in treatment and changing choice of drug.[40] In the Texas system described above, a drug usage model based on the epidemiologic concepts of sensitivity, specificity, and utility was used to determine clinical standards for antipsychotic drugs.[41]

EVALUATING CLINICAL APPROPRIATENESS

Traditional prescribing studies are a well-known approach to the evaluation of appropriate drug, dose, and combinations of drugs in clinical practice. In public psychiatry, ad hoc surveys of prescribing have been a means of assessing a health service system that generally is regarded as under-funded and lacking in quality care. Polypharmacy continues to be a concern in recent reports[42] and persists even after the publication of proscribed practices.[43] Longitudinal data on the prescribing pattern of psychotropic drugs are rare.[44] A different approach to appropriateness is taken by the interdisciplinary team review of antipsychotic orders after six months of use in severely, profoundly mentally retarded persons. This approach was reported to reduce medication (presumed favorable outcome for this population) without a significant increase in major injuries.[45]

Efficacy Methods

In the 35 years since chlorpromazine was marketed for the treatment of acute and chronic psychosis, a large body of research and clinical literature has developed supporting the effectiveness of this antipsychotic (neuroleptic) agent and the 20-odd congeners that have followed its introduction. Crane estimated that more than 250 million patients had been exposed by the end of 1970.[46] Such extensive usage has given rise to a specialty area termed "biological psychiatry."

Antipsychotics are used widely in the major psychotic disorders affecting children, adults, and elderly patients and are used less frequently in the treatment of nonpsychotic and personality disorders. Nevertheless, the efficacy of the antipsychotics continues to be the subject of reinterpretation.[35,47] Similarly, assessing the three major psychotropic classes marketed after the antipsychotics (i.e., antidepressants,[48,49] benzodiazepines,[50] lithium[51]), raises questions. These questions suggest there is a gap between the inferences based on the original efficacy data from the randomized, double-blind, controlled clinical trials and the growing populations of treatment-resistant patients. To account for the apparent gap between research findings and real-world clinical usage, it is necessary to review the research studies and consider the following limitations of the clinical trial model in applying it to evaluate behavioral outcomes of neuropharmacologic drug usage.

LIMITATIONS

Clinical trials evaluate selected patients on limited response measures in restricted settings. Population-based psychotropic drug usage is evaluated by epidemiologic survey methods of outpatient data, such as those available from the National Ambulatory Medical Care Survey (NAMCS), an annual survey of health resource utilization in the U.S.[52] These surveys provide estimates of outpatient drug usage, albeit without dose exposure information, and have provided a comparison of psychotropic drug prescribing among primary care, psychiatry, and all other specialties.[53] A sophisticated analysis demonstrated gender bias in psychiatric drug prescribing by primary care clinicians after controlling for statistically significant symptoms, physician diagnoses, sociodemographics, and health service factors because women were more likely to receive prescriptions for anxiolytics and antidepressants.[54] This study illustrates the usefulness of large database methods for generating hypotheses that can then be examined by more rigorous experimental methods. NAMCS limitations include failure to capture the full spectrum of psychiatric drug usage that includes the more severely ill patient who requires a larger dosage during the inpatient phase of a psychotic episode and then typically receives follow-up care from mental health outpatient services. In addition, psychotropic drug usage occurs among the institutionalized psychiatric or medically ill people in nursing homes, as well as the deinstitutionalized psychiatric, elderly, and developmentally disabled people living in various domiciliary care settings.[55] Among these patient populations there are distinct differences in: (1) diagnosis; (2) baseline level of intellectual, emotional, and behavioral functioning; (3) severity of illness in terms of acute target psychiatric symptoms; and (4) chronic need for supervised living arrangements, and social and occupational rehabilitation. Given the range of clinical and social factors needed to characterize patients receiving psychiatric drug treatment and the likelihood that treatment will be ongoing for many patients, the distinctions between long-term treatment outcomes and the more limited response measures of the typical clinical trial are understandable.

Clinical trials in patients with acute psychiatric disorders have reported univariate outcomes in short-term studies that do not generalize to all patients. Of the hundreds of studies reporting the remission of acute psychosis with antipsychotic drugs, the most compelling evidence was provided in two rigorously conducted studies. In the National Institute of Mental Health collaborative study, the response measure was acute symptom reduction. Seventy-five percent of the patients who received chlorpromazine (mean 700 mg/d) showed moderate or greater improvement compared with 25 percent of placebo-treated patients.[56] The VA Collaborative

Study evaluated readmissions for chronic schizophrenia and found a statistically significantly greater improvement over 12 weeks in patients treated with fixed doses of chlorpromazine 400 mg/d compared with placebo-treated patients.[57]

Current research is directed at finding efficacious treatments for the 25 percent of drug-treated nonresponders and the 25 percent of placebo responders. Studies evaluating drug therapy in nonresponders include the schizophrenic patient with negative symptoms[58] and evaluations of targeted symptom,[59] low-dose regimens,[60] and the intermittent use of benzodiazepines (e.g., lorazepam[61,62]) to control agitated and aggressive behavior in chronic schizophrenic or bipolar patients who have not been controlled by antipsychotics or antipsychotics plus lithium. The individual treatment needs of specific patient subgroups will emerge from these studies to the extent that the studies reflect good design. For example, the study should incorporate the target behaviors of the patient population in question, provide detailed drug regimen data, particularly regarding recent past and baseline adjunctive drugs and their doses, involve appropriate multidimensional outcome measurements, and provide sufficient statistical power to observe the expected differences in outcome. The lack of complete drug regimen data in empirical investigations of the mentally retarded has been cited as a major failing in the literature.[63] Failure to establish relative potency in comparative drug studies confounds outcome measures and their findings produce confusion.[64]

Clinical trials of maintenance medication for chronic psychosis sometimes fail to take into account important potential confounding factors. The evaluation of drug therapy for the maintenance phase of treatment of chronic psychotic patients relies on aggregating findings across the 30-odd maintenance or withdrawal studies.[65] In an update of this meta-analysis, 35 controlled studies (n=3500) were summarized and reported a relapse rate of 16 percent for drug-treated patients compared with a rate of 58 percent in placebo-treated patients.[36] However, numerous arguments have been raised questioning the validity of this meta-analysis.[66]

A major confounding problem in withdrawal studies concerns the recognition of a clinical syndrome associated with drug withdrawal.[67] During the first four to six weeks of antipsychotic drug withdrawal, dyskinesias may emerge that previously have been masked by the drug. Sometimes they are accompanied by cholinergic rebound effects manifested as nervousness, tremor, and gastrointestinal and flu-like symptoms and may present a clinical picture indistinguishable from clinical decompensation.[68] Thus, the extent to which the reported relapse rates of the patients withdrawn from active antipsychotic drugs were a function of the short-term withdrawal effect is unknown. Moreover, the drug withdrawal study design is limited by the fact that the experimental variable manipulated is discontinuation of the drug rather than dopaminergic function.[69] Drug withdrawal protocols that require gradual decrements over sufficient time periods for physiological and behavioral readjustment or include a prior drug-relative potency criterion among study inclusion criteria may prevent the confounding of treatment outcome by withdrawal effects.

There are additional, smaller-scale studies with results that create doubts about past findings.[70-77] For example, subgroups of schizophrenics with high premorbid functioning were demonstrated to benefit by drug therapy in one study[78] but not in another.[79] The limitations of studies with small sample sizes have been known for many years.[80] Newer studies of chronic schizophrenia have combined two or more interventions, such as drugs and psychosocial intervention, based on the stress-diathesis model. A detailed review of this major research area is available.[81] In the combined intervention studies, treatment outcome measurement usually is more comprehensive than in the older drug-alone studies, but both types of prospective parallel group studies (trials and drug withdrawal relapse studies) have design limitations. Also, most evident in a current review of the antipsychotic drug efficacy literature is the need for an integrated conceptual approach, in which combined biological and psychosocial treatment interventions are tested in rigorously designed dosing studies at the low end of the dose range to permit analysis of the relationship of drug dosage to treatment outcome in chronic psychiatric disorders.[82]

Safety Methods

Current concerns regarding the safety of marketed neuropharmacologic agents are reflected in the increasing number of case reports of neuroleptic malignant syndrome,[83,84] sudden deaths associated with antipsychotic and antidepressant usage[85,86] acute intoxications involving neuroleptics and lithium[87,88] and the increased risk associated with rapid neuroleptization.[89] Baldessarini[90] has documented and we[5] have replicated the relatively greater daily doses (chlorpromazine-equivalents) associated with the use of high-potency (low-dose) antipsychotic agents such as haloperidol and fluphenazine. This change in prescribing patterns has implications for the prevalence of chronic UDEs (e.g., tardive dyskinesia), assuming a dose-risk relationship. Efforts to revise neuroleptic dosing protocols are especially needed in order to avoid the cycle of excess dosing, leading to unrecognized behavioral toxicity misidentified as symptom worsening, and leading to an increased dose.[91,92] In addition, studies are needed to establish accurate dosing conversions from one antipsychotic to another and to incorporate these dosing rules into clinical practice.[36,93] Safety issues also are related to the appropriate downward dosage titration to avoid acute drug-withdrawal effects.[94-96]

The need for denominator-based UDE rates for marketed medications is a major thrust of pharmacoepidemiology. Inman has summarized the existing approaches to drug safety monitoring that focus on spontaneous reporting mechanisms (numerator-based); he also described the need for routine denominator-based methods.[3]

OBSERVATIONAL STUDY METHODS FOR DRUG SAFETY

Observational studies have been used to evaluate mental and behavioral symptoms suspected of being drug-induced. For example, the prevalence of drug-induced psychiatric symptoms was estimated to occur in 0.6 percent of general hospital admissions according to the Boston Collaborative Drug Surveillance Program. Computerized outpatient drug records of health maintenance organization enrollees were used as the source of a cohort study of anticonvulsant use secondary to tricyclic antidepressant therapy in order to link seizures to antidepressant use.[97] Replication of the low prevalence (<1 in 1000 exposures) in more severely ill and higher-dosed patients would be useful.[98]

In smaller, traditional, prospective clinical studies, medication-related admissions of Israeli psychiatric patients were more prevalent (7.5 percent) than is reported in studies of medical admissions.[99] Using a broader operational definition, Stewart et al. found that one-third of American psychiatric admissions were drug-related.[100] Replicating these findings in a VA setting, one-third of the admissions were attributed to licit drug intoxication, UDEs or compliance, and total drug-related admissions had significantly longer hospitalizations than those with non-drug-related admissions.[101] None of these traditional approaches addresses the problem of the unrecognized drug-induced event, that is, when drug-induced symptoms are considered to be a worsening of the underlying illness.

More recent computerized database approaches to drug UDE questions have taken advantage of the availability of Medicaid drug billing information. For example, the association of beta-blockers with depression was evaluated by observing the significantly higher frequency (23 vs. 10 percent) of tricyclic antidepressants among hypertensive patients taking beta-blockers compared with those taking methyldopa or reserpine. The finding was interpreted as supportive evidence of beta-blocker-induced depression based on a method free of the limitations of previous studies.[102] In a cogent case-control study analysis, the risk of hip fracture in elderly patients was determined to be significantly increased for Medicaid enrollees receiving hypnotic-anxiolytics, tricyclic antidepressants, and antipsychotics with long half-lives. The risk increased in relation to the dosage and the effect persisted after stratifying for dementia.[103]

The unrecognized drug-induced event is a problem of particular concern in neuropharmacology. One attempt to overcome this dilemma is the intensive drug monitoring program operating since 1979 in three German psychiatric hospitals. Randomly selected inpatients are observed by a psychiatrist drug monitor who classifies events according to a specific severity grading system. Severity is determined implicitly by rating the impact of therapy as follows: grade I–no change in medication, grade II–dosage reduction, and grade III–discontinuation of medication. After 32 months of monitoring, the grade III UDE was observed in 15 percent of patients compared with a rate of 9 percent in an organized spontaneous reporting system. The greater incidence reported in the denominator-based system supports the notion that systematic surveillance of UDEs corrects for the under-reporting bias that is believed to occur in spontaneous reporting systems.[104]

Phase III drug trials include routine monitoring of patients for UDEs. One of the most sophisticated psychopharmacologic drug assessment tools developed for this purpose is called SAFTEE and involves a generalized review of body systems. In this approach, a regular quantitative assessment is made of the frequency and severity of symptoms. Statistical analysis of the relationship between variables (e.g., symptom, severity, pattern, time of onset, drug, and dose) makes it possible to identify a UDE by statistical means, rather than by an a priori rule of clinical judgment.[105]

A simplified version of SAFTEE was developed for routine clinical practice using drug or dose changes as a trigger. The feasibility of this approach was established in a pilot test based on acute admissions units and psychogeriatric units of a state hospital population.[106] Future work entails quantifying the drug variable so that dosage can be related to symptom severity. The epidemiologic analysis that employs a statistical measure of the relationship between symptoms (putative UDEs) and drug or dose may be particularly useful in distinguishing drug-induced from illness-based behaviors. In addition, inverse statistical relationships may suggest new indications; for example, a protective effect may be hypothesized when the baseline incidence of a behavioral symptom such as depression is reduced in the presence of a drug not recognized as having an antidepressant effect.

DRUG-INDUCED VERSUS ILLNESS-BASED SYMPTOMS

A major task of the psychopharmacologist in the 1990s is the need to distinguish drug-induced from illness-based symptoms. Behavioral toxicity symptoms[9] such as akathisia[107] and akinesia[108] were the subject of considerable debate before they were accepted as drug-induced phenomena. Pharmacoepidemiologic methods permit the testing of hypotheses regarding the relationship between neuropharmacologic drug, dose, or drug combinations, and behavioral effects (selected psychological and behavioral UDEs, e.g., anxiety, agitation) in real-world patients and with medication prescribed in a customary use fashion.

Statistical Methods for Drug Decision-Making in Individual Patients and Specific Subgroups

Sackett listed five biases that may be operating when the clinician infers a causal association between a change in the patient's behavior and the introduction of a medication. These biases are spontaneous remission, regression effect, placebo effect, expectancy effect, and the obsequiousness bias.[109] Some of these problems can be minimized by following the N of 1 study method. The study is designed to evaluate the effect of a medication in a single subject (on active drug/on placebo in a randomized, double-blind design) in the customary clinical setting.[110,111] This approach can be a low-cost yet rigorous evaluation preliminary to the clinical trial for the assessment of marketed drugs for unlabeled indications. For example, the method could be useful in determining the effectiveness of carbamazepine in patients with treatment-resistant affective disorder and propranolol in treatment-resistant violent patients.

The effectiveness of a neuropharmacologic agent in specific subpopulations such as pregnant women, the elderly, and those with co-morbid conditions can be determined by epidemiologic drug assessments. Aggregate data from the longitudinal monitoring of specific subpopulations can be used to make treatment decisions for these subgroups. For example, for the depressed patient with evidence of delayed cardiac conduction time, the benefit-to-risk ratio may favor the use of electroconvulsive therapy over tricyclic antidepressant drug therapy. The decision criteria would require a longitudinal record of quantitatively recorded symptom severity, and a history of past medication exposure to determine if there were adequate trials of nontricyclic alternatives.

Despite intensive efforts of the past decade to improve diagnostic classification with the DSM-III, therapeutic choice and outcome are still poorly predicted by symptomatology except for homogeneous diagnostic categories. As an alternative to denominator-based classification, Thomsen developed an inferential classification using Bayes' formula with correction for redundancy. For example, he calculated correlations of 0.57 between two symptom patterns and low-dose antipsychotic therapy.[112] Refining his approach would involve the addition of other clinical variables such as chronicity (prior days hospitalized), employment history, and social functioning history, which previous studies have demonstrated to predict outcome.[34]

Policy Implications

There are a number of current controversies involving the use of marketed medications in treating psychiatric patients. Since the early 1970s, the right of the involuntarily committed psychotic patient to refuse nonemergency drug treatment has been developing through judicial, legislative, and regulatory decisions.[113-116] The potential impact of these decisions on institutional psychiatric practice, where antipsychotic medication is the mainstay of treatment in more than 140 000 state hospitalized patients, is great.

Reimbursement policies for psychiatric illness are being debated and numerous prospective payment schemes are under investigation. Treatments and procedures have been proposed and disputed as alternatives to the use of diagnostic categories to predict length of stay.[117] Each of these schemes has implications that extend to drug treatment variables such as drug and dose. Drug regimens that rapidly resolve symptoms and permit clinical management in the least costly environment are consistent with this model. However, this approach would have a negative impact on specific subgroups such as the low functioning, treatment-resistant chronic patient. The recent U.S. marketing of clozapine, an atypical antipsychotic for treatment-resistant chronic schizophrenia, poses important public fiscal policy questions because its financial cost is 20 times greater than currently used antipsychotic agents.[118] Policy decisions must strike a balance between concerns about equal access to the treatment and appropriateness for a given individual as well as long-term cost effectiveness and safety.

The consensus development conference is a recent activity acknowledging the underlying social and political dimensions of science and technology. The conference aims to bring together all parties with vested interests as a means of resolving clinical practice dilemmas. To the extent that each interest group can evaluate the meaningfulness of the scientific literature on the efficacy and safety of somatic and psychotherapeutic interventions as well as the short- and long-term consequences of alternative approaches, the conference can be useful in framing the individual clinical decision within the larger societal context. In psychiatry, electroconvulsive therapy[119] and drug treatment of mood disorders[120] have been subjected to the consensus process. Two controversial drug-related topics that might benefit from this review are antipsychotic drug effectiveness in the nonemergency treatment of an involuntarily committed patient who refuses drug therapy, and the management of the long-term patient by alternative treatment modalities aimed at minimizing the risk of tardive dyskinesia.

Summary

In this chapter, knowledge of drug usage in psychiatric patients was reviewed according to the organizing and analyzing principles of epidemiology. This approach is proposed as a means of increasing the validity and appropriate application of information in the clinical science of neuropharmacology.

References

1. Rector TS. Pharmacoepidemiology: emerging roles for pharmacists (letter). *Am J Hosp Pharm* 1985;42:778,783.

2. Lawson DH. Pharmacoepidemiology: a new discipline. *Br Med J* 1984; 289:940-1.

3. Inman WHW, ed. Monitoring for drug safety. 1st ed. Philadelphia: JB Lippincott, 1980.

4. Ingman SR, Lawson IR, Pierpaoli PG, et al. A survey of the prescribing and administration of drugs in a long-term care institution for the elderly. *J Am Geriatr Soc* 1975;23:309-16.

5. Zito JM, Craig TJ, Wanderling J, Siegel C. Drug epidemiology in a cohort of hospitalized schizophrenic patients. *Am J Psychiatry* 1987;144:778-82.

6. McKenna PJ, Kane JM, Parrish K. Psychotic syndromes in epilepsy. *Am J Psychiatry* 1985;142:895-904.

7. Post RM, Uhde TW, Roy-Byrne PP, Joffe RT. Antidepressant effects of carbamazepine. *Am J Psychiatry* 1986;*143*:29-34.

8. DiMascio A. Behavioral toxicity. In: DiMascio A, Shader R. Clinical handbook of psychopharmacology. 1st ed. New York: Science House, 1970.

9. Cole JO. Behavioral toxicity. In: Uhr L, Miller JG, eds. Drugs and behavior. 1st ed. New York: John Wiley and Sons, 1960.

10. VanPutten T, Marder SR. Behavioral toxicity of antipsychotic drugs. *J Clin Psychiatry* 1987;*48*(suppl):13-9.

11. Davis JM. Antipsychotic drugs. In: Kaplan HI, Sadock BJ, eds. Comprehensive textbook of psychiatry. 5th ed. New York: Williams & Wilkins, 1989:1620.

12. Eisendrath SJ, Sweeney MA. Toxic neuropsychiatric effects of digoxin at therapeutic serum concentrations. *Am J Psychiatry* 1987;*144*:506-7.

13. Wamboldt FS, Jefferson JW, Wamboldt MZ. Digitalis intoxication misdiagnosed as depression by primary care physicians. *Am J Psychiatry* 1986;*143*:219-21.

14. Hullett FJ, Potkin SG, Levy AB, et al. Depression associated with nifedipine-induced calcium channel blockade. *Am J Psychiatry* 1988;*145*:1277-9.

15. Billings RF, Stein MB. Depression associated with ranitidine. *Am J Psychiatry* 1986; *143*:915-6.

16. Goodwin FK, Bunney WE. Depressions following reserpine: a reevaluation. *Semin Psychiatry* 1971;*3*:435-48.

17. Waal-Manning HJ. Which beta-blocker? *Drugs* 1976;*12*:412-41.

18. Parker WA. Propranolol-induced depression and psychosis. *Clin Pharm* 1985;*4*:214-8.

19. Pollack MH, Rosenbaum JF, Cassem NH. Propranolol and depression revisited: three cases and a review. *J Nerv Ment Dis* 1985;*173*:118-9.

20. Nitter L, Haraldsson A, Holck P, et al. The effect of trimipramine on the healing of peptic ulcer. A double blind study. *Scand J Gastroenterol* 1977;*12*:39-41.

21. Weiner H. Psychobiology and human disease. 1st ed. New York: Elsevier, 1977.

22. Blackman DE, Sanger DJ, eds. Contemporary research in behavioral pharmacology. New York: Plenum Press, 1978.

23. Strain JJ, Taintor Z. Consultation-liaison psychiatry. In: Kaplan HI, Sadock BJ, eds. Comprehensive textbook of psychiatry. 5th ed. New York: Williams & Wilkins, 1989:1278.

24. Lieff JD. Computer applications in psychiatry. Washington, DC: American Psychiatric Association, 1987:135-248.

25. Feinstein AR. Clinical biostatistics. II. Statistics versus science in the design of experiments. *Clin Pharmacol Ther* 1970;*11*:282-92.

26. Freed CR, Gal J, Manchester DK. Dosage of phenytoin during pregnancy. *JAMA* 1985; *253*:2833-4.

27. Overall JE, Faillace LA, Rhoades HM, et al. Computer-based monitoring of clinical care in a public psychiatric hospital. *Hosp Commun Psychiatry* 1987; *38*:381-6.

28. Allgulander C. Psychoactive drug use in a general population sample, Sweden: correlates with perceived health, psychiatric diagnoses, and mortality in an automated record-linkage study. *Am J Public Health* 1989;*79*:1006-10.

29. Laska EM, Siegel C, Simpson G. Automated review system for orders of psychotropic drugs. *Arch Gen Psychiatry* 1980;*37*:824-7.

30. Siegel C, Alexander MJ. Acceptance and impact of the computer in clinical decisions. *Hosp Commun Psychiatry* 1984;35:773-5.

31. Craig TJ, Mehta RM. Clinician-computer interaction: automated review of psychotropic drugs. *Am J Psychiatry* 1984;141:267-70.

32. Zito JM, Craig TJ, Wanderling J, et al. Pharmacotherapy of the hospitalized young adult schizophrenic patient. *Compr Psychiatry* 1988;29:379-86.

33. Schwartz CC, Myers JK, Astrachan BM. Concordance of multiple assessments of the outcome of schizophrenia. *Arch Gen Psychiatry* 1975;32:1221-7.

34. Strauss JS, Carpenter WT. The prediction of outcome in schizophrenia. *Arch Gen Psychiatry* 1974;31:37-42.

35. Baldessarini RJ, Cohen BM, Teicher MH. Significance of neuroleptic dose and plasma level in the pharmacological treatment of psychosis. *Arch Gen Psychiatry* 1988;45:79-91.

36. Davis JM, Andriukaitis S. The natural course of schizophrenia and effective maintenance drug treatment. *J Clin Psychopharmacol* 1986;6:2S-10S.

37. Baldessarini RJ. Drugs and the treatment of psychiatric disorder. In: Gilman AG, Goodman LS, Rall TW, Murad F. Goodman and Gilman's the pharmacological basis of therapeutics. 7th ed. New York: Macmillan, 1985:410.

38. Cohen BM. Neuroleptic dosing in the treatment of acute psychosis: how much do we really know? *Psychopharmacol Ser* 1988;5:45-61.

39. Tardive dyskinesia. Task force report 18. Washington, DC: American Psychiatric Association, 1980.

40. Hargreaves WA, Zachary R, LeGoullon M, et al. Neuroleptic dose: a statistical model for analyzing historical trends. *J Psychiatr Res* 1987;21:199-214.

41. Overall JE, Garza-Trevino E, Rhoades HM, et al. Justifying neuroleptic drug treatment. *Hosp Commun Psychiatry* 1989;40:749-51.

42. Muijen M, Silverstone T. A comparative hospital survey of psychotropic drug prescribing. *Br J Psychiatry* 1987;150:501-4.

43. Clark AF, Holden NL. The persistence of prescribing habits: a survey and follow-up of prescribing to chronic hospital in-patients. *Br J Psychiatry* 1987;150:88-91.

44. Williams P, Murray J, Clare A. A longitudinal study of psychotropic drug prescription. *Psychol Med* 1982;12:201-6.

45. Glaser BA, Morreau LE. Effects of interdisciplinary team review on the use of antipsychotic agents with severely and profoundly mentally retarded persons. *Am J Ment Defic* 1986;90:371-9.

46. Crane GE. Clinical psychopharmacology in its twentieth year. *Science* 1973;181:124-8.

47. Carpenter WT, Heinrichs DW, Hanlon TE. Methodologic standards for treatment outcome in schizophrenia. *Am J Psychiatry* 1981;138:465-71.

48. Barreira PJ, Vogel W. The clinical vs. research paradox in psychopharmacological research. *Psychiatry Res* 1988;25:109-10.

49. Woggon B. Unsolved problems in the pharmacotherapy of depression. *Psychopharmacol Series* 1988;5:159-65.

50. Kales A, Kales JD. Shortcomings in the evaluation and promotion of hypnotic drugs. *N Engl J Med* 1975;293:826-7.

51. Schou M. Lithium prophylaxis: myths and realities. *Am J Psychiatry* 1989; 146:573-6.

52. Nelson C. The National Ambulatory Medical Care Survey, United States: 1975-81 and 1985 trends. Vital and Health Statistics, Series 13, #93, DHHS publ no (PHS) 88-1754. Washington, DC: U.S. Government Printing Office, 1988.

53. Hohmann AA, Larson DB, Thompson JW, et al. Psychotropic medication prescription in U.S. ambulatory medical care. *DICP Ann Pharmacother*, 1990 (in press).

54. Hohmann AA. Gender bias in psychotropic drug prescribing in primary care. *Med Care* 1989;*27*:478-90.

55. Avorn J, Dreyer P, Connelly K, et al. Use of psychoactive medication and the quality of care in rest homes. *N Engl J Med* 1989;*320*:227-32.

56. Cole JO, Klerman GL, Goldberg SC, et al. Phenothiazine treatment in acute schizophrenia. *Arch Gen Psychiatry* 1964;*10*:246-61.

57. Casey JF, Bennett IF, Lindley CJ, et al. Drug therapy in schizophrenia. *Arch Gen Psychiatry* 1960;*2*:210-9.

58. Carpenter WT, Heinrichs DW, Alphs LD. Treatment of negative schizophrenia. *Schizophrenia Bull* 1985;*11*:440-56.

59. Carpenter WT, Stephens JH, Rey AC, et al. Early intervention vs. continuous pharmacotherapy of schizophrenia. *Psychopharmacol Bull* 1982;*18*:21-3.

60. Kane JM. Dosage reduction strategies in the long-term treatment of schizophrenia. In: Kane JM, ed. Drug maintenance strategies in schizophrenia. Washington, DC: American Psychiatric Press, 1984:2-11.

61. Arana GW, Ornsteen ML, Kanter F, et al. The use of benzodiazepines for psychotic disorders: a literature review and preliminary clinical findings. *Psychopharmacol Bull* 1986; *22*:77-87.

62. Wolkowitz OM, Pickar D, Doran AR, et al. Combination alprazolam-neuroleptic treatment of the positive and negative symptoms of schizophrenia. *Am J Psychiatry* 1986; *143*:85-7.

63. Agran M, Moore S, Martin JE. Research in mental retardation: underreporting of medication information. *Res Dev Disabil* 1988;*9*:351-7.

64. McKane JB, Robinson DT, Wiles DH, et al. Haloperidol decanoate v. fluphenazine decanoate as maintenance therapy in chronic schizophrenic in-patients. *Br J Psychiatry* 1987;*151*:333-6.

65. Davis JM. Overview: maintenance therapy in psychiatry: I. Schizophrenia *Am J Psychiatry* 1975;*132*:1237-45.

66. Tobias LL, MacDonald ML. Withdrawal of maintenance drugs with long-term hospitalized patients: a critical review. *Psychol Bull* 1974;*81*:107-25.

67. Gardos G, Cole JO, Tarsy D. Withdrawal syndromes associated with antipsychotic drugs. *Am J Psychiatry* 1978;*135*:1321-4.

68. Lieberman J. Cholinergic rebound in neuroleptic withdrawal syndromes. *Psychosomatics* 1981;*22*:253-4.

69. Levine J, Schooler NR, Severe J, et al. Discontinuation of oral and depot fluphenazine in schizophrenic patients after one year of continuous medication: a controlled study. In: Cattabeni F, Racagni G, Spano PF, Costa E, eds. Long-term effects of neuroleptics. New York: Raven Press, 1980:483-93.

70. Leff JP, Wing JK. Trial of maintenance therapy in schizophrenia. *Br Med J* 1971;*3*:559-604.

71. Rappaport M, Hopkins HK, Hall K, et al. Are there schizophrenics for whom drugs may be unnecessary or contraindicated? *Int Pharmacopsychiatry* 1978;*13*:100-11.

72. Rosen B, Engelhardt DL. The hospitalization proneness scale as a predictor of response to phenothiazine treatment. II. Delay of psychiatric hospitalization. *J Nerv Ment Dis* 1971;*152*:405-11.

73. Saenger G. Patterns of change among "treated" and "untreated" patients seen in psychiatric community mental health clinics. *J Nerv Ment Dis* 1970;*150*:37-50.

74. Carpenter WT, McGlashan TH, Strauss JS. The treatment of acute schizophrenia without drugs: an investigation of some current assumptions. *Am J Psychiatry* 1977;*134*:14-20.

75. Paul GL, Lentz RJ. Psychosocial treatment of chronic mental patients: milieu vs. social-learning programs. Cambridge, MA: Harvard University Press, 1977.

76. Mosher LR, Menn A, Matthews SM. Soteria: evaluation of a home-based treatment for schizophrenia. *Am J Orthopsychiatry* 1975;*45*:455-67.

77. Esterson A, Cooper DG, Laing RD. Results of family-orientated therapy with hospitalized schizophrenics. *Br Med J* 1965;*2*:1462-5.

78. Klein DF, Rosen B. Premorbid asocial adjustment and response to phenothiazine treatment among schizophrenic outpatients. *Arch Gen Psychiatry* 1973;*29*:480-5.

79. Goldstein MJ, Rodnick EH, Evans JR, et al. Drug and family therapy in the aftercare of acute schizophrenic outpatients. *Arch Gen Psychiatry* 1978;*35*:1169-77.

80. Peto R, Pike MC, Armitage P, et al. Design and analysis of randomized clinical trials requiring prolonged observation of each patient. I. Introduction and design. *Br J Cancer* 1976;*34*:585-612.

81. Schooler NR, Hogarty GE. Medication and psychosocial strategies in the treatment of schizophrenia. In: Meltzer HY, ed. Psychopharmacology: the third generation of progress. New York: Raven Press, 1987:1111-9.

82. Karasu TB. Psychotherapy and pharmacotherapy: toward an integrative model. *Am J Psychiatry* 1982;*139*:1102-13.

83. Levenson JL. Neuroleptic malignant syndrome. *Am J Psychiatry* 1985; *142*:1137-45.

84. Steinberg DE. Neuroleptic malignant syndrome: the pendulum swings (editorial). *Am J Psychiatry* 1986;*143*:1273-5.

85. Craig TJ. Medication use and deaths attributed to asphyxia among psychiatric patients. *Am J Psychiatry* 1980;*137*:1366-73.

86. Zugibe FT. Sudden death related to the use of psychotropic drugs. In: Wecht CH, ed. Legal medicine. Philadelphia: WB Saunders, 1980:75-90.

87. Goldney RD, Spence ND. Safety of the combination of lithium and neuroleptic drugs. *Am J Psychiatry* 1986;*143*:882-4.

88. Miller F, Menninger J. Correlation of neuroleptic dose and neurotoxicity in patients given lithium and neuroleptic. *Hosp Commun Psychiatry* 1987;*38*:1219-21.

89. Bollini P, Andreani A, Colombo F, et al. High-dose neuroleptics: uncontrolled clinical practice confirms clinical trials. *Br J Psychiatry* 1984;*144*:25-7.

90. Baldessarini RJ, Katz B, Cotton P. Dissimilar dosing with high-potency and low-potency neuroleptics. *Am J Psychiatry* 1984;*141*:748-52.

91. Osser D. A systematic approach to pharmacotherapy in patients with neuroleptic-resistant psychoses. *Hosp Commun Psychiatry* 1989;*40*:921-7.

92. Weiden PJ, Mann JJ, Haas G, et al. Clinical nonrecognition of neuroleptic-induced movement disorders: a cautionary study. *Am J Psychiatry* 1987;144:1148-53.

93. Kane JM, Woerner M, Sarantakos S. Depot neuroleptics: a comparative review of standard, intermediate, and low-dose regimens. *J Clin Psychiatry* 1986; 47(suppl):30-3.

94. McMahon T. Anti-depressant and antipsychotic withdrawal syndromes (abstract). *Neurobehav Toxicol Teratol* 1985;7:203.

95. Noyes R, Clancy J, Coryell WH, et al. A withdrawal syndrome after abrupt discontinuation of alprazolam. *Am J Psychiatry* 1985;142:114-6.

96. Zito JM, ed. Psychotherapeutic drug manual. New York: New York State Office of Mental Health, 1989:1-6.

97. Danielson DA, Porter JB, Lawson DH, et al. Drug associated psychiatric disturbances in medical inpatients. *Psychopharmacology* 1981;74:105-8.

98. Jick H, Dinan BJ, Hunter JR, Stergachis A, et al. Tricyclic antidepressants and convulsions. *J Clin Psychopharmacol* 1983;3:182-5.

99. Hermesh H, Shalev A, Munitz H. Contribution of adverse drug reaction to admission rates in an acute psychiatric ward. *Acta Psychiatr Scand* 1985;72:104-10.

100. Stewart RB, Springer PK, Adams JE. Drug-related admissions to an inpatient psychiatric unit. *Am J Psychiatry* 1980;137:1093-5.

101. Salem RB, Keane TM, Williams JG. Drug-related admissions to a Veterans Administration Psychiatric Unit. *Drug Intell Clin Pharm* 1987;21:741-7.

102. Avorn J, Everitt DE, Weiss S. Increased antidepressant use in patients prescribed beta-blockers. *JAMA* 1986;255:357-60.

103. Ray WA, Griffin MR, Schaffner W, et al. Psychotropic drug use and the risk of hip fracture. *N Engl J Med* 1987;316:363-9.

104. Schmidt LG, Grohmann R, Helmchen H. Adverse drug reactions. *Acta Psychiatr Scand* 1984;70:77-89.

105. Systematic Assessment for Treatment Emergent Events (SAFTEE-SI). Rockville, MD: NIMH, Pharmacologic and Somatic Treatments, Research Branch.

106. Zito JM, Craig TJ, Wanderling JA, et al. SAFTEE-EPI: a pilot study of a computerized adverse drug reaction monitoring system. *Pharmacoepidemiol News* 1986;2(1/2):6.

107. Van Putten T. The many faces of akathisia. *Compr Psychiatry* 1975;16:43-7.

108. Rifkin A, Quitkin F, Klein DF. Akinesia. *Arch Gen Psychiatry* 1975;32:672-4.

109. Sackett DL. Bias in analytic research. *J Chronic Dis* 1979;32:51-63.

110. Guyatt G, Sackett D, Taylor DW, et al. Determining optimal therapy—randomized trials in individual patients. *N Engl J Med* 1986;314:889-92.

111. Porta MS. The search for more clinically meaningful research designs: single patient randomized clinical trials. *J Gen Intern Med* 1986;1:418-9.

112. Thomsen IS. Analysis of syndromes using Bayes's formula. *Acta Psychiatr Scand* 1984;69:143-50.

113 Tancredi L. The rights of mental patients: weighing the interests. *J Health Polit Policy Law* 1980;5:199-204.

114. Brooks AD. The right to refuse antipsychotic medications: law and policy. *Rutgers Law Rev* 1987;39:339-76.

115. Appelbaum PS. The right to refuse treatment with antipsychotic medications: retrospect and prospect. *Am J Psychiatry* 1988;145:413-9.

116. Zito JM, Haimowitz S, Wanderling J, et al. One year under *Rivers*: drug refusal in a New York state psychiatric facility. *Int J Law Psychiatry* 1989;12:295-306.

117. Siegel CS, Alexander MJ, Goodman AB. Alternatives to DRGs: research issues. *Psychiatry Q* 1985;57:203-16.

118. Kane J, Honigfeld G, Singer J, et al. Clozapine for the treatment resistant schizophrenic. *Arch Gen Psychiatry* 1988;45:789-96.

119. Electroconvulsive therapy, consensus conference. *JAMA* 1985;254:2103-8.

120. Consensus Development Panel. Mood disorders: pharmacologic prevention of recurrences. *Am J Psychiatry* 1985;142:469-76.

15

Drug Safety, Pharmacoepidemiology, and Regulatory Decision Making

Robert C. Nelson

Abstract

The safety of risk assessment of a pharmacotherapeutic agent begins early in its development and continues throughout its use cycle. The practice of pharmacoepidemiology is the art of using the sciences and the tools of science to generate information about pharmaceutical outcomes, including associated risks, in the postmarketing environment. A pharmacoepidemiologist must be capable of functioning with a matrix constructed of three components: a knowledge base, a conceptual framework, and an interpretive framework. From this perspective one can establish surveillance schemes, or understand a posed research question, select strategies, apply methodologies, and interpret the results of purposeful investigations. When conveyed to the risk manager, appropriately interpreted results of a properly conducted risk assessment can be used in regulatory decision making. Eight case studies are presented as pragmatic examples of this approach.

Therapeutic intervention with modern pharmaceutical agents is a mainstay of medical practice. The multiple levels of required premarket testing are very effective in identifying and eliminating potential drugs that are markedly toxic. However, every known physiologically active exogenous agent also possesses an adverse consequence profile, the components of which can remain hidden until the drug is being marketed and used in a broader population than experienced in the preapproval trials. This chapter provides an introductory view of the way pharmacoepidemiologic principles are conceptualized and have been applied to drug and biologic product postmarketing safety issues within the regulatory environment of the FDA.

A set of conceptual and methodologic approaches is presented, some that were developed in an effort to conduct meaningful epidemiologic research at the FDA. To illustrate these approaches, I have included many unpublished but public citations. The reader is encouraged to review these public citations, which are available through a Freedom of Information Act request, and to consult the references included in the other chapters or the standard references in pharmacoepidemiology.

This chapter proposes a functional framework for pharmacoepidemiology and proceeds to practical application. The latter is a set of examples in which pharmacoepidemiologic approaches were used to address drug safety concerns. A distinction is made between the function of risk assessment and decision-making risk management within the FDA.

Background

The safety or risk assessment of a pharmacotherapeutic agent is a complex task, requiring a multidisciplinary synthesis of information. This synthesis should take place early in the development of the agent and continue throughout its use cycle. Conventionally, postmarketing risk assessment for pharmaceutical agents is limited to the identification of iatrogenic morbidity (the adverse consequences of legitimate pharmacotherapy). However, given that our modern society is afflicted with pharmacophilia, a complete assessment also must include the unintended drug effects (UDEs) associated with the nonmedical use of legal drugs.

Adverse drug experience* is defined in U.S. federal regulation 21 CFR (Code of Federal Regulations) 314.80 as

> any adverse event associated with the use of a drug in humans, whether or not considered drug related, including the following: an adverse event occurring in the course of the use of a drug product in professional practice; an adverse event occurring from drug overdose whether accidental or intentional; an adverse event occurring from drug abuse; an adverse event occurring from drug withdrawal; and any significant failure of expected pharmacological action.

Figure 1 displays a conceptual framework for the UDEs of drug use intentionally consumed for therapy. UDEs may be direct or mediated by an interaction with an-

*For the purpose of uniformity, UDE is used throughout.

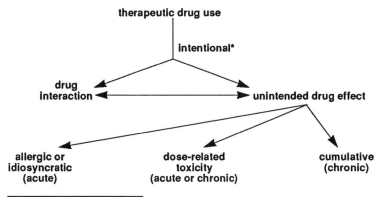

Figure 1
Relationship Between Therapeutic Drug Use and Adverse Outcomes

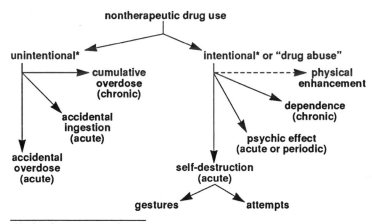

Figure 2
Relationship Between Nontherapeutic Drug Use and Adverse Outcomes

other factor. The latter factors include other concomitant medications, specific foods, the presence or absence of food, age, gender, genetics, and comorbid conditions. UDEs directly attributable to the administration of a pharmacotherapeutic agent may manifest acutely as allergic or idiosyncratic reactions, as dose-related toxicities to organ systems, or chronically due to accumulation in the body of the agent or its metabolites.

A more complex framework for the consequences of nontherapeutic drug use, which is divided as to the motive of consumption (i.e., unintentional or intentional consumption of the nontherapeutic dose of the drug) is displayed in Figure 2. Unintentional nonmedical consumption includes the erroneous acute ingestion of a drug, the chronic ingestion of an excessive amount, or the accidental acute poisoning episode. The intentional nontherapeutic ingestion of a drug is an abuse situation. The intentional ingestion for self-destruction, whether a suicide gesture or attempt, is included here as a component of a drug's safety profile. The capacity for a drug to produce psychic effects and/or induce psychologic dependence, or to lead to physical dependence are all indicative of a drug's abuse potential and are variables to be considered in risk assessment. This component of a drug's safety profile is particularly pertinent for psychoactive drugs.

The intentional consumption in a nontherapeutic mode model has recently undergone a revision to include use for "physical enhancement." The anabolic steroids and, most recently, human growth hormone are two such agents. All UDEs associated with the use of legal pharmaceuticals fall within the regulatory mandate of the FDA.

The potential limitations of the UDE data obtained from clinical trials have been discussed extensively in the literature,[1,2] and are addressed by Rogers in Chapter 5. The UDE rates derived from clinical trial data are reported to be more conservative than those derived from formal Phase IV studies for the more common and generally less serious reactions and usually are not useful for low incidence reactions.[3] However, these clinical trial data are used in the FDA-approved final printed labeling (i.e., the package insert), which accompanies the drug product to the healthcare marketplace. All industry-generated advertising of the product, whether verbal (i.e., through detailmen) or written, must conform to approved labeling. Because most practicing physicians learn about new drug products from the manufacturer, the importance of the labeling information is evident. The labeling can be revised when new UDEs are detected in the postmarketing arena.

Prescription drug labeling may lag behind the practice of medicine for beneficial new events (i.e., indications) because inclusion is contingent upon demonstration by the drug's sponsor of substantial evidence of both safety and efficacy. The labeling usually is more current for new UDEs. That is not to say that the addition of a UDE to a product label is easy and straightforward. The detection of a UDE and its attribution to a drug product is more difficult in the postmarketing era than during premarketing. Confounders abound in the open or uncontrolled environment. A UDE may be due to the drug product, the indicated underlying disorders, a spontaneously generated disorder, irrational prescribing, a patient compliance problem, an interaction with food or another drug product, or an individual variation. Clearly, the relationship between a drug and a UDE often appears to be casual rather than causal.

The preceding chapters have explained the breadth and the scope of pharmacoepidemiology, and have introduced the reader to theory, algorithms, and the wide variety of data sources that can or could be tapped for study. However, the conversion of data into information, and the proper weighting of abstract knowledge into a decision-making equation concerning the safety of a pharmacotherapeutic agent, currently defy predictive modeling. Skill, logic, a healthy dose of ingenuity, and a degree of pragmatism are required, especially if one is forced to function within a regulatory environment with its inherent timelines. Safety issues are not absolute; they must be evaluated in light of competing risks, benefits associated with the drug's approved indication(s), and competing benefits from other forms of therapy.

FDA's Regulatory Mandate

The FDA shares with the product manufacturer the responsibility for the initial and continual assessment of drug safety. The FDA's authority to affect the conditions of marketing for drugs and biologic products comes from the Food, Drug and Cosmetic Act (1938) as amended, the Public Health Service Act (1904) as amended, and Section 201 of the Controlled Substances Act (1971), the CSA. FDA's regulatory role is placed in the proper perspective when one understands that the FDA does not approve drugs or biologics. Rather, these existing U.S. statutes and regulations provide the basic requirements for determining the safety and efficacy of new drug products. The process includes the development of safety and efficacy data during the investigational new drug (IND) phase, and the submission of these data in support of a marketing application (the new drug application, NDA). The FDA approves a drug product or a biologic for a specific indication if adequate and well-controlled clinical trials support its safety and efficacy for the specific indication.

The Division of Epidemiology and Surveillance (DES) within the Center for Drug Evaluation and Research (CDER) is FDA's functional pharmacoepidemiology unit, i.e., the risk assessors. This Division houses the Spontaneous Reporting System (SRS), manages the cooperative agreements with extramural sources for epidemiologic data, and employs epidemiologists and other health professionals to assess drug safety in the postmarketing arena. Interaction with the regulatory component of CDER is vital. The new drug product review division within the Office of Drug Evaluation I (ODE I) and the Office of Drug Evaluation II (ODE II) are the functional regulatory decision-making units, that is, the risk managers.

In addition to informal communication pathways, the main forum for interaction is the monthly safety conference. Key individuals of the DES staff, coordinated by the epidemiology team leaders, meet separately with each of the nine drug product review divisions to discuss issues of safety. The three general areas for discussion at these safety conferences are any important new UDE signals received through the SRS, consultations from or areas of regulatory concern to the ODE I/II divisions, and recent literature reports and relevant epidemiologic studies. Normally, an individual from DES, referred to as a reports evaluator, identifies and researches a new UDE, which, if of substance, is then referred to as a signal. The strength of this signal is contingent upon both the quantity and quality of the SRS reports. Usually, two or three well-documented reports make up the minimal data set. In a rare case, causality may be attributable from a single well-documented rechallenged report.[4] The data supporting this new signal then are presented to the regulatory divisions either for their information or as an action item depending on the strength of the case. The DES staff, as advisors and consultants to ODE I and II, prepare epidemiologic reports on areas of regulatory concern and present these results at the safety conferences. The goal is, whenever possible, to narrow the regulatory decision gap with a well-conducted safety assessment. Although it is generally recognized that the most concentrated postmarketing effort should be placed on the detection and verification of new, unexpected, and serious reports, they compose only a small portion of the total amount of safety and relative safety issues that arise.

The FDA must address all the safety issues brought to its attention and make a decision as to the action necessary; the actual research questions are varied in nature and importance. High-quality and accessible data sources used by well-skilled risk evaluators increase the likelihood of reliable and timely risk assessments.

When a new drug (hereafter referred to as a drug product) enters the FDA review process, it receives a priority designation based on its chemical uniqueness and a prediction of its eventual medical utility (see Chapter 4). In an ideal situation, the DES epidemiology staff monitors the inhouse progress of the NDA. When the situation warrants, formal Phase IV programs should be planned by the ODE staff, with advice from the DES staff, as early in the drug development process as possible. The DES staff obtain advanced information (usually a draft of the Summary Basis of Approval, SBA) on the new molecular entities and other designated drug products of special concern from the reviewing division before they are marketed, so that an efficient and effective postmarketing surveillance effort can be set in place. If residual concerns about safety remain at the potential approval point, a formal, Phase IV safety study can be negotiated with the manufacturer. In either case, the postmarketing risk assessor requires full knowledge of the new drug product which includes the drug's pharmacokinetic profile, the UDE profile seen in the Phase III clinical trials, data from foreign marketing experience, and knowledge of the UDE profile of pharmacologically similar marketed drugs, in order to increase the probability of predicting the problems that may occur in the marketplace. The ideal goal of postmarketing surveillance is to bring the time of discovery of a major proportion of new information as close to the time of marketing of the new drug as possible.[5]

Functional Frameworks

Pharmacoepidemiology, an epidemiologic specialty, requires a synthesis of multidisciplinary information, and its practice is the use of the sciences and the tools of science to generate information about pharmaceutical outcomes. In an enlargement upon this theme, the practice of pharmacoepidemiology in a regulatory environment is the art of using the sciences and the tools of science to generate information that is then used as part of the basis for regulatory decisions that impact the public health by their effect on drug therapy.

A pharmacoepidemiologist must be capable of functioning with a matrix constructed of three distinct frameworks: a knowledge framework made up of the information on drugs and disease states, as well as clinical and general medical care principles; a conceptual framework for understanding, orientation, and direction, which includes the epidemiologic principles and methodologies; an interpretive framework that relies heavily on logic and the elimination of alternative explanations. Knowledge and understanding of the availability and validity of data sources are required across all parts of the matrix.

The knowledge framework is based firmly when the pharmacoepidemiologist has obtained a sense of understanding of the research question from the relevant medical and scientific disciplines involved. An epidemiologist should not begin any form of information syntheses until this understanding is obtained. One must know when, why, and under what circumstances a drug is actually used. A full understanding of the pharmacology, pharmacodynamics, and pharmacokinetics of both the drug of concern and the other members of its pharmacologic and/or therapeutic class is required. A full understanding of the pathological process for which the drug is indicated is also necessary.

The conceptual framework will be discussed most extensively in this section. When referring to the UDEs of drug use, one can envision a five-segment continuum in the pharmacoepidemiologic approach: (1) the detection of an event (often referred to as a signal or signalling), (2) generation of a hypothesis, (3) description, (4) assessment of the strength of an association, and (5) testing of a hypothesis.

These segments appear in Table 1, with the latter two segments distinguished by the validity of underlying statistical assumptions. The conceptual framework for pharmacoepidemiologic techniques as presented in Table 1 has been modified from the frameworks developed by Jones.[5,6] This framework allows one to organize the many approaches and data sources available for the study of drug effects. The two main conceptual categories, ascertainment by drug and by event, were originally described by Finney,[7] but are presented here in a revised and modified form. The strategies in each category are those in current use and are not exhaustive listings.

These two conceptual categories differ in directionality, in the time lapse until functional, and in their usage. Each category contains a number of strategies or methods employed either in a surveillance mode or in addressing a specific research question. The ascertainment by drug category begins with the drug, and then identifies and evaluates the adverse pharmaceutical outcomes. This addresses the question: What UDEs are associated with this drug? In a larger sense, this is not limited just to UDEs, but includes new beneficial ones. This concept is similar to that which underlies the practice of clinical epidemiology: the evaluation of the consequences of therapeutic intervention. The ascertainment by drug category has three components that vary in function: monitoring, numerator analysis across events, and the cohort study design. The first two do not have the advantage of controls.

The primary surveillance mode, i.e., monitoring, is practiced through the use of the FDA-SRS and the medical literature. In general, this large-scale operation is used to detect new events, or signals. When the signal is an unexpected one from the perspective of biologic plausibility, or one for which the interpretation is controversial, additional confirmation is necessary, and a hypothesis is generated. A numerator analysis (across events without denominators, and without controls) can present a qualitative and a quasiquantitative description of a drug's safety profile. For example, reported UDEs can be plotted across physiologic body systems, then at a finer level, across diagnostic terms within a body system. The comparison of these profiles among drugs within a pharmacologic class often is informative and may lead to new signals and/or new hypotheses. The formally designed prospective cohort study with a control group can be used to assess the strength of an association or as a formal test of a hypothesis.

A reversal of directionality yields ascertainment by event. This addresses the question: What are the pharmaceutical risk factors for this UDE? The four methods

Table 1
Conceptual Framework for Pharmacoepidemiologic Techniques

	Detection or Signaling	Hypothesis Generation	Description	Strength of Association	Hypothesis Testing
Ascertainment by drug					
A: monitoring (without controls)	A-1 yes	A-2 yes	A-3 no	A-4 no	A-5 no
B: numerator analysis—across events (without controls)	B-1 yes	B-2 yes	B-3 yes	B-4 no	B-5 no
C: cohort study (with controls)	C-1 no	C-2 no	C-3 no	C-4 yes	C-5 yes
Ascertainment by event					
D: numerator analysis— event-specific (without controls)	D-1 yes	D-2 yes	D-3 yes	D-4 no	D-5 no
E: single drug-event analysis (with denominator) (without controls)	E-1 no	E-2 yes	E-3 yes	E-4 no	E-5 yes*
F: comparative proportional analysis (with internal controls)	F-1 no	F-2 yes	F-3 no	F-4 yes	F-5 no
G: case-control study design (with controls)	G-1 no	G-2 yes	G-3 no	G-4 yes	G-5 yes

*With external or historical controls.

in the conceptual category are: numerator analysis (event specific, without denominators, and without controls), single drug-event analysis (with denominators, without controls), comparative proportional analyses (with denominators, internal control) and, the case-control study design. The event-specific numerator analysis can be used to examine which drugs have been associated with a specific UDE (e.g., hepatotoxicity). The single drug-event analysis can examine the context in which the events occur through a content analysis of the data. Comparative proportional analyses assess the strength of associations relative to other members of a comparable drug group. The formally designed case-control study can be used to generate hypotheses, but is most valuable when used to test a hypothesis. The integration of existing data sources into this conceptual framework is illustrated in the next section.

The interpretive framework concerns interpretation, utilization, and decision making. An axiom of empirical research says that the more well controlled and internally valid the study design, the more straightforward, statistically valid, and less judgmental the interpretation of the results. At best, a properly designed analytical epidemiologic study, which is based on observational data, that did not have the benefit of random allocation and other design features of prospective controlled trials, is difficult to interpret. The open research methods often used to address pharmacoepidemiologic questions contain most, if not all, of the threats to internal validity listed by Campbell and Stanley.[8] Interpretation of such results usually requires the use of additional outside sources of information, such as multiple databases, to eliminate or assess the relative likelihood of alternative explanations. The most important source of information used in the interpretation of pharmacoepidemiologic findings is the previously described knowledge framework. Overall, this medicological form of interpretation could be called the art of epidemiologic diagnosis.

Utilization of the results of epidemiologic research requires information dissemination. The DES staff submits inhouse reports on its risk assessment efforts to the ODE I/II divisions for regulatory decision making and elective dissemination in regulatory media. For selected issues, publication in the medical literature is also sought.

The phrase "regulatory decision making" is used in this context to differentiate it from scientific, or clinical, decision making. Scientific decision making includes decisions concerning what to study and how to study it, and then infers deductive logic and the refutation of the null hypothesis through formal testing. The diagnosis and treatment of the individual based on a well-established knowledge framework characterizes the sphere of clinical decision making. Regulatory decision making, like the forms discussed above, often occurs in the environment of uncertainty. In the postmarketing arena the decision gap, that is, the difference between the amount of information one has and the amount required for a comfortable determination regarding drug safety, may be quite large. The interpreted pharmacoepidemiologic results are of regulatory value to the extent that they serve to narrow this gap for the risk component of the benefit-to-risk decision that must be made in a timely manner to protect the public health.

In order to establish an effective postmarketing system for the evaluation of drug safety, a network of data sources must be supported and maintained. Selection of the appropriate types of sources is contingent upon a clear understanding of needs and goals. Early detection and reliable and valid assessment are the general goals. The assessment goal, however, often is elusive due to the many forms a drug safety research question can take.

Application of Pharmacoepidemiology Strategies

The first line of defense is ascertainment by drug through active use of the passive case report monitoring system, the FDA-SRS, and published reports in the medical literature. Use of spontaneously submitted case reports can be considered both an inherently limited and an abundantly useful endeavor. Proper use of the submitted reports is somewhat like panning for gold: valuable nuggets can be found among the massive quantities of common matter, but diligent panning by the DES staff can actualize the potential of the SRS. Changes in the UDE reporting regulations, made in August 1985, have increased the efficiency of this mining process.[9] Also, the receipt of complete and well-documented reports (via FDA form 1639) from health professionals can increase the potential.

The next challenge for the pharmacoepidemiologist is to find strategies that maximize the quality and value of risk assessment, given a signal and/or a specific research question. At this point we can integrate the strategies for functioning within the conceptual framework (Table 1) with the methods and data sources that are available. Many of the currently available data sources are described in Chapter 8. Some of those sources, as they represent specific research methods, and a variety of research methods used with the FDA-SRS database, are listed in Table 2. The annotations in the primary and secondary function columns in Table 2 refer to the cells in Table 1. It is readily apparent from the tables that the primary function of many of these methods is detection of events, or signalling (cell A-1). It is fortunate that their value often is not limited to these indicated functions.

Alerting, now referred to by the DES as a monitored adverse reaction, implies the hands-on review by an inhouse health professional of a 15-day (i.e., serious and unlabeled) or a direct (from a healthcare provider) SRS report. Algorithms for causality assessment are used in this review.

Automated surveillance refers to the computer-controlled screening of all received reports. Programmed output reports are used to screen for large changes in type or frequency of labeled reactions, and those unlabeled reactions that fall short of the serious outcome criteria outlined in the revised regulations (CFR 314.80).

Database or Method	Primary Function	Secondary Functions
"Alerting"	A-1	A-2
Automated surveillance	A-1	B-3, A-2
SRS "safety profile"	B-3	B-1, B-2
SER-type analyses	F-4	F-2
Registries	D-3	D-1
Medical literature	A-1	C-5, G-5
Medicaid	C-4	B-2, G-4
Puget Sound (BCDSP)	G-5	C-5, E-3
DAWN	A-1	B-3, F-4
SEU	G-2	G-5

Table 2
Relationship of
Current Databases
and Methods to
the Conceptual
Framework

BCDSP = Boston Collaborative Drug Surveillance Programs; DAWN = Drug Abuse Warning Network; SER = standardized event rate; SEU = Slone Epidemiology Unit; SRS = Spontaneous Reporting System.

An SRS safety profile refers to numerator analysis of all events, clustered by a meaningful unit of examination, e.g., a body system, reported for a specific drug. Such profiles are informative and more so when compared with those of the other drugs in a pharmacologic or therapeutic class.

A standardized event rate (SER) type of analysis is a form of a comparative proportional analysis. Essentially, it examines whether the observed reporting rate for a specific drug-event pairing is greater than would be expected in a set of comparable drugs, given that it is an event reported with use of the compared drugs. No causality assessment is conducted here. SER is used to examine the relative strength of an association using the reporting event rates for the comparable drugs as an internal control.

Registries, such as the FDA-supported ophthalmology and dermatology registries, are ascertainment by event vehicles used to describe the spectra of drugs reported to be associated with the outcome events of emphasis. Occasionally, a new drug-event pairing is detected from these sources.

The medical literature is a rich but often underutilized source of data and information. The information available in the medical literature ranges from single case reports of UDEs (usually in the form of letters to the editor), through the formal reporting of the results of an epidemiologic or randomized investigation, to relevant research results from other disciplines and sciences, especially those that shed light on the pharmacokinetics or pharmacodynamics of a drug of interest or the pathogenesis of the disease under treatment as well as the one being characterized as the UDE.

Medicaid records form the largest, but probably the most complex and confounded source of pharmacoepidemiologic data. Although the most common use of these data is for formal cohort studies, case-control studies have been conducted using them. Broad-based screening by drug also has been tried with these data.

Components of the medical database at the Puget Sound health maintenance organization are under the management of the Boston Collaborative Drug Surveillance Program (BCDSP). This arrangement provides data linkage suitable for a variety of study methodologies, especially the case-control design.

The Drug Abuse Warning Network (DAWN), currently managed by the National Institute on Drug Abuse (NIDA), is one of a few useful drug abuse indicator systems. These data have been used to describe the abuse situations associated with specific psychotropic drugs, and to perform a variety of comparative proportional analyses. The Slone Epidemiology Unit (SEU) in Boston maintains a case-control surveillance program to generate hypotheses about drug-event associations, and to test specific research questions.

Monitoring through ascertainment by drug is an effective means of detection or signalling; however, the nature of the research question, the nature of the drugs of interest, the availability of data sources, and the working time frame determine the optimal research methods used for risk assessment. Less than a full understanding of any of these factors can lead to a flawed and misleading evaluation.

Case Examples

This section illustrates the varied nature of drug safety research questions and demonstrates the impact some recent epidemiologic risk assessments have had on regulatory decision making. The case example format provides a pragmatic approach. Full details of the methods used are contained in the literature referenced for the cited unpublished documents.

Each of the cases is, by necessity, presented in abbreviated format. The relationship of the three underlying frameworks, while present, may not be readily apparent as a consequence of this brief outline format. However, the importance of the frameworks in organizing and conducting inquiries in response to a drug safety research question cannot be overstated.

CASE EXAMPLE 1—AMOXAPINE TOXICITY UPON OVERDOSE

Signal: A literature report based on poison control center data observed a greater likelihood of lethality from an amoxapine overdose relative to the tricyclic antidepressants. More seizures were also reported.[10]

Purpose: Support or refute the conclusions of the literature report. Assess the relative toxicity and seizure profile of the marketed antidepressants upon overdose.

Data Sources: FDA–SRS, DAWN, FDA–Poison Control Center Data (PCC), National Disease and Therapeutic Index (NDTI), National Prescription Audit (NPA), and the medical literature.

Methods: Relative case fatality rates were calculated for each antidepressant from a number of the above databases. For example, a DAWN case fatality rate was estimated as DAWN Medical Examiner (DAWN–ME) mentions per 1000 DAWN Emergency Room (DAWN–ER) mentions. They then were rank-ordered and compared. Consistent support was obtained from similar calculations performed independently on data from the PCC and FDA–SRS databases. Therapeutic ratios also were calculated, after a content analysis of the SRS reports, and compared.

Results: No substantial difference in lethality on overdose was found between amoxapine and the standard tricyclic antidepressants. Amoxapine was found to differ in the clinical manifestations of overdose, most notably the presence of intense seizure activity. A potential selection bias was alleged for the PCC data used in the original literature reports.[11]

Action: No regulatory action was considered necessary regarding the relative lethality issue. The overdose section of the label was revised as to the presence of seizures as a major symptom and recommended an aggressive course of treatment. Physicians were encouraged to contact their local poison control center for the latest overdose treatment advice.

Follow-up: Monitor and reassess periodically.

Comment: Strategies from Table 1 used in this case include cells D-3, E-2, E-3, and F-4. The consistency in results on multiple measures across multiple databases provided a sufficient level of certainty for decision making. However, all the event measures were from unvalidated data sources; therefore, continual reassessment and external validation are still necessary.

CASE EXAMPLE 2—TRAZODONE: OVERDOSE TOXICITY VS. PRIAPISM

Signal: Continuing concern over a previous signal regarding priapism and the contrasting allegations that trazodone was less toxic on overdose then other drugs used to treat depression.

Purpose: The regulatory division was weighing the need to recommend, via the labeling, that trazodone use be considered second-line due to the occurrence of priapism. The DES was asked to assess the risks associated with trazodone overdose relative to its class, and contrast that to the risk of the unique reaction of priapism.

Data Sources: SRS, PCC, DAWN, NDTI, NPA, and the medical literature.

Methods: Similar to that used in example 1, but on a more recent time frame.

Results: Overdoses with trazodone appeared less likely to be lethal in this initial analysis. Seventy percent of the overdose episodes were in women. Priapism in men is estimated to occur about once per 7000 trazodone exposures.[12]

Action: Labeling was modified with new information. A second-line drug status was not conferred upon trazodone, although use in men should be only with a clear understanding of the risk for priapism.

Follow-up: Periodically monitor and reassess the overdose profile.

Comment: When this analysis was conducted trazodone had been marketed for a brief time. Confirmation is still needed. However, the suggestion that it may be less likely to be lethal on overdose was sufficient to retain its full indication.

CASE EXAMPLE 3—MAPROTILINE AND SEIZURES

Signal: British Committee on the Safety of Medicines (CSM), FDA-SRS, and the medical literature.

Purpose: Seizures have been reported with the use of most antidepressants. However, the signal suggested a higher frequency with maprotiline exposure. The DES was asked to assess whether seizures that occur while on therapy are more strongly associated with maprotiline than with comparable antidepressants.

Data Sources: SRS, NPA, NDTI, and the medical literature.

Methods: SERs were calculated for a comparison of events for maprotiline, amoxapine, and trazodone. Seizures in overdose situation were excluded from the analyses.

Results: Seizure events were associated more strongly with maprotiline than with therapy with comparable antidepressants.[13]

Action: Label was modified. A "Dear Doctor" letter was required.

Follow-up: Two hypothesis testing studies utilizing Medicaid data were commissioned. Those results were inconclusive. External support for these findings appeared in a subsequent report.[14]

Comment: Strategies from Table 1 included cells D-3 and F-4. This innovative analysis was used to test for substantial differences in a specific event across a group of comparable drugs. It addresses a manufacturer's claim that all drugs in a class are associated with a specific event already in the labeling. Proper use requires the acceptance of a set of assumptions and adjustment for known biases in the SRS data.

CASE EXAMPLE 4—PIROXICAM AND UPPER GASTROINTESTINAL EVENTS

Signal: CSM, SRS, Health Research Group's Citizen Petition, and the medical literature.

Purpose: To assess whether piroxicam was more strongly associated with upper gastrointestinal events than the other drugs in the nonsteroidal antiinflammatory (NSAID) group. The signal was seen for the older age group.

Data Sources: FDA–SRS, NPA, NDTI, the medical literature, Boston Collaborative Drug Surveillance Program, and Vanderbilt University's Medicaid Database.

Methods: SER calculation adjusted for a variable secular reporting trend over the past decade.

Results: When adjusted for known biases and trends in the SRS database, then adjusted for drug use, an SER analysis showed that piroxicam was not substantially different from other NSAIDs for gastrointestinal-associated morbidity and mortality. Findings from the other cited databases were supportive of this finding.[15]

Action: The Health Research Group's petition was denied. At present, no labeling changes have been ordered.

Follow-up: Continual monitoring.

Comment: This was the most extensively researched drug safety question of the past few years. Some of the extramural data sources supported by the FDA were consulted with high priority due to the high visibility of this issue. Their input supported the SER analysis performed by inhouse staff.

CASE EXAMPLE 5—HUMAN GROWTH HORMONE AND CREUTZFELDT-JAKOB DISEASE

Signal: Three 1639 case reports of Creutzfeldt-Jakob disease were submitted to the FDA for the NIH-sponsored treatment IND.

Purpose: To assess whether these three reports of this very rare neurologic disorder were more than expected.

Data Sources: National Center for Health Statistics mortality data, and exposure data from the IND.

Methods: The observed rate was compared with the expected rate to test the hypothesis of no difference.

Results: A rate of 3 per 10 000 exposed was significantly greater than could be expected in the population.[16]

Action: The production and distribution of pituitary-derived human growth hormone was halted. A recombinant product received FDA priority, under orphan drug status, and was soon thereafter approved for use in human growth hormone-deficient conditions. A Health and Human Services Task Force was created to identify and monitor the balance of the exposed individuals.

Follow-up: A Health and Human Services Task Force will monitor and conduct a National Death Index-based study.

Comment: A simple but innovative analysis was sufficient to allow a confident decision. This analysis is best described as a special case of strategy E-5 (Table 1), with a firm denominator and external control from the National Center for Health Statistics data.

CASE EXAMPLE 6—IMPACT OF NALOXONE ON PENTAZOCINE ABUSE

Signal: An internal FDA request from our drug abuse staff.

Purpose: To assess the impact of a regulatory action taken about three years prior, when the narcotic antagonist naloxone was added to the oral tablet formulation of pentazocine.

Data Sources: DAWN, NPA, the medical literature, and FDA–SRS.

Methods: A hypothesis testing trends analysis of DAWN emergency room and medical examiner data over NPA retail prescription data that compared data before and after the addition of naloxone to the oral tablet dosage form of pentazocine.

Results: There was a significant decrease in the number of drug abuse mentions per reporting quarter in each of the DAWN system parameters since the addition of naloxone.[17]

Action: No additional regulatory action was warranted. The intervention appeared successful to date.

Follow-up: Analysis to be repeated if a new signal requires another examination.

Comment: The strategy is a special case of cell E-5 (Table 1) using a historical control to test the hypothesis of no change in trend. This assessment of a prior regulatory action clearly demonstrated a public health impact. The original agreement to add naloxone illustrated a constructive spirit of cooperation between industry and government (FDA, DEA, and NIDA).

CASE EXAMPLE 7—WITHDRAWAL SEIZURES WITH ALPRAZOLAM

Signal: FDA–SRS, and the medical literature.

Purpose: To describe the condition under which seizures occur and to assess whether they are more strongly associated with any specific benzodiazepine anxiolytic.

Data Sources: FDA–SRS, the medical literature, NPA, NDTI.

Methods: Content analysis of FDA–SRS reports.

Results: Seizures secondary to withdrawal from benzodiazepine anxiolytics are rare events. They are reported most frequently for the potent benzodiazepines alprazolam and lorazepam. The data were plotted as dose against duration of therapy. Risk appeared dependent upon sufficient exposure to produce a physical dependence state. For alprazolam, higher doses appear to decrease the time to risk. These data support the pharmacologic theory of cumulative exposure.[18] The data on lorazepam were insufficient to draw a defensible conclusion. A more recent analysis of these data were presented to an FDA advisory committee in the fall of 1989. Further exploration and confirmation is still needed.

Action: Awaits additional supportive data.

Follow-up: Continued SRS monitoring.

Comment: Strategies D-2 and D-3 were used (Table 1). A comparative proportional analysis could not be conducted because the NDTI data demonstrated that alprazolam had a unique usage pattern (i.e., more often prescribed by psychiatrists for affective and panic disorders). Therefore, there were no comparable drugs. Additionally, an appropriate denominator for this contingent event was not available. The generated hypothesis awaits testing. The conduct of confirmatory studies will be difficult, however, because these type of data are outside the scope of all of the usual postmarketing databases.

CASE EXAMPLE 8—ISOTRETINOIN AND BIRTH DEFECTS

Signal: Centers for Disease Control (CDC) December 1987 correspondence to the FDA based upon a cluster of reports from the New Jersey Birth Defects Surveillance Program.

Purpose: To quantitate the magnitude of the occurrence of this previously documented drug-outcome relationship.

Data Sources: CDC, FDA–SRS, Medicaid, NDTI, NPA, National Health and Nutrition Examination Survey (NHANES)

Methods: This multidatabase evaluation[19] included an estimate (obtained via NHANES) of severe cystic acne in women of childbearing potential, an estimate (via NPA, NDTI) of drug usage and prescriber information, a risk estimate (via Medicaid) in a population, a content analysis and an estimate of the degree of underreporting in spontaneous reports (via FDA–SRS). Foreign experience, literature reports, and estimates of contraceptive failure also were important data sources.

Results: Use of this potent teratogen was 15–20 times greater than the estimate of severe recalcitrant cystic acne in women. This disease is 4–5 times more prevalent in men. Between 70 and 85 percent of isotretinoin was prescribed by dermatologists. Medicaid data illustrated that pregnancy exposure was substantial. An extrapolation of these data provides an estimate of 900–1300 severe birth defects that have occurred since the 1982 introduction of isotretinoin. The FDA–SRS, however, only had about 60 reports. The CDC estimated that 25 percent of pregnancy exposures brought to term would produce birth defects.

Action: The most extensive product relabeling and repackaging effort ever requested of a drug manufacturer was required. In addition, an extensive prescriber and consumer education campaign, plus an intervention assessment survey, were launched.

Follow-up: The FDA formed an internal multidisciplinary Accutane Monitoring Group to monitor compliance with the new regulatory action, the epidemiologic data, and the progress of the intervention assessment efforts. The firm is required to submit a quarterly update on all components of the program, then meet with the Accutane Monitoring Group to review and discuss the findings.

Comment: Soon after marketing began in 1982, reports of congenital defects were received by the FDA. The FDA conducted a limited epidemiologic evaluation at that time. This topic was discussed at public advisory committees in 1983 and 1984. Professional labeling was modified to include a boxed warning regarding the association of the drug with human birth defects. After receipt of the CDC query in 1987, the FDA-DES began a comprehensive epidemiologic assessment of the issue. The strength of those results were the basis for the May 1988 regulatory action.

This case illustrates the importance of an in-depth comprehensive multidatabase assessment that includes the use of natural history and drug use data. In addition, the formation of an active monitoring group that will continually assess this issue and the success of the regulatory interventions will prevent this important public health issue from once again losing priority.

It is important to understand that the regulatory actions cited in the case examples were not taken solely upon the results of the postmarketing risk assessments. The new findings are added to the existing knowledge database and the benefit-to-risk equation is recalculated or more correctly rejudged by the risk manager. Decisions are based upon consideration of the aggregate information available.

Summary

Risk assessment of a new drug is a continual process. Pharmacoepidemiologic risk assessment is the postapproval stage of the continuum. Postmarketing risk assessment strategies should be guided by the cumulative experience with the new drug to that point. Phase IV safety studies should address specific residual concerns.

Responsibilities for assessing postmarketing risk and for the application of these to the risk management and regulatory functions exist in different organizational components of the FDA. The postmarketing decision makers are the same functional units who worked with the drug throughout its entire development process.

The practice of pharmacoepidemiology is not amenable to a standardized or cookbook approach. This chapter explains the concepts and foundation of the art in pharmacoepidemiology so that thinking, creative individuals can apply them as the research questions warrant. It is important to reemphasize that each new research question requires a different individualized approach, and that there are more exceptions than methodologic rules. The only valid rules in this field are those of research logic. The need for mastering a conceptual framework and a solid knowledge base cannot be stressed too strongly. Diverse data sources are required to address the breadth of potential questions that arise in this field. Due to the secondary and imprecise nature of most of the available data, multiple data sources should be examined for each research question so that consistent and confirmatory findings are generated. Unfortunately, current extramural databases are utilized only on a limited scale to address FDA-initiated research questions. Clearly, there is much room for improvement. Each question posed to the FDA must be addressed in a timely manner. However, not all questions can currently be answered and additional data sources are needed.

Epidemiologic data on drug safety in the postmarketing arena are valuable in the regulatory environment when they can be used to form an interpretable risk assessment that can narrow the often very-large decision gaps and aid rational regulatory decision making. Regulatory adjustments made by the FDA impact public health by affecting patient care through prevention and or minimization of unsafe drug therapy.

The sponsors bear responsibility for identifying and characterizing actual and potential safety issues associated with the use of *their* products in the postapproval environment, as well as prior to approval. The new drug sponsors need to develop pharmacoepidemiologic capabilities so they can meet their responsibility. The FDA views pharmacoepidemiologic assessment of risk as a necessary component of its public health mission . . . a mission that does not end when an approval (to market) letter is issued.

The FDA will continue to refine its program and will assess risks using the best techniques and data sources possible. Better sources of epidemiologic data will increase the probability that the decision the FDA has to make on safety issues will be rational and correct.

An earlier version of this chapter was presented at the 4th International Conference on Pharmacoepidemiology, September 1987, and was published in its proceedings.

References

1. Gross FH, Inman WHW, eds. Drug monitoring. New York: Academic Press, 1977:1-16, 79-89.

2. Faich G. Adverse drug reaction monitoring. *N Engl J Med* 1986;*314*:1589-92.

3. Rossi AC, Knapp DE, Anello C, et al. Discovery of adverse drug reactions. A comparison of selected Phase IV studies with spontaneous reporting methods. *JAMA* 1983;*249*:2226-8.

4. Temple R, Jones JK, Crout JR. Adverse effects of newly marketed drugs (editorial). *N Engl J Med* 1979;*300*:1046.

5. Jones JK. Broader uses of post-marketing surveillance. In: Wardell WM, Velo G, eds. Drug development, regulatory assessment and post-marketing surveillance. New York: Plenum Press, 1981:203-16.

6. Jones JK. Regulatory use of adverse drug reactions. In: Skandia International Symposia. Detection and prevention of adverse drug reactions. Stockholm: Almqvist & Wiksell International, 1984:203-14.

7. Finney D. Statistical logic in the monitoring of reactions to therapeutic drugs. *Methods Inf Med* 1971;*10*:237-45. Revised and updated. In: Inman WHW, ed. Monitoring for drug safety. Lancaster: MTP Press, 1980:383-400.

8. Campbell DT, Stanley JC. Experimental and quasiexperimental designs for research. Boston: Houghton Mifflin, 1963:5-6.

9. U.S. Code of Federal Regulations, Part 314.80.

10. Litovitz TL, Troutman WG. Amoxapine overdose: seizures and fatalities. *JAMA* 1983;*250*:1069-71.

11. Nelson RC. Amoxapine toxicity on overdose. Unpublished report. Rockville, MD: Food and Drug Administration, Office of Epidemiology and Biostatistics, 1984.

12. Baum C, Nelson RC. Trazodone toxicity on overdose. Unpublished report. Rockville, MD: Food and Drug Administration, Office of Epidemiology and Biostatistics, 1985.

13. Nelson RC. Maprotiline and seizures. Unpublished report. Rockville, MD: Food and Drug Administration, Office of Epidemiology and Biostatistics, 1984.

14. Jabbari B, Bryan GE, Marsh EE, Gunderson CH. Incidence of seizures with tricyclic and tetracyclic antidepressants. *Arch Neurol* 1985;*42*:480-1.

15. Rossi A, Hsu JP, Faich GA. Ulcerogenicity of piroxicam: an analysis of spontaneously reported data. *Br Med J* 1987;*294*:147-50.

16. Piper J. HGH & CJD. Unpublished report. Rockville, MD: Food and Drug Administration, Office of Epidemiology and Biostatistics, 1984.

17. Baum C, Hsu JP, Nelson RC. Impact of the addition of naloxone on the abuse of pentazocine tablets. *Public Health Rep* 1987;*102*:426-9.

18. Nelson RC, Barash D, Graham D. Intense abstinence syndromes and the newer benzodiazepine anxiolytics. Unpublished report. Rockville, MD: Food and Drug Administration, Office of Epidemiology and Biostatistics, 1985.

19. Graham D. Maternal exposure to Accutane. Unpublished report. Rockville, MD: Food and Drug Administration, Office of Epidemiology and Biostatistics, 1988.

16

Risk Analysis and Pharmaceuticals: A Guide for Decision Makers

Harry Otway

Abstract

Chapter 15 focused on the regulatory assessment of drug risks; this chapter examines the broader question of what factors determine whether not only drugs but many other potentially risky activities or products can be acceptable. An outline of risk analysis is provided, and the usual stages of the process are discussed. Psychosocial factors influencing risk perception (including drug risks) are analyzed. Because judgments of acceptability are strongly dependent on their particular context, it is suggested that risk analysis usually provides no simple answers to the question of what is an acceptable level of risk. However, qualitative criteria are proposed that can be used by drug policy makers in decisions to develop, market, promote, or withdraw a drug, and to supplement and critically evaluate quantitative risk analysis.

Outline

A ctions to regulate potentially dangerous activities usually are taken only after the consequences have become visible in the form of accidents or unanticipated health or environmental effects. The idea that regulations or other risk management measures should be based on theoretical analyses and should precede permission being given for the activity is relatively new. Although this idea is still somewhat controversial and subject to criticism, its application is gaining wider acceptance.

The main scientific support for this anticipatory form of regulation has become known as risk analysis (or risk assessment). Risk analysis is the use of available data, supplemented by calculation, extrapolation, theory, and expert judgment, to define the risks to people due to their exposure to hazardous materials or operations. This approach to identifying and quantifying risks has been applied to a number of activities with varying results.

Quantitative risk analyses have proven useful in helping planners to understand better the potential risks of their proposals, and as supporting documentation for licensing applications. But risk estimates, even when predicting low risks as compared with the ordinary risks of daily life, have not proven convincing to public groups concerned about the hazards of large-scale technologies, such as nuclear power, and newer ones, such as biotechnology. This has given rise more recently to an expansion in the scope of risk analysis to include social science-based investigations of how people perceive different risks and what their expectations are about what should be done, and by whom, to manage these risks.

The availability of systematic methods for estimating risks and for measuring public perceptions has perhaps led to over-optimistic expectations on the part of expert communities about their applicability to policy decisions. Quantitative estimates of risk magnitudes and people's perceptions of risks may seem, at first glance, to constitute a rational basis for policy formation. However, it ignores the fact that it is the risky technologies or activities themselves, not their risks taken out of context, that will be accepted or rejected. Moreover, in democratic societies these decisions are based on cultural, social, and political considerations as well as analytical data.

The assessment of pharmaceutical risks is covered by Nelson in Chapter 15; the present chapter discusses qualitative criteria that can be used by policy makers to supplement and evaluate critically the use of quantitative risk analyses in decisions to market a new drug. The focus here is on risks to public health and safety.

Outline of Risk Analysis

It should be realized that although formal risk analysis is a relatively new concept, most of the methods used are not new. Risk analysis is based on a collection of methods drawn from fields as diverse as engineering, toxicology, epidemiology, economics, and the social sciences. Its originality lies primarily in promising a comprehensive approach to examining the hazards of new activities or products. However, analysts tend to focus on variables that are amenable to analysis; thus the completeness and comprehensiveness of risk analysis often depend on the degree to which the problem under consideration can be described accurately in quantifiable variables.

Applications or risk analysis are usually iterative. The sequence of steps depends on the activity considered and the way in which it presents itself. Obviously a proposed activity for which there is no prior experience will be analyzed differently than one discovered because of some adverse, unanticipated health effect believed to be caused by a pharmacologic agent. In general, the process of risk analysis can be broken down into the following stages:

Identification. What are the possible negative unintended effects of the drug (UDE) and the likely exposure pathways? Who may be at risk?

Estimation (Quantification). What is the probability of a UDE occurring? What are its expected consequences? How uncertain is the relative scientific knowledge base?

Evaluation. What is the significance of the expected consequences? Are the risks to health and safety meaningful in an absolute sense? Are they reversible? How are the technologies and agents that produce the risks, and the risks themselves, perceived by those at risk? Are wider social, community, cultural, or health values affected?

Management. What options are there to control risk levels, their relative costs, and social acceptability? How enforceable are they? What are the alternatives to the proposed action? It is important to emphasize that these are *studies* of possible management strategies, not actual risk management decisions.

Risk analysis stops here and *may* begin to interact with the policy process—may, because policy decisions can be made without analysis, and often are. Sometimes decisions are driven primarily by political or economic considerations; sometimes risk analyses are performed because the results are expected (for various reasons) to support preconceived decisions; and sometimes (but seldom) risk analysis reveals a decision acceptable to all involved—regulatory agency, pharmaceutical industry, and patients.

Qualitative Aspects and the Decision Context

Policy-making processes select the strategies to be followed, based not on analytical results alone, but also informed by knowledge of the unquantifiable social, cultural, political, and organizational factors that form the context for the particular decision. The plural form, processes, is used because, depending on the setting, these decisions are taken at different levels and by different actors (e.g., company management, regulatory agency, or at the political level).

The particular context in which a decision is made determines the relative importance of the risk analysis stages (e.g., estimation versus evaluation). For example, three aspects in which decision contexts may differ are:

Public Awareness. Sometimes public groups who have something at stake are aware that a decision is being taken that will affect them. This may be the case in decisions about the licensing of drugs of doubtful efficacy that are already being taken by patients who believe in them (e.g., laetrile, ribavirin). Here the understanding of risk and benefit perceptions is more important. This may lead to public hearings which, in effect, turn the decision into a political bargaining process. In other cases involving new pharmaceuticals, the public may not be involved at all and the regulatory agency simply evaluates the information provided by industry and other sources and decides what level of risk should be acceptable.

Opportunities for Intervention. For some decisions, the opportunity for intervention by opposition groups is such that implementation of the decision can be frustrated, or at least made difficult, such as opposition to the siting of a hazardous facility or, at the individual level, travel to a foreign country to acquire an unlicensed drug that is legal there. In other cases, however, there is little focus for opposition except the regulatory agency itself. For example, although biotechnology is an important topic of public concern, this research can be carried out on a very small scale with rather limited resources; the opposition to a new drug can hardly be demonstrated effectively at thousands of retail pharmacies, and a large, multinational pharmaceutical company can choose to produce a new drug at any of a number of existing facilities.

Risk Increase Versus Risk Reduction. Some of the decisions mentioned earlier impose new risks on the public, thus increasing the potential for controversy. Other decisions may deal with the reduction of existing risks, such as the decision to take a pharmaceutical off the market or to clean up an existing toxic waste dump. Although risk reduction decisions may also be controversial, the decision maker is in a stronger moral position with regard to justification than in situations where the imposition of a new risk is the outcome. The earlier example of laetrile and ribavirin may be seen as risk reduction decisions because their use implies the risk of foregoing more effective conventional treatment.

Risk analysis could be more useful to policy makers if its results were supplemented by qualitative information, much of which is available but too often neglected either because analysts are not sensitive to it or because it does not fit the analytical framework chosen. In the following sections some qualitative (subjective) aspects of risk analysis are presented which are frequently obscured when results are reported.

Qualitative Aspects of Risk Identification

The identification of health and safety risks, especially of new products, is an art. It depends on the professional experience and judgment of the analyst, and also on human creativity—the ability to imagine effects never before seen, sometimes even contrary to the conventional wisdom of one's discipline.

Average levels of risk are potentially deceptive because particular subpopulations with exceptionally high exposures may be present. Thus, once the risks and exposure pathways have been identified, the risk analyst must identify the subgroups at highest risk, either because they are preferentially exposed (e.g., because of preexisting disease) or because they are more sensitive to the particular agent (e.g., children exposed to radioactive iodine in milk, or elderly persons who may suffer toxic effects from the standard dosage of a drug).

Beyond this, it is necessary to be aware of possible synergistic effects, where two or more exposures, perhaps individually tolerable, can combine to create a risk much greater than the sum of the individual exposures (e.g., two drugs that produce a dangerous interaction when administered together; smokers, who are at much higher risk when exposed to asbestos than nonsmokers).

Although synergism may not be involved, there is the need for "risk mapping," a systematic effort to identify risks to which patients are already exposed before proposing to add a new risk (a patient at risk of renal failure who has indication for a drug that undergoes renal clearance; a group at risk due to releases from a proposed industrial facility might also be at risk from an upstream dam). But the analyst also must go beyond considerations of physical health and safety to examine possible risks to intangibles such as social, community, and cultural values.

The decision maker must be convinced, through careful study of the analysis or by interrogation of the risk analyst, that a comprehensive risk identification has been done. The most careful quantification of risks will be useless if the most important element has been excluded.

Qualitative Aspects of Risk Estimation

Every risk analysis begins with assumptions about the problem under study. According to philosophers of science, the problem statement used to condense and represent what is initially perceived as an amorphous problem situation predetermines the set of possible solutions that can be found.[1] This applies also to risk analysis with respect to the assumptions implicit in the framework chosen by the analysts. Among these assumptions are what sources of data are considered valid and how they will be analyzed, how risks are defined and aggregated, what models and which techniques are to be used, and how the system is limited and defined to make it simple enough to be analyzed. Taken together, these assumptions effectively bound the outcome of analysis.

The reliability of the data on which analyses are based may vary from one kind of risk to the next. This goes beyond the mere accuracy of handling data (which can also be a problem), and the difficulty of imagining all possible failure modes and their consequences, to the inherent uncertainty, and the uncertainty about the uncertainty, or data derived by quite different means and, often, from different sources. For example, risk estimates may be based on:

1. fairly hard evidence, such as statistics on deaths, disease prevalence, and injuries, although definitional differences can arise among countries, or even among departments in the same country, as to the exact criteria for attributing a death to a given cause (e.g., number of days after an accident that death occurs, cultural bias against reporting deaths by suicide);
2. soft evidence such as the number of excess cancers in a population, as estimated from epidemiologic data;
3. controversial interpretations of data where there is no scientific consensus, so opposing experts can argue with integrity and conviction to support different positions (e.g., Bendectin and congenital defects; lung cancer and passive smoking); and
4. "inspiration," rather than established scientific theory, thus yielding highly uncertain estimates (e.g., the risks to industrial facilities from sabotage or terrorism).

Further, risks can be defined and aggregated in different ways, for example:

1. mortality is usually chosen as the risk measure although injuries or other nonlethal side effects more difficult to estimate may be more important when options are compared;
2. the age at which death occurs is not often considered in technical analyses, even though a risk that preferentially affects the young cannot be compared directly with one that affects the elderly; and
3. risks are often reported in terms of average (or total) life shortening in the exposed population (e.g., counting the loss of 50 years of life by a 20-year-old the same as if 50 70-year-olds each lost one year of life).

Qualitative Aspects of Risk Evaluation

One of the first tasks of a policy maker presented with quantitative risk estimates is to determine if the levels predicted are too high. This may be done by comparison with other risks that people are exposed to in their everyday lives. However, even if the proposed new risk seems to be of reasonable magnitude, this does not necessarily mean that it will be found acceptable by those who will be exposed to it. In fact, even if the regulator finds a risk to be too high on this basis, it may still be quite acceptable to the public. The artificial sweetener debate in the U.S. is an example of this, where a diet-conscious public opposes the banning of suspected carcinogens. Another example is the case of unproven "wonder" drugs, the efficacy and safety of which are contested by the medical community and regulatory authorities, but which are nevertheless bought on the black market by people made desperate by disease.

One of the more serious errors committed by policy makers is to assume that if predicted risk levels are low on a comparative basis then the policies should be accepted by the public. Public opposition to technologies with apparently low predicted risks has sometimes even been called "irrational" or "inconsistent" by those in authority, adding fuel to already overheated debates.

People may perceive risks as being higher or lower than they really are because of ignorance of actual risk levels or because of the way questions about risks are asked. However, there are many values associated with the attributes of risk-bearing activities, and with risks themselves, that affect how they are perceived. Research repeatedly has shown that people characterize activities and their risks by many dimensions, so risks cannot be properly compared only on the single dimension of physical risk. The factors listed below were developed in a review paper.[2]

Psychological factors that tend to cause risks to be perceived as more serious than indicated by quantitative estimates are:

1. involuntary exposure to risk as opposed to risk-taking by choice (involuntary exposure to second-hand smoke for a nonsmoker, voluntary exposure to injury for a skier);
2. lack of personal control over the outcome of risk exposure (no control for an airline passenger, skill-based control for a skier);
3. uncertainty about the outcome of exposure (whether it is well understood, even by experts);
4. no personal experience of risk (fear of the unknown);
5. difficulty in conceptualizing or imagining the risk (originates from processes difficult for lay people to understand);
6. association of the risk with technological failure, causing feelings of helplessness, as opposed to risks of natural hazards, which we do not expect to control (empirically verified as a source of stress);[3]
7. delayed effects occurring after the direct risk exposure has ceased (increased stress levels have been empirically measured in people who believed they were exposed to radiation in the Three-Mile Island accident and in those who felt they had been victimized by leaking toxic waste dumps) (unpublished observation, Dr. I. Fleming, Battelle Northwest, 1987);
8. future generations being affected because of congenital malformations due to exposure during pregnancy or because of damage to genetic material;
9. the benefits of the risk-bearing activity not being highly visible or else being received by a group different from the one at risk; and
10. the possibility of large-scale, low-probability accidents that could affect large numbers of people.[2]

An activity or product also may be perceived as having social and political attributes associated with it. The list below is based primarily on research related to the perception of hazardous industrial technologies, but similar attributes related to moral, ethical, and social values also apply to the perception of new medical technologies and pharmaceuticals (e.g., surrogate motherhood, contraceptive drugs that act by causing very early abortion, preconception sex selection, euthanasia, diagnosis of congenital abnormalities in the womb). The following attributes may either enhance or diminish acceptability, depending on the values of the individual, if that person believes the technology will:

1. provide benefits corresponding to real (as opposed to frivolous) needs;
2. increase the standard of living;
3. create new jobs;
4. stimulate economic growth;
5. enhance national prestige and allow independence from foreign suppliers;
6. cause dependency on small groups of elite people;
7. require strict physical security measures or special police powers; and
8. lead to centralization of political and economic systems.

These lists of psychological and sociopolitical attributes of risks and technologies are not meant to be complete. Rather they demonstrate the complexity of how activities may be perceived and the difficulties inherent in trying to make comparisons based only on physical risks. Indeed, such lists can never be complete because the attributes that are relevant to judgment of an activity can be anything that people have learned to associate with the activity.

In agreement with the Royal Society study on risk, it can be concluded that "there is not, and cannot be, a single acceptable level of risk" as a generalizable number or mathematical relationship.[4] Nor can there be a threshold value of risk below which social acceptability can be assumed. The acceptance of risk is determined by the acceptance of the activities that cause them. This, in turn, depends on the information people have chosen to believe; the values they hold; the social experiences they have had access to; how they combine experience, information, and values to imagine the future; the dynamics of interest groups; the political process; and the historical moment.

Qualitative Aspects of Risk Management Studies

A study sponsored by the U.S. National Academy of Sciences found that instead of alleviating regulatory conflicts, risk analysis often became the focus of debate.[5] Part of the controversy surrounding the use of risk analysis as a basis for policy decisions results from confusion between the theoretical world of risk management studies and "real world" decision making. This confusion has given rise to overly optimistic expectations, with analysts sometime seeming to believe that, in a rational world, the policies selected would be those policies favored by risk studies.

Risk management studies take a wide variety of forms because the information deemed sufficient for policy analysis depends very much on the discipline of the analyst, the interests of the study's sponsor, and the decision making style assumed. A technical risk analyst might recommend the option with the lowest risk, regardless of other aspects not included in the analysis; an economist might favor the most cost-effective solution. Analytical approaches to risk management often imply a single decision maker, thus ignoring organizational and institutional influences on decision outcomes as well as other nonanalytical factors.

Organizational realities mean that decision makers often operate within rather narrowly fixed limits: "horizontally" in terms of the remit which they have, and "vertically" in terms of the financial and staff resources available to them. For example, an agency may have a remit in the safety area that does not allow it to formally consider mental health aspects of decisions. Limited resources may force the agency to choose which problems to address among a variety of possibilities, all of which fall within its remit. In a similar manner, comparison of risks may be irrelevant to an agency responsible for managing only one type of risk; the argument that money might be better spent on drug information is pointless if the agency's remit is water quality. Not only are risk comparisons unconvincing to many lay people, they are also institutionally meaningless in many cases. A decision to act on a risk problem may depend less on the magnitude of the risk than on the organizational possibilities for action.

Risk management studies require the analyst to know the goals of the decision maker so that options can be developed to best satisfy them. There is a general problem with goal elicitation: it is not that decision makers do not know what their objectives are, but rather that their true objectives often cannot be stated for organizational or personal reasons. One goal of organizations is to ensure their continued existence. An organization will not happily accept a decision that will benefit a competing agency at their own expense, especially if the underlying scientific basis for the decision is seen to be "soft." Likewise, individual managers and politicians have career goals that may be favored by one option and hurt by another. Risk studies sometimes are undertaken to legitimize the implementation of decisions already made in private, an objective that cannot be openly admitted.

Having discussed the limitations of risk management studies, it should be emphasized that the studies can be useful by giving decision makers a range of options to consider. However, to be effective they should:

1. consider the alternatives to the proposed action, including the use of other, perhaps less glamorous, technologies or procedures to achieve the same benefit;
2. investigate the effects of cancellation of the action as an alternative, bearing in mind that unemployment and its consequences for physical and mental health can sometimes be one of the risks of not taking risks;
3. evaluate the cost of risk reduction for each alternative;
4. carefully examine the equity issues involved, such as who bears the risks, who received the benefits, and who must pay for risk reduction measures;

5. examine the problems of implementation and enforcement of risk reduction measures; and
6. consider the institutional dimensions of the particular situation, recommending only actions that are consistent with organizational remits and resources.

Experts

Policy decisions about risk-bearing activities have the paradoxical quality that they are likely to be most urgent just where scientific knowledge is the most uncertain. The origins of the problems addressed by risk analysis guarantee their relative insolubility because they are either discovered as unexpected and unwanted side effects of an existing technology or are theoretical projections of the side effects of a new and untested technology. The scientific basis needed tends to be fragmentary or nonexistent, drawing on relatively new or underdeveloped fields such as epidemiology or molecular biology. The data that do exist often have been produced for other purposes and are therefore less appropriate and reliable when used in a different context. Even methods of investigation may be uncertain and open to debate.

Facts do not exist independently of people. There is an intrinsic human element in knowledge, in contrast to what is often thought of as a dry, passionless search for abstract truths. The legitimate differences of opinion that exist in all scientific fields (and especially in immature fields where uncertainties in the scientific materials are larger, and institutional and professional relationships are still evolving) are magnified by the fact that the resulting debates, where policies are at stake, often take place in public arenas employing forensic rules of evidence poorly suited for discussions of this type. When decisions involve the power to influence policies and cannot wait for the delayed emergence of scientific consensus, the informal means by which scientific communities enforce quality control and standards of behavior are ineffective. Without the constraint of unambiguous scientific results, experts representing diverse interests can support their positions with sincerity, conviction, and integrity. This is further complicated by role ambiguity due to the experts' dual loyalties to those they advise and to their own disciplines.

Rip concluded that expert advisers should consider the social and political impact of their advice and that those who use expert advice should expect more uncertainty and instability in the advice given. The myth of absolute scientific objectivity should be discarded and expert advice seen as a support in clarifying issues and evolving pragmatic solutions to problems rather than as a clear and unambiguous basis for decisions.[6]

Suggestions for Decision Makers

It would be presumptuous, as well as impossible, to propose a rigorous checklist specifying the attributes of a "good" risk analysis. This is partly because what constitutes a good analysis depends on the context in which it is to be used, and also because my discussion of the qualitative aspects of risk analysis is itself subjective and obviously reflects my values. However, decision making informed by analysis is preferable to having no analysis at all *if* the limitations and assumptions of the analysis are clearly understood by the decision maker. An analysis that meets the criteria below is likely to be better, in the sense of being more complete and more informative, than one that does not. The questions that follow should be answered in the affirmative.

Does the discussion of risks include mention of possible synergistic effects? Is the distribution of risks among differing age, regional, occupational groups, and so forth, reported? How are threats to a sense of community, well being, values, and so forth, treated?

Are alternative models of risk-producing processes mentioned? Are the uncertainties in the underlying data explained as well as uncertainties in the calculation itself? Are areas of scientific controversy clearly identified? Are results given using alternative risk measures? Is the absolute magnitude of possible severe reactions given instead of the probability-weighted expected value of risk from them?

Are psychological and social attributes of risk that may affect public perceptions discussed (e.g., voluntariness, control, visibility, dependence on technical elites)? Does the study avoid predicting public acceptance based on numeric comparisons of different risks?

Does the policy portion of the study avoid assuming simple decision-making objectives? Does it consider alternatives (including cancellation) to the proposed activity? Are the costs of risk reduction (including effects on employment) evaluated? Are the equity aspects of all alternatives examined? Are problems of implementation and enforcement discussed? Are the social and institutional contexts of decisions considered?

In addition to asking these and other questions about the analysis, decision makers should entertain a few questions about the analysts (and the expert advisors).

Might the analysts be wearing "disciplinary blinders," causing them to favor some specific technology or procedure?

Have the analysts made an "ego investment," through past work that might lead them to prefer a particular alternative or method of analysis?

Who sponsored the study, and what are their interests?

From what sources have the analysts been funded in the past?

Where differences exist within the scientific community, are they clearly described and the implications of alternative theories explained?

Qualitative analysis can be just as rigorous and informative as quantitative analysis, especially if the quantitative study is incomplete or based on unexamined assumptions and soft thinking.

References

1. Ravetz J. Scientific knowledge and its social problems. Harmondsworth, England: Penguin, 1973.

2. Otway H, Von Winterfeldt D. Beyond acceptable risk: on the social acceptability of new technologies. *Policy Sci* 1982;*14*:247-56.

3. Baum A, Fleming R, Davidson LM. Natural disaster and technological catastrophe. *Environ Behav* 1983;*15*:333-54.

4. Risk assessment: a study group report. London: The Royal Society, 1983.

5. Risk assessment in the federal government: managing the process. Washington: National Academy of Sciences, 1983.

6. Rip A. Experts in public arenas. In: Otway H, Peltu M, eds. Regulating industrial risks: science, hazards and public protection. Boston: Butterworths, 1985:94-110.

17

The Role of Epidemiology in Pharmaceutical Research, Development, and Marketing

Harry A. Guess

Abstract

Suggesting scientifically and commercially promising targets for drug discovery, providing background information for market forecasts, reducing drug approval times, improving safety monitoring, and supporting health economic studies are among the potential contributions of epidemiology to pharmaceutical research and development. Because the type of epidemiologic research needed to aid pharmaceutical development is often unlikely to attract government funding, it should be funded by the pharmaceutical industry. Epidemiology contributes to clinical trial planning by providing knowledge on the natural history of the disease to be treated and scientific justification for the use of surrogate endpoints. To be effective, epidemiologic studies should be started very early in the development process, even before specific drug candidates have entered Phase I trials. Given the marketing value of public fascination with health risk estimates, epidemiologic information on disease morbidity is helpful in explaining the benefits of drugs to the public, to governmental panels, and to healthcare organizations.

Outline

T here is a widespread perception within both the pharmaceutical industry and the epidemiologic community that pharmacoepidemiology is the only area of epidemiology relevant to the pharmaceutical industry and that, for all practical purposes, epidemiology means postmarketing surveillance. In keeping with this, it is a common but serious mistake to begin epidemiologic planning only shortly before anticipated market approval. This chapter explains how other areas of epidemiology have contributed to drug approval and suggests how pharmaceutical companies can more effectively target research in epidemiology to support drug development.

Epidemiology has been defined as "the study of the distribution and determinants of health-related states and events in [human] populations."[1] It is the focus on populations rather than individual patients that distinguishes epidemiology from other medical sciences. In contrast to this dry definition, the results of major epidemiologic studies typically generate broad public interest and coverage in the popular press because people are interested in their health and their odds of getting or avoiding some dreaded disease. Governmental agencies also are beginning to demonstrate some responsiveness to epidemiologic findings, particularly when they relate to the cost and quality of medical care.

In Chapter 1, pharmacoepidemiology is defined as "the application of epidemiologic knowledge, methods, and reasoning to the study of the effects (beneficial and adverse) and uses of drugs in human populations." Thus, epidemiology refers to the study of health in populations and pharmacoepidemiology is the branch of epidemiology that studies the uses and effects of drugs in human populations. In both cases the emphasis is on populations rather than individuals; the distinguishing feature of pharmacoepidemiology is the focus on drugs and their effects. Just as a clinician must understand what potential complications to anticipate when treating patients with a given disease, an epidemiologist who sets out to study drug effects in patients with a given disease must understand the epidemiology of the disease. In other words, epidemiology is a prerequisite to pharmacoepidemiology.[2]

Epidemiology in the Discovery and Approval of Lovastatin

It is helpful to examine a section of the lovastatin (Mevacor) package insert for some idea of what other areas of epidemiology have done for the pharmaceutical industry.

Epidemiological studies have established that high LDL (low-density lipoprotein) cholesterol and low HDL (high-density lipoprotein) cholesterol are both risk factors for coronary heart disease. The Lipid Research Clinics Coronary Primary Prevention Trial (LRC-CPPT), coordinated by the National Institutes of Health (NIH), studied men aged 35–59 with cholesterol levels 265 mg/dL or greater, and triglyceride levels not more than 300 mg/dL. This seven-year, double-blind, placebo-controlled study demonstrated that lowering LDL cholesterol with diet and chole-styramine decreased the combined rate of coronary heart disease death plus non-fatal myocardial infarction.

Mevacor has been shown to reduce both normal and elevated LDL-cholesterol concentrations. The effect of lovastatin-induced changes in lipoprotein levels, including reduction of serum cholesterol, on cardiovascular morbidity or mortality has not been established.[3]

Lovastatin was approved for the treatment of hypercholesterolemia on the basis of double-blind, randomized clinical trials showing that it lowered cholesterol. A coronary heart disease prevention trial was not required for approval, because of the strong epidemiologic evidence (including clinical trial evidence with another drug) that lowering cholesterol lowers cardiovascular disease. Thus cholesterol reduction was accepted as a "surrogate endpoint" in place of the actual endpoint of cardiovascular disease reduction. If the epidemiologic evidence linking cholesterol and coronary heart disease had been lacking, it is unlikely that cholesterol reduction alone would have been accepted as evidence of efficacy for purposes of approval. If marketing approval had been delayed until completion of long-term cardiovascular disease prevention trials with lovastatin, availability of the drug would have been delayed for five or more years, preapproval development costs would have increased by tens of millions of dollars, and the net present value of the drug would have been much lower. Thus, epidemiology literally made lovastatin possible.

This example illustrates the most economically important application of epidemiology to drug approval: the potential to accelerate drug approval times by as much as several years by justifying the use of surrogate endpoints (e.g., blood pressure and cholesterol reduction) that can be measured in short-term trials instead of having to demonstrate a reduction in clinical endpoints (e.g., stroke, coronary heart disease) whose measurement would require trials lasting many years. One lesson which should not be drawn from this example is that the pharmaceutical industry can continue to count on government funding of the epidemiologic research needed to support drug development. Since research into cardiovascular disease has a high priority for research funding by the NIH, virtually all of the epidemiologic research contributing to the early approval of lovastatin was funded by government research grants. For many other diseases NIH funding priorities are lower; if research is to be done, private companies will have to support targeted epidemiologic research, just as they now support biochemical and molecular biologic research to discover new drug candidates.

Cardiovascular epidemiology contributed to lovastatin's discovery as well as its timely approval, by providing much of the rationale for undertaking the biochemical research to develop a specific inhibitor of cholesterol synthesis. Hence, the example of lovastatin also illustrates how epidemiologic research into disease etiology can suggest scientifically and commercially promising targets for drug discovery and development. In addition, it illustrates the marketing value of public fascination with health risk estimates, that is, with epidemiologic information.

Epidemiology in Marketing Research

The decision to undertake research in a new therapeutic area depends on an assessment of the potential for both scientific and commercial success. It is in the latter area that unpublished epidemiologic data from government surveys often are underutilized by pharmaceutical companies, despite being readily available on computer tapes at the cost of making the tapes. Examples of some government surveys are the National Medical Care Utilization and Expenditure Survey, the National Ambulatory Medical Care Surveys, and the National Hospital Discharge Surveys. All of these surveys provide data on medical care utilization and the first two also include data on prescribed drugs. There are two National Health and Nutrition Examination Surveys (NHANES I and NHANES II) which provide interview data and medical examination and laboratory results on the same individuals. A subset of the individuals enrolled in NHANES I has been followed in the Epidemiologic Followup Study. The National Health Interview Surveys (NHIS) provide only interview data, but subjects interviewed in 1984 who were 70 years of age and older have been followed in the Longitudinal Study of Aging. More detailed descriptions of these tapes and others are available in the Catalog of Public Use Data Tapes from the U.S. Department of Health and Human Services. NHIS tapes can be obtained from the Division of Health Interview Statistics, National Center for Health Statistics, 3700 East-West Highway, Hyattsville, MD 20782 (301/436-7087). All other tapes can be ordered from the National Technical Information Service, U.S. Department of Commerce, Springfield, VA 22161 (703/487-4650). To make use of these tapes it is necessary to have basic knowledge of epidemiologic and biostatistical principles, working knowledge of standard packages (e.g., SAS or SPSS) for computer-based data analysis, the background to follow the data analysis instructions supplied with the tapes, and an understanding of what kinds of conclusions can and cannot validly be drawn from such data.

Just as pharmaceutical companies sometimes neglect government data, academic researchers in departments of epidemiology sometimes are insufficiently aware of the excellent information on drug utilization developed by marketing research companies such as IMS America, Ltd. (660 West Germantown Pike, Plymouth Meeting Executive Campus, Plymouth Meeting, PA 19462, 215/834-5000). This valuable source of epidemiologic data on utilization of pharmaceutical products is well known to pharmaceutical companies.

Epidemiology in Planning Clinical Trials

The most valuable contribution of epidemiology to clinical trial planning lies in providing scientific justification for the use of a surrogate endpoint, as noted in the lovastatin example. For a surrogate endpoint to be acceptable for purposes of drug approval, one must be able to provide convincing evidence that improving the surrogate endpoint (e.g., lowering blood pressure in patients with hypertension) would be expected to improve a clinically important endpoint (e.g., lowering the incidence of stroke) which the clinical trial is too limited in scope and/or duration to measure. Thus, the surrogate endpoint must be accepted as causally related to the actual clinical endpoint. There also must be some assurance that improvement in the surrogate endpoint produced by the study drug is not accompanied by negative effects that could outweigh the beneficial effects. Entire textbooks have been written on the subject of causal inference[4,5] and numerous research papers have been written on criteria for deciding what sort of evidence is sufficient to justify acceptance of a surrogate endpoint. The reader is referred to selected publications for an introduction to the literature on this subject.[6-12]

Epidemiologic data have many other uses in planning clinical trials, especially in new therapeutic areas where methodology is not well established, definitions and choices of endpoints are unclear, rates of disease progression among untreated patients are poorly known, or important prognostic variables have not been determined. Under such conditions, which are common in clinical trials of breakthrough drugs in new therapeutic areas, epidemiologic information may contribute to more efficient clinical trial design, provided that the studies are carefully designed to answer specific questions and that they can be completed quickly. To obtain such data in a timely manner, the epidemiologic studies should be started very early in drug development. This is not always feasible; however, it can be done in therapeutic areas where a company has made a major research commitment to discover and develop new drug candidates. In such cases, it would make sense to begin epidemiologic studies even before there is a specific drug candidate. Such is already the practice in vaccine development and in the long-term coronary heart disease trials funded by NIH; however, it is not yet common in pharmaceutical company drug development.

Clinical research into prevention and treatment of osteoporosis provides an example of how epidemiologic data can be useful in planning clinical drug trials. Criteria for defining and quantifying the progression of vertebral fractures are not standardized enough to permit their use in the clinical trial of a drug to retard progression of preexisting vertebral fractures. To define such standards would require analyzing existing cross-sectional epidemiologic data to develop age-specific norms for vertebral body shape. Once such standards have been developed, the rates of fracture progression can be determined as a function of age and other baseline factors. These rates can be used to help decide upon entry criteria and to sharpen sample size calculations. The age-specific norms can be used in defining clinical trial efficacy endpoints.

Epidemiology in Investigating Rare, Serious Adverse Events

Epidemiology can be particularly useful in assessing the significance of one or two isolated cases of a rare disorder encountered in clinical trials of a new drug.

Because of the limited number of patients who are treated prior to market approval, the most likely outcome for many rare adverse events is for no cases to occur prior to marketing. The next most likely outcome is for one or two isolated cases to occur under circumstances where it is easy to find explanatory factors other than the study drug. The FDA recognized this problem in a draft guideline prepared several years ago to assist manufacturers in presenting the clinical data section of a new drug application.

> The serious, potentially life-threatening events that are not known to be drug-related should be searched for clues to an unexpected drug-relationship. It has historically been easy to consider as intercurrent illness, or as related to the underlying disease, events that in retrospect were drug-related. It should be appreciated that in most treatment populations of 1000–2000, screened at baseline for major abnormalities and basically well except for a specific illness, such events as acute hepatitis, acute renal failure, aplastic anemia, agranulocytosis, thrombocytopenia, seizures, ventricular tachyarrhythmias, gastrointestinal hemorrhage, stroke, pulmonary embolism, acute myocardial infarction, peripheral arterial obstruction, or sudden death are unusual and will usually not occur in the course of a several month period of observation. Any such events deserve close scrutiny, comparison between treatment groups, and if possible, comparison with historical series of the same patients.
>
> Obviously, certain populations will be predisposed to some such events, but the extent of such predisposition should be evaluated with available data, not assumed.[13]

The suggestion to consider historical control comparisons to document claimed predispositions encourages the use of epidemiologic data in the investigation of serious adverse events. Although the limitations of historical comparisons are well known, such comparisons can be helpful in getting an idea of just how unexpected a certain type of adverse event may be when considered in light of the number and types of patients treated and the duration of treatment. Certainly, a combined clinical and quantitative assessment is more convincing than the more common approach of generically dismissing each case with an assertion that such events are to be expected in seriously ill patients with the type of disease studied.

Relevant epidemiologic data frequently are available in the medical literature. It often is possible to use these data to provide responses to regulatory inquiries within a matter of days, provided that adequate computer programming and statistical support can be made available. In the few instances in which data are totally lacking, a separate study may be needed. For example, when seizures were reported during noncomparative clinical trials of the antibiotic imipenem-cilastatin, it was found that the information was lacking on the relative importance of the many potential seizure risk factors in seriously ill hospitalized patients. A small retrospective study was undertaken to obtain this information[14] and a retrospective study of risk factors for seizures among clinical trial patients treated with imipenem-cilastatin was made.[15] This work led to changes in the package insert regarding dosage adjustments in patients with impaired renal function. Other published examples of safety problems that have been addressed, with specialized analyses of clinical trial or postmarketing study data done by the Epidemiology Department at Merck Sharp and Dohme Research Laboratories, include the time-dependent nature of the risk of angioedema among patients treated with enalapril[16] and the association of steroid therapy with varicella-like rashes among children with leukemia treated with the varicella vaccine in clinical trials.[17]

Investigations of drug safety problems are examples in which pharmacoepidemiology makes use of the results obtained in other areas of epidemiology. There is a clear parallel with occupational epidemiology, where findings in cancer epidemiology, cardiovascular epidemiology, and reproductive epidemiology are all used in studies of employee health and safety.

Epidemiology in Marketing

One of the lessons that has been learned repeatedly in developing vaccines for adult immunization is that disease awareness is a prerequisite to vaccine acceptance. In other words, information about the morbidity and risk of the disease can be helpful in explaining the benefits of the vaccine to an audience which normally does not think of vaccination. The same lesson applies to conditions, such as hypercholesterolemia, which for the first time have an effective form of drug therapy. In addition to being useful to marketing in a traditional sense, epidemiologic information on disease morbidity is helpful in explaining the benefits of pharmaceutical products to governmental panels and to health maintenance organizations.

Epidemiology Is a Prerequisite to Health Economic Studies

With the increasing pressure by government agencies and third-party payers to contain healthcare costs, there has been an increasing interest of the pharmaceutical industry in health economic studies. Any mathematical model of the economic consequences of an illness and how they are predicted to be affected by medical therapy is necessarily based on epidemiologic data, whether available from existing sources or obtained in studies. Thus, epidemiology is a prerequisite to health economic studies. Much of the epidemiologic data in the U.S. regarding cardiovascular epidemiology is available; therefore building the health economic model can start from a comparatively solid base. With many other diseases in which new drugs are being developed, relatively little epidemiologic information is available and so targeted studies must be undertaken. This is a further reason why planning for epidemiologic needs must begin early in drug development. In summary, any plan for health economic studies must address the needs for epidemiologic data and how they will be met. A comprehensive plan for obtaining such data in a timely manner must be developed and adequately funded.

Summary

Epidemiologic research can contribute to pharmaceutical research and development in such diverse areas as suggesting new targets for drug discovery, providing background information for market forecasts, reducing drug approval times by providing the scientific support to permit use of a surrogate endpoint (e.g., cholesterol reduction) in place of a clinical endpoint (e.g., reduction in coronary heart disease), improving safety monitoring, and supporting health economic studies. The type of epidemiologic research needed to support pharmaceutical development is not likely to attract government grant funding except when the disease is one for which established grant funding priorities exist (e.g., cardiovascular disease, AIDS). For this reason epidemiologic research in support of drug research and development should be funded by the pharmaceutical industry. To be effective, epidemiologic research should be started very early in the development cycle. When a company has made a major research commitment to discover and develop drugs in a particular area, it would make sense to begin targeted epidemiologic research even before specific drug candidates have entered Phase I. In that way clinical trial planning and product development can proceed from a more sound knowledge of the natural history of the disease to be treated.

Epidemiology has contributed to many areas of the pharmaceutical industry, from basic research to marketing. Although much of the epidemiologic research into cardiovascular diseases has been funded by the government, this cannot be expected in most of the newer disease areas where pharmaceutical research is now active. The need for industry-funded targeted epidemiologic research probably will increase over the next ten years as drugs are developed to prevent and treat osteoporosis, benign prostatic hyperplasia, and other chronic disease which, until recently, were considered to be an inevitable part of the aging process.

References

1. Last JM. A dictionary of epidemiology. Oxford: Oxford University Press, 1983.

2. Guess HA, Stephenson WP, Sacks ST, Gardner JS. Beyond pharmacoepidemiology: the larger role of epidemiology in drug development. *J Clin Epidemiol* 1988;41:995-6.

3. Physicians' desk reference. 44th ed. Oradell, NJ: Medical Economics, 1990.

4. Susser M. Causal thinking in the health sciences. Oxford: Oxford University Press, 1973.

5. Elwood JM. Causal relationships in medicine—a practical system for critical appraisal. Oxford: Oxford University Press, 1988.

6. Kowey PR, Fisher L, Giardina EG, et al. The tPA controversy and the drug approval process. The view of the Cardiovascular and Renal Drugs Advisory Committee. *JAMA* 1988;260:2250-2.

7. Ellenberg S, Hamilton JM. Surrogate endpoints in clinical trials: cancer. *Stat Med* 1989;8:405-13.

8. Wittes J, Lakatos E, Probstfield J. Surrogate endpoints in clinical trials: cardiovascular diseases. *Stat Med* 1989;8:415-25.

9. Hillis A, Seigel D. Surrogate endpoints in clinical trials: ophthalmologic disorders. *Stat Med* 1989;8:427-30.

10. Prentice RL. Surrogate endpoints in clinical trials: definition and operational criteria. *Stat Med* 1989;8:431-40.

11. Norris RM, White HD. Therapeutic trials in coronary thrombosis should measure left ventricular function as primary end-point of treatment. *Lancet* 1988;1:104-6.

12. Horwitz RI. The experimental paradigm and observational studies of cause-effect relationships in clinical medicine. *J Chronic Dis* 1987;40:91-9.

13. U.S. Food and Drug Administration. Draft guideline for the format and content of the clinical data section of an application [docket no. 85D-0467]. January 1986. Available from: Center for Drugs and Biologics, Office of Drug Research and Review (HFN-100), Food and Drug Administration, 5600 Fisher's Lane, Rockville, MD 20857.

14. Guess HA, Resseguie LJ, Melton LJ, et al. Factors predictive of seizures among intensive care unit patients with gram negative infections. *Epilepsia* (in press).

15. Calandra G, Lydick E, Carrigan J, Weiss L, Guess H. Factors predisposing to seizures in seriously ill infected patients receiving antibiotics: experience with imipenem/cilastatin. *Am J Med* 1988;84:911-8.

16. Slater EE, Merrill DD, Guess HA, et al. Clinical profile of angioedema associated with angiotensin converting-enzyme inhibition. *JAMA* 1988;260:967-70.

17. Lydick EG, Kuter BJ, Zajac BA, Guess HA, and the NIAID Varicella Vaccine Collaborative Study Group. Association of steroid therapy with vaccine-associated rashes in children with acute lymphocytic leukemia who received Oka/Merck varicella vaccine. *Vaccine* 1989;7:549-53.

18

Standards of Postmarketing Surveillance: Past, Present, and Future

Bert Spilker

Abstract

The standards (i.e., the scientific principles that underlie commonly accepted practice) of postmarketing surveillance (PMS) activities are discussed specifically in the context of relationships between regulatory authorities and pharmaceutical companies. The current state of PMS within most companies should be interpreted as representing important progress, and not as being an ideal state. The cardinal rule for using multipurpose databases is that patient diagnoses must be confirmed; the same validation principle applies to other types of studies. Standards for other innovative designs and the British guidelines for PMS are discussed. Developing new standards for pharmacoepidemiologic studies may contribute to the discipline reaching adulthood by the turn of the century.

Outline

here are few fields of medicine that have evolved as rapidly over the last 15 years as postmarketing surveillance (PMS). Evolution is evident in the methods, standards, and results of this scientific discipline. It is informative to examine and compare the status of PMS as it existed at the dawn of the last decade, as it exists today (at the dawn of the 1990s), and also as it will most likely look in ten years, at the dawn of the next century. The standards of PMS are defined briefly and discussed in terms of their development, after which the following selected issues are discussed.

1. Principles governing relationships between regulatory authorities and companies
2. Reporting unintended drug effect (UDE) data to regulatory authorities
3. Organizing PMS activities within companies
4. Standards for establishing UDE causality
5. Standards of methodology for PMS studies
6. Establishment of standards and guidelines for conduct of PMS activities
7. Standards for regulatory agency conduct regarding PMS

Definition of Standards and How They Are Developed

Standards are defined operationally in this chapter as the scientific principles that underlie commonly accepted practice. Standards are not immutable; rather, they evolve over time, as scientific practices and professional behavior change. Pharmacoepidemiologic standards are established and influenced by a variety of groups involved in conducting studies, reporting UDEs, writing about this area, and developing the practice of the field in other ways.

Standards probably are influenced most strongly by regulatory authorities when they pass regulations or promote guidelines to influence current conduct and practice. Government task forces and committees outside the aegis of regulatory authorities also have played a role in this field, as described later in this chapter. Pharmaceutical companies influence the standards, particularly when they determine that obtaining the best data possible makes good business sense and this goal is encouraged. Academicians who are active in this field also influence standards.

Another group that affects the form standards take are professional societies. The recently formed International Society of Pharmacoepidemiology has members from academia, industry, regulatory authorities, and various other institutions and plays an important role in the development of PMS standards. Professional trade associations (e.g., Pharmaceutical Manufacturers Association) also have played a major role in influencing both the direction and growth of this field. Finally, there are many individuals associated with pharmacoepidemiology who influence standards through their writings, speeches, and peer pressure.

Principles Governing Relationships Between Regulatory Authorities and Companies

It is difficult to generalize about relationships in this area, but a few basic principles are evident, the most important being cooperation between regulatory authorities and pharmaceutical companies. This principle existed in the past and will continue into the future. What does change over time is how well this principle is fulfilled through the standards of PMS practice and through the spirit of cooperation. Fortunately, positive interactions are occurring.

A marked degree of cooperation has existed between several of the larger regulatory authorities (e.g., in the U.S. and France) and corporate sponsors. Although some disagreements previously existed, currently exist, and probably will continue to exist, both groups approach most issues with a positive attitude toward seeking agreement and improving standards.

Most regulatory authorities have begun to allow earlier marketing of important new medicines in exchange for sponsor guarantees to conduct adequate PMS studies. The most well-known example to date is zidovudine (Retrovir, Burroughs Wellcome). The early marketing of zidovudine is an important event for future breakthrough medicines. All companies would like to see this approach expanded to include most new medicines. Given current trends, however, I believe that this will not occur significantly by the year 2000. Some skeptics state that more rapid approval of breakthrough medicines has occurred at the expense of all other medicines. The data to prove or disprove this assertion are not yet available.

Reporting UDE Data to Regulatory Authorities

Ten years ago, few regulatory authorities in industrialized countries had requirements about what types of UDEs they wanted reported and at what frequency the reports should be made. Practice was governed by impressions and inferences of regulators and the regulated, but was not widely codified in regulations outside the U.S. and the United Kingdom. Practices such as whether or not labeled (i.e., included in the package insert) or only unlabeled UDEs were reported within a short, specified period often differed within a country, as well as from country to country. The allowable time for reporting UDEs after they occurred also differed among countries, but most large regulatory agencies primarily were concerned with UDEs that occurred within their borders.

The situation today is quite different, and some regulatory authorities (e.g., Sweden, West Germany) want to learn about all serious UDEs of medicines marketed in their country, regardless of where the UDEs occur. This change has been relatively rapid and, even within the short span of ten years, has gone through several phases. Ten or more years ago, each interested regulatory authority began to evolve its own rules for types of UDEs to report and how frequently to report them. Each authority designed its own forms and created its own definitions. This increasingly complex situation was becoming a nightmare for pharmaceutical companies. Some described PMS as building a Tower of Babel. It became rapidly apparent that cooperation between regulatory authorities and companies could resolve many unnecessary complexities and benefit both groups as well as physicians and, ultimately, patients.

The Council for International Organizations on Medical Sciences (CIOMS) is an informal coalition of medical associations (e.g., American Medical Association), trade associations (e.g., International Federation of Pharmaceutical Manufacturers Associations), and regulatory authorities. The CIOMS is a neutral forum where form, format, and content of UDE reports are discussed. A working group of regulators and industry representatives initially convened in 1987 under the auspices of CIOMS and made several recommendations. A pilot test of these recommendations for alert reporting has been judged as successful. This effort originally involved regulatory authorities from six countries and manufacturers from seven. Uniform forms in English were designed to promote rapid and efficient submission of relevant UDE data from manufacturers to regulators. The primary goal of this program is to facilitate postmarketing reporting using common definitions and uniform reporting forms, categories, and frequencies. A second phase is focusing on the content, format, and timing of reports for important UDEs that are labeled and not serious. This program is another example of extraordinary cooperation in the PMS field that has benefited all groups.

Future needs for collaborative efforts include steps to minimize, if not eliminate, variances between the forms, format, frequency, and content of all types of periodic UDE reports. This is part of European Economic Community harmonization that hopefully will occur over the next decade and may be based, in part, on the CIOMS model. A more distant goal relates to the formalization and harmonization of epidemiologic studies on a worldwide basis.

Organizing PMS Activities Within Companies

To gather, assemble, and report on UDEs, most research- and development-based companies have established PMS departments over the last decade. In 1980 there were extremely few departments in the industry, although many, if not most companies, had specific professionals to correspond with physicians who reported UDEs. This early precursor of the modern PMS department is as different from the large computer-assisted PMS groups of today as are the accounting scribes sitting on high stools, carefully writing numbers in a ledger book in a Dickensonian novel from computer-assisted financial departments today. The modern PMS group designs a specific PMS program for each investigational medicine during Phase III. This package of studies is designed to obtain important medical data as early during the postmarketing period as possible, which may be considered to begin during Phase IIIb (i.e., after the regulatory submission has been made, but prior to the drug's initial approval). The current state of PMS organizations within companies should be interpreted as representing important progress, and not as being an ideal state.

DATABASES WITHIN COMPANIES

Numerous problems remain to be resolved in the area of PMS. One of these is how to determine whether a pharmaceutical company with two (or more) UDE surveillance sites should use a single, worldwide database or whether they should have separate databases in each site and share information on an open and periodic basis. The pros and cons of each approach are not presented here.

It is predicted that in ten years almost all pharmaceutical companies will have centralized their UDE data reporting facilities for ease of operations. Most companies will use a single worldwide database, despite a number of important limitations and potential problems with this approach (e.g., combining UDE data of differing qualities). Subsetting the data within the database according to its quality and validity undoubtedly will occur. Data also may be partitioned based on country of origin, or according to any other factor that can be flagged as the data are entered into the computer.

Standards for Establishing UDE Causality

Causality is the assessment of a cause and effect relationship between two associated events. The likelihood of the cause and effect relationship usually is expressed in such terms as definite, probable, possible, unlikely, and definitely not. Causality assessments may be viewed on several levels. For individual patients it is often critically important to determine whether a medicine is the cause of the patient's UDE. The specific causality assessment helps determine whether or not the drug should be discontinued. For individual clinical trials, the causality assessment often determines whether the trial itself must be prematurely terminated. For individual companies, it usually is critically important to be aware of causal relationships between medicines and serious UDEs that are reported. This assessment often plays a major role in the company's decision to continue or terminate the drug's development.

For large PMS studies, and UDE evaluations, the assessment of causality usually is not relevant for interpreting the data, because it usually is not possible to obtain sufficient information on reported UDEs. Information obtained is often fragmentary, unverified, and of variable quality. It often is impossible to obtain sufficient additional data to answer questions. The interpretation of such data, even from many large, well-known databases, is subject to substantial error if the data are analyzed too finely (i.e., to assess causality). Although causality has been found to be an important, and even critical, tool for Phase I and other clinical trials, it is less valuable, and sometimes even counterproductive, to evaluate causality in PMS studies.

TOOLS USED TO ASSESS CAUSALITY

The tools available to assess causality have evolved over 20 years from an emphasis on global introspection (i.e., assessment by an expert using clinical judgment, experience, and data on the specific case), to the use of algorithms (i.e., simple or complex preestablished questions that lead to an answer), to formal Bayesian logic and, finally, to the use of natural history registries to establish background rates.

Up to the mid-1970s, global introspection was the method most widely used to establish causality between a drug and a UDE. This approach was criticized by various professionals who were able to demonstrate lack of agreement among experts who used these methods. Global introspection approaches also have been criticized by proponents of algorithms as being a less scientific and less valid method for establishing causality.[1]

Ten years ago, we were at the height of the "algorithm phase" for establishing the causality of purported drug-induced adverse reactions. At least 15 separate algorithms, many of which with a highly logical approach, were developed and published. It is no accident that many algorithms were developed by individuals trained as scientists and not by practicing clinicians.

During the 1980s a sense of frustration developed with algorithms, particularly when insufficient clinical data were available to utilize the algorithm as designed. This was particularly common with complex (i.e., elaborate) algorithms that posed many questions. Algorithms are utilized retrospectively, often when some important information either is unavailable or was never obtained. Algorithms are not patient-specific and are not necessarily correlated with medical decision making. The more simple algorithms proved easiest to use.

A group of active professionals in this area developed a Bayesian approach to the causality issue during the mid-1980s using concepts of formal logic. This methodology is probably as capable as any other method of yielding a definitive answer to the cause and effect issue. The method is well suited for assessing causality for individual patients and, therefore, could assist clinical treatment. This approach is unsuitable, however, for medicines for which a great deal of data are unavailable, because the method requires a substantial amount of prior knowledge. Therefore, the method is useful only for medicines in Phases III and IV. This method is also extremely time consuming and is not appropriate except when the importance of the clinical question justifies the use of a relatively large amount of resources.

At present the need to assess causality during clinical trials differs from the need to assess it during PMS. Clinical trials must consider it. In the future, as well as today, when serious unlabeled UDEs arise in clinical trials, a sponsor might want to use both global introspection and a moderately simple/complex algorithm. If results differ, I would place more reliance on the former method to establish the strength of the association of the event with the medicine.

There will be an increased demand for natural history epidemiology in PMS studies. This means that registries of the natural history of diseases will be used more in the future to establish the background rate of UDEs in patients with that disease. This information will be compared with medicine-induced rates. Comparing the rates for UDEs with rates obtained in natural history registries will be more important for PMS evaluations than focusing on the attribution of individual adverse events with the drug.

Several registries that gathered UDE data in selected therapeutic areas were founded prior to the 1980s. In the U.S. this includes the National Registry of Drug-Induced Ocular Side Effects, Registry of Tissue Reactions to Drugs, and Hepatic Events Registry. The Dermatological Adverse Drug Reaction Reporting System was begun in 1980.

Standards of Methodology for PMS Studies

Several large and costly PMS cohort studies (e.g., prazosin, cimetidine) had been mounted by 1980 with a goal of enrolling approximately 10 000 patients each. This number had a somewhat mystical connotation and often was described as representing a balance between the minimum size necessary to observe most rare UDEs (i.e., those with an incidence of less than 1 in 3000) and the maximum size that could be managed practically by a single company. Standard methods of assembling large cohorts of patients (e.g., conducting multicenter studies) were used for these PMS studies. These methods usually were applied to all medicines for which prospective PMS was considered, rather than custom designing different approaches for particular drugs. PMS studies sometimes involved retrospective analyses of data already collected, to look for increased incidence rates of UDEs in specific groups of patients.

The balance between conducting retrospective and prospective studies has switched over the last decade from a preponderance of large, prospective, cohort studies to a preponderance of studies involving a retrospective or mixed examination of data in large multipurpose, automated, linked databases. The pendulum also has swung from most information and signals about possible UDEs coming from passive intelligence gathering to a greater proportion of signals coming from active searching of published literature and more active solicitation and evaluation of spontaneously generated reports.

The most important single change in PMS over the last decade has been the development and use of large, automated, multipurpose databases to evaluate purported drug-induced UDEs. The cardinal rule today for using these multipurpose databases for record linkage studies is that patient diagnoses *must* be confirmed. Without this essential step, erroneous interpretations and conclusions based on misclassifications of patients are possible.

The same principle of validation also applies to other types of studies, such as those of clusters of UDEs. This situation is well known to public health investigators. For example, a report that 50 people who had emesis at a dinner party all ate the chicken salad, or that 50 people who lived in a polluted environment developed cancer, must be checked carefully. It may turn out in the former case that there was a contact psychological reaction that began when someone was overheated and felt nauseous; and in the latter case, many of the people involved may have had unassociated types of cancers or may have only recently moved to the area.

The discipline of PMS is currently in the midst of a substantial effort to develop additional and broader large automated, linked, multipurpose databases. Without sufficient linkages within each database and without a sufficient number of databases, it is impossible to adequately address relevant PMS questions and important issues. Risk Assessment of Drugs–Analysis and Response (RAD–AR, initiated by Ciba-Geigy) is an important industry-wide group that helps build sufficient database capacity for pharmacoepidemiology, and helps clarify the relationship between medicine benefits and risks. This group has four major functions or goals:

1. to explore and support the appropriate role of epidemiology in the pharmaceutical industry,
2. to serve as a forum for exchanging epidemiology and related information,
3. to serve as a coordinating group for intercompany activities relating to epidemiology, and
4. to act as a liaison between the pharmaceutical industry and other organizations (e.g., regulatory agencies, universities) for epidemiology-related activities.

One of RAD–AR's first projects was to assemble and issue a four-volume series titled "International Drug Benefit/Risk Assessment Data Resource Handbook."[2] The four volumes cover North America, the United Kingdom, Japan, and West Germany/The Netherlands/Switzerland. These volumes are the most complete list of sources of databases and available information. RAD–AR has achieved success at both the national and international levels. At the national level, numerous groups have evaluated pharmacoepidemiologic methods, standards, and capacity within their own country. At the international level, RAD–AR has achieved a network of many national groups and has helped foster the formation of the International Society of Pharmacoepidemiology.

Major pharmaceutical industry resources are being spent to evaluate current databases in terms of validity of diagnoses and data, as well as completeness and linkability. Numerous large automated databases with record linkage currently exist, primarily in the U.S. (see Chapter 8). By the year 2000 many more probably will have been established in most other countries where new medicines are developed. One of the keys to developing more large linked databases outside the U.S. is their endorsement by large international health organizations (e.g., World Health Organization), which would encourage some countries to overcome their current reluctance to build such databases. This reluctance often is based on the perceived need to protect the privacy of individuals.

These large databases will become more efficient in the future as they are used to address important PMS questions. Most of the existing databases are available to companies on a contractual basis. These include databases of health maintenance organizations, states, Medicaid, consortiums of hospitals, and selected registries. It should be noted that these databases were not designed with pharmacoepidemiology studies in mind, and they differ significantly from each other in the data they collect and their ability for linking different types of data. As a result, there are numerous pros and cons of using each database from a pharmacoepidemiologic viewpoint.

Current major experiments in PMS methodology include Prescription Event Monitoring (PEM) by the Drug Safety Research Unit (DSRU) in England. This technique involves systematic sampling of up to a million prescriptions per year, chosen (from 350 million written) because of the medicine prescribed. Each of the prescribing physicians of these million prescriptions is sent a green form requesting information on whether the prescription involved a new diagnosis, referral, unexpected improvement, change of treatment, and whether any UDE occurred. The goal of the DSRU is to conduct PEM on all new major chemical entity medicines used within the National Health Service. Eventually, PEM may also be used to test specific hypotheses in England (Wales, Scotland, and Ireland are not included in this survey).

Data obtained through PEM must be interpreted with a great deal of caution because (1) patient diagnoses are not confirmed and validated, (2) a causal relationship of a UDE cannot actually be established, and (3) a high reporting rate of UDEs may falsely suggest that the medicine is less safe than others. For example, if a new drug is promoted as being *less* liable than others to cause a certain UDE, physicians will tend to place more of their high-risk patients (for developing that UDE) on the medicine. Thus, a higher rate of that adverse experience may be noted with the drug, but may not reflect a true incidence figure for UDEs.

Results of PEM and other population-based methods are expected to differ from data obtained in drug development studies sponsored by pharmaceutical companies. This is because the UDE profile of a relatively healthy or select group of patients receiving a medicine, in a study conducted in a limited patient population (e.g., in clinical trials), will differ from the UDE profile obtained in all patients in a large population who receive the medicine. However, many physicians do not return any data on their patients to the DSRU, and the data returned may not represent a true cross-section of what is occurring. Even if physicians return data to the DSRU, the validity is uncertain. Moreover, the background incidence of most

UDEs measured is unknown. Thus, without population controls, excesses in frequency are difficult to interpret. The type of patients who are prescribed new medicines is also unknown. One final drawback of PEM is that it requires a minimum of several months to gather sufficient data, whereas a multipurpose automated database may take only one hour or even less to obtain suggestive PMS results.

Epidemiologic intelligence from sentinel sources, such as physician observations in letters sent to pharmaceutical companies, regulatory agencies, and the literature will remain an important source of information for identifying UDEs that should be further evaluated. Allegations from the media of important medical risks from marketed medicines will also remain a mechanism to trigger responses in both companies and regulatory agencies.

Establishment of Standards and Guidelines for Conduct of PMS Activities

There were no guidelines or standards for PMS studies prior to establishment of the Joint Commission on Prescription Drug Use. The U.S. Congress established the Commission in 1976 "to describe a postmarketing surveillance system that could be used to detect, quantitate, and describe the anticipated and unanticipated effects of marketed drugs, and to recommend a means by which information on the epidemiology of prescription drug use in the U.S. could be distributed regularly to interested parties in the United States."[3] The commission's final report was issued on January 23, 1980, and contained five major recommendations:

1. A systematic and comprehensive system of PMS should be developed in the U.S.

2. Such a system should be able to detect important UDEs that occur more frequently than once per thousand uses of a drug, to develop methods to detect less frequent reactions, and to evaluate the beneficial effects of drugs as used in ordinary practice. New methods will have to be developed for the study of delayed drug effects, including both therapeutic and adverse effects.

3. An integral function of the PMS system should be to report the uses and effects of new and old prescription drugs.

4. Recognizing the progress that the FDA has made in the area of PMS in the last three years, the Commission recommends that PMS should be a priority program of the FDA and that the FDA should continue to strengthen its program in this area.

5. A private, nonprofit Center for Drug Surveillance should be established to further the development of a PMS system in the U.S. This Center should foster cooperation among existing PMS programs, develop new methods for carrying out surveillance, train scientists in the disciplines needed for doing PMS,

and educate both providers and recipients of prescription drugs about the effects of these drugs.

The first four recommendations have been initiated to a large degree by the FDA and the pharmaceutical industry in the U.S., working jointly as well as independently. The last recommendation has not been implemented, but the need for a national center certainly could be debated.

In the United Kingdom, an analogous group to the Joint Commission on Prescription Drug Use was the Graham-Smith Working Party. There are currently no formal requirements, however, that serve as standards for PMS studies in either country.

Many regulatory agencies believe that there should be formal criteria or decisional standards to determine what medicines require tests, what types of studies are needed, and how PMS studies should be established, monitored, and reported. In other words, many groups believe that the postmarketing period of a drug's life should be evaluated as systematically and carefully as the premarketing period. There are generally well-designed standards for the premarketing period of new chemical entities and these are being reviewed in a search for appropriate PMS standards.

No guidelines existed for PMS in 1980. Ten years ago, the data used and combined in PMS often contained contaminants (inaccurate or incomplete data), and data were not validated for accuracy. The few studies conducted were mainly designed by clinical groups without training in epidemiologic methods. There were no guidelines at regulatory agencies to decide which drugs should be subject to PMS studies.

A set of 19 guidelines for PMS were proposed by a joint committee of the Association of the British Pharmaceutical Industry (ABPI), the British Medical Association, the Committee on Safety of Medicines, and the Royal College of General Practitioners. These guidelines were developed particularly for observational cohort studies sponsored by pharmaceutical companies. These 19 points are primarily principles and managerial guidelines rather than scientific guidelines or standards useful for the design and conduct of PMS studies. The British guidelines include a definition of PMS and describe basic principles underlying most studies (e.g., there should be a valid medical reason for undertaking the study). The guidelines state that studies should not be designed solely for promotional purposes, and that any breaches of this guideline are to be reported to the Code of Practice Committee of the ABPI. Another guideline is that appropriate fees may be paid to physicians for completing data forms, but no other financial inducements may be offered.[4] These guidelines might best be viewed as starting points for the development of scientific guidelines.

Investigational new drug and new drug application rewrites, plus regulatory commentary and additional guidelines written by the FDA during the 1980s, indicate gradually increasing and clarified regulatory requirements on what UDE data to report. This pertains to UDEs that occur in clinical trials as well as after the drug is marketed. The frequency and timing of these reports also are more precisely specified, both for short-term serious, unexpected, and unlabeled UDEs, and for those included in quarterly or annual reports.

In the U.S., the Emerging Epidemiological Monitoring Techniques Committee of the Pharmaceutical Manufacturers Association is actively and aggressively exploring the development of standards for the field of PMS equivalent to Good Laboratory Practices. Forty companies are participating in discussions on this topic. In sharing their problems and perspectives, they have followed the public health approach encouraging multiple groups to work together to help protect the well-being of patients using pharmaceutical products. Many practices that were standard five years ago are no longer acceptable today.

Most research and development-based pharmaceutical companies are opposed to the establishment of regulatory guidelines for the postmarketing period. They do not believe that the FDA has the regulatory authority or mandate to put forth these guidelines. Thus, no guidelines currently determine which medicines require PMS studies in the U.S. and what types of studies to perform. These decisions are handled on an individual basis between the sponsor and the regulatory agency. The European Economic Community is looking for harmonization with the U.S. and it is hoped that a general consensus between these groups can be reached. As a general principle, any guidelines enacted should consider the ability of sponsors to conduct PMS studies with available methods and databases, and should not force sponsors to adopt standards and methods that are beyond current capabilities.

More formal PMS guidelines undoubtedly will exist in the future. It is hoped that these scientific guidelines will be put together as a consensus of all interested parties and will represent state-of-the-art scientific principles that are realistic to achieve. Setting standards that are unrealistic in terms of methodologies or resources required to meet those standards will be counterproductive and not in the best interests of patients, the ultimate group for whom standards are created.

Standards for Regulatory Agency Conduct Regarding PMS Studies

An undesirable pseudoscientific practice of the past has been termed the "fishing expedition." In this method, someone at a regulatory agency or academic center with access to a large database would punch into his or her keyboard the name of a drug and a number of adverse medical events to determine whether any association existed. If an academician found, in the initial evaluation, a higher rate of UDEs associated with a medicine than anticipated, then an academic paper or a letter to the editor often resulted. The report could be picked up by the media or a regulatory authority and pursued further. If regulatory people conducted this fishing expedition, they would ask the relevant company how they intended to respond to any associations found. This letter might require the company to conduct a survey or study, but at the minimum would require that the company respond. Because of the ease of deriving possible associations by looking at one UDE across multiple drugs or by examining various patient populations and multiple UDEs for a single medicine, a single individual could potentially keep the entire pharmaceutical industry busy investigating such associations. This could occur despite the fact that most, or almost all, of these associations were not meaningful and could not be confirmed.

Obviously, the actual situation never deteriorated to this extent, and it is currently scientifically unacceptable for causality assessments to be derived in this nonscientific manner. Associations that should (or must) be analyzed usually arise from case studies, in the literature, or from reports received by a company or regulatory authority from physicians, sales representatives, or other sources.

Both the FDA in the U.S. and the Department of Health in the United Kingdom periodically publish reports of purported associations. For example, if either agency receives an increased frequency of blood dyscrasia reports occurring with a particular medicine, they often will include those data in the newsletter that all physicians receive. Their intention, to alert physicians about a potential problem and to seek additional data to define better the numerator and denominator of its incidence, is quite worthwhile. Unfortunately, this method may have the effect of eliciting many additional reports that complicate rather than simplify the assessment of a drug's benefits and risks.

In the future, perhaps all regulatory agencies will adopt a more logical and scientifically sound approach to increased frequencies of reports of known UDEs or to reports of serious new UDEs. The first step should be to contact the medicine's sponsor, manufacturer, or distributor and to notify them of the purported UDE. One company's response may be to dispatch trained monitors to visit the sites where the reported cases occurred and to evaluate all available data. At the same time, both the company and regulatory agency would review their existing databases to determine what cases were reported previously and the details of those cases. These assessments could better establish the importance of the signal, evaluate whether specific risk factors were involved in the cases, and describe any characteristics common to two or more of the cases. Benefit-to-risk assessments would be determined and a meeting would be arranged (if necessary) to plan the next stage of follow-up.

Any one or more of the following additional steps could be taken. A group of experts from academia and/or the government could be brought together to review the data and make recommendations. The regulatory authority or sponsor could issue a notification to all physicians in the country, in order to seek further information (i.e., examples). At this point, it would have to be determined if the name of the specific drug or only the chemical or therapeutic class should be identified. The latter approach would prevent biasing physicians against a single medicine, and would also minimize the chance of a "fishing expedition." This approach would determine more fairly whether the UDE was characteristic of an entire class of medicines. Large, automated, multipurpose databases could be used to evaluate the hypothesis. Other types of epidemiologic studies also could be conducted. Additional prospective epidemiologic studies could be undertaken to evaluate the UDE. Finally, if specific risk factors were identified and the benefit-to-risk consideration dictated that specific patients should not receive the medicine, then package labeling changes could be negotiated and the new data disseminated using a variety of techniques.

Summary

This brief discussion illustrates some of the vast changes in PMS that have evolved over the last 15 years and indicates a number of potential future trends. The field has moved from its own Dark Ages of the 1970s, when little consensus and no standards existed, into the light of the 1990s. Pharmacoepidemiology needs to continue to move forward and further develop and refine the scientific standards and guiding principles that represent signs of a more mature discipline. Practitioners of pharmacoepidemiology should accept this challenge either individually or through appropriate organizations. Let us hope that the scientific growth of the field of PMS and the development of standards for its conduct continue, and that the once fledgling and fragmented field reaches adulthood by the turn of the next century.

The author gratefully acknowledges fruitful discussions with Michael Joseph, M.D., and Hugh Tilson, M.D., Dr.P.H., both of whom kindly reviewed the manuscript.

References

1. Kramer MS. Assessing causality of adverse drug reactions: global introspection and its limitations. *Drug Inf J* 1986;*20*:433-8.

2. Pharma Corporation and the Degge Group. International drug benefit/risk assessment data resource handbook. Basle, Switzerland: CIBA-Geigy, 1988.

3. Melmon K. Final report of the Joint Commission on Prescription Drug Use. U.S. Senate Committee on Labor and Human Resources. Subcommittee on Health and Scientific Research. Washington, DC: U.S. Government Printing Office, 1980.

4. Joint Committee of ABPI, BMA, CSM, and RCGP. Guidelines on post-marketing surveillance. *Br Med J* 1988;*296*:399-400.

19

Pharmacoepidemiology: The Future

Hugh H. Tilson

Abstract

The future of pharmacoepidemiology, like all other futures, is not entirely clear. However, major forces exist that are driving the agenda for pharmacoepidemiology. This chapter reviews and weighs factors such as technology, data sources, healthcare delivery, public expectations, liability insurance systems, and epidemiologic intelligence. The roles of the major related actors (particularly physicians, pharmacists, patients, government, academia, and industry) are also analyzed. The pharmacoepidemiologic future lies partially in the progressive reduction of uncertainty both in the making of therapeutic decisions at the individual level and in the development of public policy decisions regarding therapeutics. Like all health futures, the future of pharmacoepidemiology can be influenced positively by responsible contributions, particularly by the pharmaceutical community.

Outline

P
redicting the future in any field is hazardous work, given the complexities of human endeavor and the weaknesses of our predictive tools. In epidemiology, predicting the future is all in a day's work, as the epidemiologist searches for trends within various components of the living equation—trends that are leading or contributing to the outcome. One could call these trends risk factors, confounding variables, or causes.

Predicting the future of the field of pharmacoepidemiology is equally challenging, perhaps more so for the epidemiologist, because the data are mostly lacking or soft. This chapter looks at the trends in pharmacoepidemiology and addresses the extent to which they point toward the future.

The trends seem to be convergent, relatively powerful, and, on balance, quite positive for a bright and exciting future for pharmacoepidemiology. The technology is burgeoning; the capacity is expanding; the public and private expectations, even demands, seem unrelenting; and the commitments of those critical actors in the field appear progressively positive. By the year 2000, we will find ourselves still negotiating over improvements, obligations, determinants, and constraints, and still struggling with an uncertain methodology to predict the year 2020. But, clearly, we will be more than 20 years into the era of pharmacoepidemiology by the year 2000.

The Factors

TECHNOLOGY

Perhaps the strongest single trend leading toward the era of pharmacoepidemiology is the evolving capacity to monitor society's transactions through large, automated databases. As the cost of memory core and other hardware decreases, as software becomes more user-friendly, and as the contributions of automated systems to cost containment and service effectiveness become progressively better understood and more clearly proven, the computer, in some form, will be as central to the healthcare transaction as are the stethoscope, ballpoint pen, and pill-counting trays today. Naisbitt, in *Megatrends*, describes a trend toward "high-tech, high-touch" in which the human side of our transactions will catch up with the technological side.[1] This trend will define the computer as partner, not successor, to the healer.

Part of the compelling trend is the emergence of a new method for studies of drug effects: record linkage.[2] How simple in concept is the new methodology, and yet how ancient. The model involves, first, the establishment of a marker (e.g., a unique identification number or code for each patient) that can be attached to each patient. Second, the linkage model involves finding a way to capture information on all healthcare transactions. Record linkage can be achieved by manually compiling all prescriptions, even hard copy, and combining these into cohorts. In the next step, all accompanying medical records can be manually searched to find all events or health problems associated with exposure to the drug in question; rates of events can be compared with one or more comparable nonexposed, similarly linked cohorts or groups.

However, the miracle of automation shortens the multiyear tedium for countless clerks and student research associates to a few hours of programming data that have been downloaded from automated pharmacies, and linking these data via a patient identification marker to the coded computerized hospital discharge file. At least, that is how record linkage pioneers, such as Hershel Jick of the Boston Collaborative Drug Surveillance Program (BCDSP), were able to achieve pharmacy record and medical chart linkage with the Group Health Cooperative (GHC) of Puget Sound in Seattle, WA. The skeptic should read one of the more than 50 published reports resulting from this extraordinary collaboration.[3] The health maintenance organization (HMO) is not the only data source of such linkages. Third-party payment programs and reimbursement schemes also contain medical and prescription data with potential for record linkage, e.g., provincial health plan data from Saskatchewan and U.S. data from state-level Medicaid programs.

Linkage methodology made possible and effective through the support of computer technology will not simply be understood, but rather embraced as central to the logic of pharmacoepidemiology in the future. Concerns about confidentiality that have limited our progress are being successfully addressed. New techniques must be used to protect against conspiracies that misuse confidential information and compromise our ability to get the most out of the power of the computer. The computer can identify important details about us that our physicians, pharmacists, and we ourselves never even understood, much less remembered, and we must be mindful of the sensitivities of people who have the right to demand their privacy.

We are entering an era in which the various components of our personal health, including pharmaceuticals, important medical diagnoses, healthcare behaviors, hospital utilization, and vital statistics, are entered into the same computer, all using our health master identification number. Microfiche and microchip technology probably will be extended so that we will carry vital medical information on our wrists or maybe even as implants, allowing us to plug in each time there was a new transaction and have our chip updated. Likewise, population databases will be central stores from which physicians deduce treatment strategies for the individual and introduce prevention plans to the community.

CONCEPTUALIZATION

Of course, all the previously discussed new methodology and technology available by 2000 will require the education and training of pharmacoepidemiologists—pharmacists, physicians, nurses, and other health professionals literate in computer-assisted data analysis techniques—who can bring about the revolution toward the database and away from hands-on techniques. In earlier times, epidemiologists spent at least half of their time trying to figure out clever ways to collect data on the form with the most convenient format, asking the right question of the right respondent. In addition, it took inordinate amounts of time from busy practitioners who did not like research and did not understand how to get observational data without an experiment or from confused patients who did not wish to be our guinea pigs. Then we developed complicated ways of entering the data and manipulating the numbers from ad hoc studies in ad hoc computer files, only then to begin thinking about how we analyzed them. Having large amounts of data available in a structured and retrievable form is changing our approach to conducting pharmacoepidemiologic studies. Currently, with all the data stored in the computer, the data collection phase for many record linkage studies is completed before the study is even proposed. At the outset we must formulate creative hypotheses; proper controlling, qualifying, and structuring will be aided by the design of the database. In fact, what seems revolutionary today, such as the application of multivariate analysis techniques that rely on computers to simulate the loading of various factors, will be central to the education of every decision maker by the year 2000, not only epidemiologists.

Additionally, methodologies that take into account the complex dimensions of cost-benefit and effectiveness analysis and routinely provide computer-assisted risk/benefit comparisons using all of the available data against all of the available alternative scenarios will be common in our society. In a practice application, a physician will be able to key individual patient risk factors and desired outcomes into an online computer system at the office work station; the physician can then have these matched against the benefit-to-risk algorithms tempered for (stratified by) the patient's specific risk category for computer-assisted therapeutic decision making. The policy maker will likewise use the same simulation methodologies at the population level to assess relative merits and proper indications (placement) and balance these against the risks of various therapeutic modalities.

In 1990, when difficult decisions needed to be made, a common approach was to get all of the facts and then "sit around together and think hard," to paraphrase David Eddy, noted policy analyst from Duke University.[4] A next logical step is to identify the variables that are important in our decision analysis and consequently quantify these by assigning a probability score to them. By the year 2000, drug epidemiology will have introduced computer-assisted decision algorithms, not to replace thinking hard, but to help us quantify the extent to which our thinking hard is in fact governed by information that may reduce our level of uncertainty. Translated into the positive, the epidemiology future lies in progressive incremental reduction of uncertainty both in the making of therapeutic decisions at the individual level and in the development of public policy decisions regarding therapeutics.

HEALTHCARE DELIVERY

A third dimension of change to factor into the equation predicting our pharmacoepidemiologic future is reflected in the movement of Western cultures into organization-based delivery of health services: in medicine, the marriage of profession and business, or at least the change from individual entrepreneurship to organized management structure as the way of healthcare delivery. Within large healthcare organizations, innovative means of financing healthcare are characteristic. Basing the reimbursement system for Medicare patients in hospitals on the diagnosis-related group (DRG) system has changed individual department in the hospital from profit centers to cost centers. However, reducing cost in one department may increase to a larger proportion the cost in another department. If, for example, the pharmacist is being instructed to cut costs, the pharmacist may actually increase overall costs by substitution of a more costly surgical or medical alternative for a cost-effective pharmaceutical product, effectively shifting the pharmacy cost to the cost of the medical department. The classic example of this occurs when the formulary committee turns down an innovative drug because it is too expensive without considering the costs of the emergency room visit that could have been shortened, the intense monitoring that could have been offset, or the earlier discharge that the marginally better innovator could have made possible.

When working together, the various elements of the structured system can keep costs down and can, in fact, obtain the synergy inherent in any system. The pharmacoepidemiologist will benefit from the evolution of large healthcare organizations that will inevitably bring not only more computerization but also the application of the technology and methodology described above to more enrolled populations. The greater the population covered by the databases, the greater the power to detect important associations through linkage methodology.

Several automated systems supporting healthcare organizations are already in some stage of readiness to complement the linkage capacity of the BCDSP at GHC with its ten years of data on more than 300 000 people. Notable among these systems are several of the Kaiser-Permanente Health plans (e.g., Kaiser-Portland with over 300 000 patients and Kaiser-Los Angeles with over 2 million people).[5] The HMO concept means efficiency; efficiency means computers; and computers may mean yet another population that can be added to the denominator of potential users of a new pharmaceutical, and may up the power for such linkage efforts to detect rare events. Indeed, one of the great challenges to the pharmacoepidemiologic community will be to make ourselves actively involved in the design of the database to ensure that, when health plans become automated, the systems that develop are compatible with the public policy imperatives of data linkage and are suitable for pharmacoepidemiologic research.

Among other changes, healthcare organizations will emphasize prevention not solely as a method of cost containment but as a value in itself, the benefits of which are probably better documented than are the benefits of many therapeutic interventions now covered by traditional medical insurance plans. With this change will come greater demand for more preventive medicines—drugs used by healthy people to promote health or counteract risk factors. The healthier the patient, the less acceptable are risks of severe although rare complications of treatment and the greater the demand to find any such problems early in the drug regimen.

PUBLIC EXPECTATION

The demand for monitoring will not wait for the era of preventive medicine. One of the major forces driving the pharmacoepidemiology movement is an evolving public intolerance in America, western Europe, and Japan to any risk, including that of injury from unintended drug effects (UDEs), and this intolerance promotes consumer advocacy programs that respond to public demand for monitoring and responsible corporate action. The emerging technology will reinforce the prevention incentive. As more data sets become available and affordably accessible, we will all know more, sooner. It seems highly unlikely that a new chemical entity would escape vigorous monitoring in structured data sets, in as large a population as available, simply to reduce the time required between the generation of a signal of a potential problem, e.g., through voluntary, spontaneous UDE reports, and the making of public policy decisions.[6]

LIABILITY

Important forces increasing the interest in and commitment to rigorous structured monitoring of drug safety following approval are two current major public policy crises: burgeoning malpractice costs and crumbling liability insurance systems. As a symptom of society's unwillingness to tolerate risks, coupled with major dysfunctions in the tort liability system, injury settlements for people with drug- and vaccine-associated UDEs have become major threats to the ability of drug companies to obtain insurance protection. Both have driven up the cost of doing business: in 1985 A.H. Robins, a major U.S. drug manufacturer, was forced to file for reorganization under the bankruptcy laws because of litigation surrounding UDEs associated with one of its contraceptive products, the Dalkon Shield; and Merrell Dow Pharmaceuticals was forced to remove from the market Bendectin, a product used to treat incapacitating nausea of pregnancy, because it could no longer afford defense against litigation, despite the lack of evidence for causal association between that product and any of the congenital defects involved in the litigation. This trend will precipitate in the 1990s a major push for tort liability reform, including limitation of settlements, limitation of punitive damages, and a reevaluation of contingency fees for plaintiff's lawyers. Although difficult to predict, recent congressional debate suggests that it will lead to some form of "workmen's compensation model" to support claims of injured parties. The need for development of an actuarial base for such a fund will surely lead to the development of still greater demand for better epidemiologic information regarding the likelihood and extent of injury for estimates of the contributions of coexisting risk factors.

EPIDEMIOLOGIC INTELLIGENCE

In pharmacoepidemiology, truly rare events must currently be, and perhaps always will need to be, detected through a global monitoring and signaling system, which is the pharmacologic equivalent of the epidemiologic intelligence network for detecting communicable disease epidemics. Under this system, physicians, pharmacists, and nurses are asked to report voluntarily to the manufacturer or the regulatory authority (e.g., FDA) any adverse medical experiences in association with use of pharmacologic agents. Such voluntary reporting is at once the strongest and the weakest of such systems—strongest because it uses as its denominator the entire population of treated people, weakest because it uses as its numerator reports generated by busy practitioners with little experience with the system and little incentive to provide the report. This, too, will change with the advent of better-informed consumers, organized healthcare settings in which ancillary staff can complete the regulatory requirements, and evolution of automation in the practice setting. The more user-friendly the computer support system becomes for office practice, and particularly the faster the retrieval on various dimensions (e.g., epidemiologic reporting of communicable diseases, chronic disease events, and drug-associated events) becomes, the more likely the busy practitioner will participate in such sentinel nets. Efforts of the FDA in cooperation will several state health departments to enhance physician reporting emphasize the inadequacies of the existing system and the need for a responsive (easy) system to improve reporting.[7]

The Actors

THE PHYSICIAN

Every medical educator in epidemiology/preventive medicine hopes that the last decade of the twentieth century will present an educational atmosphere that demands rather than tolerates rigorous epidemiologic content in curriculum and expects rather than accepts rigorous epidemiologic competence among graduates.[8] The ability to understand and apply the lessons of pharmacoepidemiology to the choice of the proper balance between risk and benefit in the individual patient's case represents one end product of pharmacoepidemiology, perhaps one as important as the public policy outcome of society's ability to review, approve, and regulate such products. In the last analysis, the intelligent use of medicines must lie in the hands of intelligent users.

Prediction. Physicians in the era of pharmacoepidemiology will understand and apply the findings of pharmacoepidemiologic studies. Warning: They won't if we don't teach them.

THE PHARMACIST

The evolving role of the pharmacist in the pharmacoepidemiology era remains unclear. Reading from recent trends is discouraging, as we see the pharmacist relegated to the business office behind an opaque wall. However, several positive trends emerging in pharmacy may reverse this negative trend: reimbursement either for dispensing or nondispensing, rather than making a living as overhead (e.g., as a proportion of the price of the product sold); the availability of consulting fees; the development of computer-supported drug profiling; direct computer links between the physician's office and the pharmacy; and a resurgent patient demand for better drug information. The evolution of the computer-supported pharmacy hold great promise in the pharmacoepidemiology sector. In many of the large HMOs, the pharmacist has been at the center of the new technology. Computerized pharmacy develops the automated cohorts that permit rigorous computer data linkage studies. For development of large populations, one questions is whether, under large non-HMO population-based reimbursement mechanisms, similar automation can be harnessed for similarly affordable and efficient cohorting. In the mid-1980s, 20 percent of community pharmacies were computerized; in 1995, almost all pharmacies will be computerized. This provides enormous potential for developing an ambulatory-care database. Pharmacy networking for economic reasons (e.g., buying groups) may be an impetus to use the same broad-based data for epidemiology purposes.

All pharmacy computer programs can screen for drug–drug interactions, allergies, and so forth. These systems are currently rudimentary because they cannot estimate accurate probabilities and predict the probability of clinical significance of the event. Patient prescribing profiles are currently pharmacy-based. As more clinical pharmacists and drug information specialists participate in direct patient care, there will be increased demand for better risk and benefit data to complement their consultation in pharmacokinetics and pharmacodynamics.

Also, an encouraging trend is shown in several experiments in automation of the hospital pharmacy as a method for developing drug exposure cohorts. These cohorts can be linked to automated discharge summaries in the same hospital, using the patient hospitalization number, to advance the intensive inpatient monitoring systems pioneered by the BCDSP. Several data management organizations have already emerged to explore pooling such data among dozens of hospitals. Under the leadership of pharmacist/epidemiologist Thaddeus Grasela in Buffalo, an ad hoc computer-supported network of hospital pharmacists is collaborating to test signals and/or erect cohorts for prospective searches. With better electronic communication among colleagues, such networks will expand and increase their contribution.[9,10] An important challenge for the next decade will be to link these cohorts with an initial hospital exposure to some form of longitudinal community-based follow-up system. Put these trends into the equation and the future looks bright.

Prediction. Pharmacists in the era of pharmacoepidemiology will understand and apply the findings of pharmacoepidemiology studies. Warning: They won't if we don't teach them.

The Patient

The individual who benefits from the medication is the reason for the many pharmacoepidemiologic efforts. As the population of the developed world achieves better economic and healthcare success, it is becoming progressively older; projected growth in the population segment over 65 years is from 25 million today to 55 million by the year 2030. With age will come more chronic illnesses, more need for potent medicines, and more demand than ever for responsible safety monitoring. The population will change, and its needs and expectations will change, as will the role the patient can play in systems designed to address drug safety concerns.

During the 1980s, we saw the development of several pharmacy-based programs that invited the patient to enroll voluntarily in a monitored follow-up system. Take as an example the medication monitoring program sponsored by The Upjohn Company, which successfully recruited thousands of patients into programs in which the exposed cohort of volunteers was followed by a structured telephone interview and, if needed (and with their consent), by a physician follow-up.[11] Similar programs are under development, perhaps most notably one at Purdue University under Stephen W. Schondelmeyer in which the patient can build his own link (personal communication, S.W. Schondelmeyer, Ph.D., Purdue University, 1986). This direct link system may close a critical information hole in the drug epidemiology net by providing data on more subtle drug-associated problems and in those for which no hospitalization occurs and no hospital computer-stored diagnosis exists.

Prediction: Patients in the area of pharmacoepidemiology will better understand preventable risk and uncertainty and demand the use of both. Warning: they won't if we don't simplify our message.

THE GOVERNMENT

In America, public policy follows public expectation and capacity in its mandates, but may lead both in its incentives. Thus, in the decade to come, in the face of all these trends, we will see first incentives and then mandates for pharmacoepidemiologic monitoring of known and potential drug-associated events, outcomes, and problems. Incentives will fall into three broad categories: (1) system- and capacity-building efforts, currently embodied in the FDA Extramural Contracts Program; (2) incorporation of epidemiologic planning into discussions with the FDA during investigational stages of product development (Phases II and III) and into consideration governing approval of new drug applications (NDA); and (3) FDA receptiveness to epidemiologic data for ongoing assessments of postmarketing drug safety, particularly in labeling negotiations.

The Extramural Program of the FDA has already amply demonstrated the first incentive. Although presently constrained by national balanced budget incentives, this program already has been effective both in developing new capacity for pharmacoepidemiologic monitoring (e.g., Vanderbilt University, Harvard University, and University of Pennsylvania, exploring methods of harnessing drug exposure and disease diagnosis data from the automated billing files of Medicaid programs) and in maintaining other more established programs (e.g., national registries, the Boston University Drug Epidemiology Unit, the pioneer in pharmacoepidemiology through its work with the GHC database, the BCDSP). Development of cooperative funding mechanisms to ensure continued support is a critical policy issue that will require attention by all sectors.[12]

There is much discussion of postapproval epidemiologic studies as part of the drug development process, not as substitutes for the best achievable and acceptable safety assurance at the time of approval, but as catalysts for speeding the transition following NDA submission to approval. This postsubmission preapproval hiatus reflects a period of residual anxiety in which no further structured drug development studies are to be expected, and yet the level of assurance from the data on-hand may be too low for comfort. Extending or adding more trials in the late phases of preapproval drug development (Phase III) or creating a "Phase III$^{1}/_{2}$" study seem to be less acceptable options than does adding more affordably the structured assurance of good science and even larger numbers after approval.

Evolving approaches to product labeling represent the third incentive to good drug epidemiology. Recent FDA Advisory Committee debates about the non-steroidal antiinflammatory drugs have set the tone for acceptance of properly conducted, large-scale, nonexperimental, observational studies to determine exact frequencies that can be incorporated into the education of health professionals and into the approved labeling itself.

The exact timing and nature of any specific mandate for inclusion of pharmacoepidemiologic studies as part of the approval of an NDA is difficult to predict. In the mid-1980s several products were conditionally approved upon the manufacturer's willingness to complete studies that included major programs in pharmacoepidemiology, and a recent Office of Technology Assessment study suggested that the power to ensure proper studies following approval may not require any legislation.[13]

The emergence of dramatic collaborative efforts between government, industry, and practice to develop and distribute new drugs for life-threatening conditions, particularly in the face of the epidemic of AIDS during the 1980s, has increased emphasis upon epidemiologic, observational studies in the preapproval phases. For a "fast-track" review, a treatment IND system requires epidemiologic monitoring of open treatment for broader availability of a drug during the period of preapproval final reporting of clinical trials and FDA review.[14] Further, an extensive program of postapproval epidemiology studies often is offered to help to "fill-in-the-gaps" left by the urgency of rapid development and shortened NDA review time. The 1990s will see these efforts expand as new therapies for AIDS are developed and new applications of fast-track and enhanced availability approaches (e.g., the parallel track) are brought to bear on other life-threatening illnesses.

On the international level, there is strong emerging consensus that postapproval epidemiology must include more than spontaneous voluntary UDE report monitoring. The development of data linkage capacity similar to that in North

America is a high priority for nations entering the European Common Market in 1992, starting with important efforts in the United Kingdom with the automated medical records supporting outpatient medical practice (e.g., VAMP and AAH Medical) and a record linkage scheme bridging prescription pricing authority documented dispensing and automated hospital discharge information (e.g., the medication events monitoring program, MEMO, in Dundee, Scotland).

THE ACADEMY

The 1980s witnessed the emergence of academic university-based programs in pharmacoepidemiology supported by the extramural program of the FDA already mentioned and by substantial industry contributions. This trend will continue as three inevitable forces continue to influence the sector: progressive erosion of "core" funds and "hard money" in academia, and with it, a progressive dependence of academic units on ad hoc and project-specific funding for their survival; a progressive realization on the part of other factors in the sector that freedom of intellect and independence of thought are most likely to result in epidemiologic projects that are scientifically credible and independent of proprietary or vested interests; and emerging recognition within academia itself that this specialized field of epidemiology is not simply important but also scientifically meritorious in comparison to other scholarly pursuits. The development of trained professionals in the field, however, will take concerted effort over the next decade. Funding for postgraduate training (residency and fellowships) will be needed, and curriculum time will be necessary to ensure that no physician, nurse, or pharmacist can graduate without orientation to the fundamental principles of pharmacoepidemiology.

THE INDUSTRY

Perhaps the most extensive and encouraging of trends among the actors in this field is the assumption of responsibility by the pharmaceutical manufacturer for rigorous scientific monitoring in the postapproval period. This explosion of interest is reflected in the creation of a strong body of industry scientists meeting regularly under the aegis of the Pharmaceutical Manufacturers Association (The Clinical Safety Surveillance Committee) which involves more than 40 research-based pharmaceutical companies. Internationally, the Risk Assessment Detection Analysis and Response (RADAR) working groups in many nations are providing leadership for development of the sector.[15] By 2001 there will be no question about the need for and desirability of pre- and postapproval epidemiology. Departments of pharmacoepidemiology in the major drug companies will couple traditional (passive) surveillance techniques (e.g., collection of UDE reports) with the epidemiologic quasiexperimental design (active) observational study. Decisions regarding exactly which approach to use and at what time in the life of the drug will be based upon rational criteria, possibly even algorithm application, balancing the need to know more than can be known at the time of preapproval experimentation with the costs of obtaining that knowledge. These decisions will be made according to feasibility. Here again, prompting this trend toward industry responsibility are the pressures of unwillingness to accept risks and uncertainty and the opportunity posed by decreasing costs of obtaining data occasioned by large automated data sets.

Summary

The fundamental goal for the future of the field must be to strike the balance between the early and aggressive use of needed new medications and the prevention of preventable drug injury (i.e., the optimization of therapeutic intervention).

The fundamental strategic question to be confronted by future decision makers regarding the conduct of pharmacoepidemiologic studies will be how far they can justify the costs of knowing that which is potentially knowable, so that we may do that which is potentially "doable." The availability of large automated data sets with their store of drug exposure information, coupled with the growing demand to prevent human suffering by early detection, will likely lead to progressively more complicated and extensive studies.

Perhaps the best point to end this glimpse into the future is with a statement of an axiom in this field: the occurrence of UDEs is an undesirable aspect of the practice of medicine, including pharmaceutical medicine. This aspect should be reduced to an irreducible minimum in the pursuit of benefit. In the area of drug safety, then, the interests and concerns of industry are no different from the interests and concerns of practice, of academia, and of regulation: to know as much as possible as soon as possible and as accurately as possible, to help bring about the best possible therapeutic decision making for humanity at all levels of policy making—individual, institutional, and national. This is the commitment of the future. The new era of pharmacoepidemiology brings this promise substantially closer to today's reality.

References

1. Naisbitt J. Megatrends. New York: Warner Books, 1982:39-53.

2. Lawson DH. Pharmaco-epidemiology: a new discipline. Br Med J 1984;289:940-1.

3. Jick H, Madsen S, Nudelman PM, Perera DR, Stergachis A. Postmarketing follow-up at Group Health Cooperative of Puget Sound. Pharmacotherapy 1984;4:99-100.

4. Eddy DM. Presentation at the annual meeting of the American College of Preventive Medicine, April 1986, Atlanta, GA.

5. Inman WHW, ed. Monitoring for drug safety. 2nd ed. Lancaster, UK: MTP Press, 1986.

6. Committee on Safety of Medicines. Adverse Reactions Working Party Report. Part 1. Limitations of ADR System, June 1983; Part 2, July 1985. Department of Health and Social Services, London, England.

7. Scott HD, Thacher-Renshaw A, Rosenbaum SE, et al. Physician reporting of adverse drug reactions: results of the Rhode Island Adverse Drug Reaction Reporting Project. JAMA 1990;263:1785-8.

8. Cooperative agreement between the National Centers for Disease Control and the Association of Teachers of Preventive Medicine, 1985.

9. Grasela TH Jr, Schentag JJ. A clinical pharmacy-oriented drug surveillance network: I. Program description. *Drug Intell Clin Pharm* 1987;21:902-8.

10. Grasela TH Jr, Edwards BA, Raebel MA, Sisca TS, Zarowitz BJ, Schentag JJ. A clinical pharmacy-oriented drug surveillance network: II. Results of a pilot project. *Drug Intell Clin Pharm* 1987;21:909-14.

11. Luscombe FA. Methodologies issues in pharmacy-based post-marketing surveillance. *Drug Inf J* 1985;19:269-74.

12. Faich GA. Adverse drug reaction monitoring. *N Engl J Med* 1986;314:1589-92.

13. U.S. Congress, Office of Technology Assessment. Post-marketing surveillance of prescription drugs. Congressional Board of the 97th Congress. Washington, DC: U.S. Government Printing Office, 1982.

14. U.S. Department of Health and Human Services: new drug and antibiotic regulations. Section 312.42. Investigational new drug (IND) applications (treatment IND). *Fed Reg* 1987; May 22.

15. Tilson H, Bruppacher R. A Working Group on Epidemiology in the Pharmaceutical Industry (EPI): a new force in the field. *J Clin Res Pharmacoepidemiol* 1990;4:91-7.

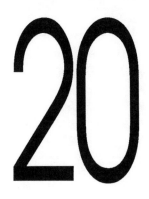

An Annotated
Bibliography on
Pharmacoepidemiologic
Studies

Abraham G. Hartzema
Donald C. McLeod

his bibliography on pharmacoepidemiologic studies was compiled after an extensive survey of the literature through early 1990. A structured approach was taken in compiling a master list of pharmacoepidemiologic studies published in the scientific literature. The two major databases, MEDLINE of the National Library of Medicine, and *International Pharmaceutical Abstracts* of the American Society of Hospital Pharmacists, were explored as provided by the database vendor BRS/Saunders Colleague. Using the string search capability available through the database vendor, the titles, key words, and abstracts were searched for terms relevant to pharmacoepidemiologic methods and cross- referenced with the term *drug*. The Medical Subject Headings (MeSH) and corresponding MeSH tree numbers are included in Table 1.

For searching the *International Pharmaceutical Abstracts*, the terms *epidemiologic methods, cross-sectional studies, longitudinal studies, cohort studies, case-control studies, product surveillance,* and *postmarketing surveillance* were used in combination with the search terms *drug* and *medication*. We did not search the literature on the term *clinical trial* because clinical trials are used mainly to study the effectiveness of the drug for its primary indication. Some clinical trials appeared in search results but were omitted from this bibliography.

The references obtained were downloaded in a master file and sorted by date of reference and author's name; duplicate entries were omitted. In the next step, a second database was created to contain selected references from the first database. The selection criteria included the following: authors' names were included; anonymous articles were excluded; articles as indicated by the title that had no relationship to pharmacoepidemiology were omitted, as were case studies, clinical trials examining the efficacy of a drug product or the comparative efficacy of two compounds, pharmacokinetic studies, and animal or human toxicology studies.

The content of the remaining articles was reviewed representing a pharmacoepidemiologic study based on the description of the methodology applied. Studies using pharmacoepidemiologic methods were abstracted and the following characteristics included in the annotation: drug name, drug category, drug dosing criteria, treatment duration, validation of exposure, study methodology, population selection criteria, sample frame limitations, total number of subjects enrolled, number of cases, number of controls, comparability of controls, drug event, validation of outcome, rule out alternative explanations, and findings.

In addition, an index of the studies was compiled using the annotations. The number following the index term refers to the reference number of the article. The bibliography was compiled to demonstrate the research efforts in the area of pharmacoepidemiology and to stimulate such efforts. References were selected to reflect the spectrum of pharmacoepidemiologic study types as well as the different study methods used. To illustrate the strengths and limitations of existing studies, some references have been cited despite their methodologic weaknesses. Other studies that merited inclusion may have been unintentionally omitted. Although we provide a comprehensive overview of the pharmacoepidemiology literature, it is not

Subject Headings	Tree Numbers	Table 1
Epidemiologic methods	E5.318	Medical Subject Headings and Tree Numbers Used in the MEDLINE Searches
cross-sectional studies	E5.318.150	
longitudinal studies	E5.318.420	
follow-up studies	E5.318.420.390	
prospective studies	E5.318.420.820	
retrospective studies	E5.318.420.820	
population surveillance	E5.318.533	
sampling studies	E5.318.821	
Epidemiologic methods	G3.850.520	
Drug	D	
Drug therapy	E2.319	

complete. The citations included are listed chronologically by year and alphabetically by first author's name within the year of publication. The bibliography is accompanied by a structured annotation system. In the annotation and indexing of the study methodology, drug exposure, and categorization of unintended effects, the terminology of the authors was adhered to wherever logical.

In addition, some articles of pertinence known to the authors, but not identified by the above computer search, were included in the bibliography.

The authors thank Pat Tennis for her contribution in developing the annotation indexing terms; Ralph Raasch for his assistance in reviewing the nomenclature; and Cathy Hardee and Jenny Hebert for their help in editing and formatting the bibliography. Further, this bibliography would not be here without the many hours spent in the library by my student research assistants, Lea Ann Walker and Melodie Bowen.

INDEX OF DRUG/DEVICE CATEGORIES

Drug/Device Category–Reference Number

YY:NN   YY = Year of publication

NN = Sequence number of article sorted by author's name within year of publication

See also Drug Names

toxins in food 82:3
tuberculostatics 69:1; 86:8
vaccines 76:4; 85:1; 87:6
vitamins 89:11

INDEX OF DRUG EVENTS

Drug Event–Reference Number

YY:NN   YY = Year of publication

      NN = Sequence number of article sorted
      by author's name within year of
      publication

aching 76:4
adenoma, hepatocellular 79:7; pituitary 79:3
agranulocytosis 88:8; 89:9
alkaline phosphatase, elevated 89:12
amenorrhea 69:2
anticholinergic toxicity 83:2
aplastic anemia 46:1; 69:5; 88:8; 89:9
arrhythmia following myocardial infarction
    81:3
arthritis 85:8
arthropathy 85:8
aspartate aminotransferase, elevated 89:12
bacteriuria, 78:1
birthweight, low 89:3
bleeding, gastrointestinal 87:2; 87:3; 87:9; 88:4;
    89:2; intravascular hemorrhage 86:6; mater-
    nal 89:8; subarachnoid hemorrhage 79:6
blood urea nitrogen, elevated 89:12
bone marrow depression 85:2
breast tumor, benign 83:7; 85:3; 75:1
cancer 77:4; 79:9; 83:4; 84:6; adenocarcinoma
    86:3; biliary 85:7; blood 87:1; breast 74:1; 79:8;
    80:2; 80:5; 80:6; 80:9; 81:2; 81:7; 82:6; 83:11;
    84:5; 84:9; 84:10; 84:11; 86:7; 86:9; 86:10; 86:12;
    89:1; 89:10; 89:13; 89:23; 89:24; breast, con-
    tralateral 88:6; cervical 77:1; 77:5; 89:22; en-
    dometrial 77:3; 79:1; 79:4; 80:4; 83:10; 85:6;
    86:11; 89:14; gastric 82:4; melanoma 84:7;
    ovarian 82:5; 82:7; primary liver 82:3; skin
    87:1; thyroid 80:3; urinary tract 87:1; 89:19
cardiac defects, congenital 81:5; 89:25
cardiovascular disease 81:1
cataract 86:15; 88:5
cholecystitis, acute 80:7
cholecystectomy 86:4; 88:7
congenital malformation 62:1; 76:3; 76:5; 77:6;
    77:7; 78:2; 81:5; 83:8; 83:9; 83:12 85:5; 85:9;
    86:5
creatinine, serum, elevated 89:12
cytogenetic abnormalities 89:7

death 74:2; 88:3; 89:5; after cimetidine use for
    peptic ulcer 83:3; after hospital admission
    69:3; cardiovascular 75:4; from asthma 89:5;
    from myocardial infarction 75:2; from peptic
    ulcer complications 87:5
depression 86:1
diabetes mellitus 80:1
dizziness 90:1
Down's syndrome 82:8
dysgenesia 85:2
dysplasia, colon 89:12
edema, pedal 90:1
encephalopathy 85:1
eosinophilia in treatment of rheumatoid arthri-
    tis 83:14
fetal/neonatal adverse outcomes 89:8
fibrocystic breast disease 76:1
flank pain syndrome 89:21
flushing 90:1
fracture, distal radius 79:5; hip 79:5; 81:4; 87:7;
    89:17; 89:18; proximal femur 89:18
galactorrhea 69:2
gallbladder disease 75:1; 86:14
gastrointestinal effects, adverse 89:7
gonorrhea, relapse 84:1
headaches 90:1
hemoglobin, depressed 89:12
hepatitis 86:8
human growth hormone, alteration in levels
    79:2
hypersensitivity reactions 88:9
hypertension 77:2; 83:5
hypospadias 82:8
IgE-dependent anaphylactic reactions 88:1
infection, relapse 86:2
jaundice 74:2; 83:6
lactic dehydrogenase, elevated 89:8
leukemia 67:1; 87:4; 87:10; 90:2; lymphocytic
    87:8; myeloid 90:3; nonlymphocytic 87:8
limb-reduction deformities 82:8
malaise 76:4
multiple sclerosis 76:4
myocardial infarction 75:3; 76:2; 78:3; 80:8; 81:6;
    89:16; death 75:2
nausea, vomiting 85:4
neoplasms 82:8
neutropenia 84:4
oral clefts 81:5; 83:12
osteoporosis 83:13
palpitations 90:1
pelvic inflammatory disease 81:8
phocomelia 62:1
platelets, depressed 89:12
preeclampsia 82:2

INDEX OF STUDY METHODOLOGIES

Study Methodology–Reference Number

YY:NN   YY = Year of publication
          NN = Sequence number of article sorted
              by author's name within year of
              publication

Legend: OR = odds ratio; CI = confidence interval; RR = relative risk

46:1   Custer RP. Aplastic anemia in soldiers treated with atabrine (quinacrine). Am J Med Sci 1946;212:211-24
Drug Name: quinacrine hydrochloride; *Category:* antimalarial
Dosing Criteria: average 100 mg/d prophylaxis; *Treatment Duration:* 1–34 months; most cases 4–14 months
Validation of Exposure: military medical records, enforced compliance in all troops
Study Methodology: retrospective, population-based, cohort
Population Selection Criteria: U.S. Army troops in Pacific-Asian theater, World War II, 1943–45
Total Number of Subjects: incidence per 100 000 reported; *Control Subjects:* other U.S. Army troops in European-Mediterranean weather. Only occasional cases of quinacrine use.
Drug Event: aplastic anemia
Validation of Outcome: pathology reports
Findings: peak incidence per six months about 2.8:100 000 in Pacific-Asian weather versus 0.2:100 000 in European-Mediterranean weather

62:1   Taussig HB. A study of the German outbreak of phocomelia. JAMA 1962;180:1106-14
Drug Name: thalidomide; *Category:* antianxiety agents, antiemetics, sedatives
Dosing Criteria: none; *Treatment Duration:* during early pregnancy
Validation of Exposure: prescription and hospital records, patient and physician interviews
Study Methodology: accumulation of spontaneous case reports and review of records of selected pediatric clinics in Germany and Britain
Population Selection Criteria: none
Total Number of Subjects: not known; *Control Subjects:* none, only anecdotal series of cases or patients managed by selected physicians
Drug Event: phocomelia
Validation of Outcome: retrospective case review and medication history
Findings: tremendous increase in cases of phocomelia in 1960–61 in Germany and later in Britain, Australia, and other countries. Retrospective investigation showed great majority of mothers had taken thalidomide during early pregnancy.

67:1   Fraumeni JF. Bone marrow depression induced by chloramphenicol or phenylbutazone—leukemia and other sequelae. JAMA 1967;201:828-34
Drug Name: chloramphenicol, phenylbutazone; *Category:* analgesics, antibiotics, nonsteroidal antiinflammatory drugs
Dosing Criteria: none; *Treatment Duration:* none
Validation of Exposure: patients previously in aplastic anemia unintended drug effect registry
Study Methodology: follow-up survey of patients' physicians
Population Selection Criteria: registry patients with aplastic anemia due to chloramphenicol or phenylbutazone
Total Number of Subjects: 151 (124 chloramphenicol, 24 phenylbutazone, 3 both)
Control Subjects: none
Drug Event: leukemia
Validation of Outcome: pathology reports
Findings: inadequate evidence that either drug is leukemogenic (three chloramphenicol patients developed leukemia, but only one with apparent cause-and-effect relationship)

68:1   Vessey MP, Doll R. Investigation of relation between use of oral contraception and thromboembolic disease. *Br Med J* 1968;2:199-205
Drug Name: oral contraceptives; *Category:* estrogens/progestins
Validation of Exposure: patient charts, home interviews
Study Methodology: retrospective, case-control
Population Selection Criteria: women 16–40 years old diagnosed with thromboembolic disease during 1964–66 in 19 large British hospitals
Total Number of Subjects: 174; *Cases:* 58; *Control Subjects:* 116
Comparability of Controls: matched for age, marital status, parity, date of hospital admission, and absence of predisposing causes of thromboembolic disease
Drug Event: thromboembolism
Validation of Outcome: medical diagnosis
Findings: RR 9.0

69:1   Evans C, Devadata S, Fox W, et al. Five-year study of patients with pulmonary tuberculosis treated at home in a controlled comparison of isoniazid plus PAS with 3 regimens of isoniazid alone. *Bull WHO* 1969;41:1-16
Drug Name: aminosalicylic acid, isoniazid; *Category:* antibacterials, tuberculostatics
Dosing Criteria: panaminosalicylic acid 10 mg/d with isoniazid 200 mg or isoniazid alone
Treatment Duration: five years
Validation of Exposure: administered in study
Study Methodology: prospective, cohort
Population Selection Criteria: newly diagnosed patients from the Tuberculosis Chemotherapy Center
Total Number of Subjects: 315; *Cases:* 315
Drug Event: tuberculosis
Validation of Outcome: remission diagnosed by physician and pathology reports
Findings: proved value of home therapy outpatient treatment for tuberculosis

69:2   Friedman S, Goldfien A. Amenorrhea and galactorrhea following oral contraceptive therapy. *JAMA* 1969;210:1888-91
Drug Name: oral contraceptives; *Category:* estrogens/progestins
Treatment Duration: pathology studies and physician visits
Validation of Exposure: patient interviews
Study Methodology: prospective, cohort
Population Selection Criteria: patients with amenorrhea, mean age 24.5 years
Total Number of Subjects: 21
Drug Event: amenorrhea, galactorrhea
Rule Out Alternative Explanations: physical examination, X-ray, and laboratory studies
Findings: no increased risk

69:3   Inman WHW, Adelstein AM. Rise and fall of asthma mortality in England and Wales in relation to use of pressurized aerosols. *Lancet* 1969;2:279-85
Drug Category: beta-agonist bronchodilators, bronchodialators
Validation of Exposure: IMS Ltd. data
Study Methodology: population-based, cohort
Population Selection Criteria: mortality statistics published by the Registrar General (Great Britain)
Drug Event: death after hospital admission
Validation of Outcome: mortality, hospital inpatient inquiry
Findings: high correlation between mortality attributed to asthma and use of aerosols

69:4   Sartwell PE, Masi AT, Arthes FG, Greene GR, Smith HE. Thromboembolism and oral contraceptives: an epidemiologic case-control study. *Am J Epidemiol* 1969;*905*:365-80

Drug Name: oral contraceptives; *Category:* estrogens/progestins
Validation of Exposure: patient interview
Study Methodology: retrospective, case-control
Population Selection Criteria: patients discharged within past 32 years from 43 hospitals, free of chronic conditions and fertile
Total Number of Subjects: 350; *Cases:* 175; *Control Subjects:* 175
Comparability of Controls: matched for hospital, age, race, residence, time of hospitalization, marital status, parity, and pay status
Drug Event: thromboembolism
Validation of Outcome: final diagnosis of thromboembolism in chart upon discharge
Findings: RR 4.4

69:5   Wallerstein RO, Condit PK, Kasper CK, Brown JW, Morrison FR. Statewide study of chloramphenicol therapy and fatal aplastic anemia. *JAMA* 1969; *208*:2045-50

Drug Name: chloramphenicol; *Category:* antibiotics
Dosing Criteria: nontopical (i.e., systemic) use; *Treatment Duration:* average drug exposure estimated at 4.5–7.5 g
Validation of Exposure: medical record review
Study Methodology: retrospective, statewide (California), cohort
Population Selection Criteria: all cases of death due to hematologic disorders mentioned on death certificates
Total Number of Subjects: 70; *Cases:* 60 deaths due to aplastic anemia, 10 had received chloramphenicol; *Control Subjects:* gross population control
Drug Event: aplastic anemia, fatal
Validation of Outcome: expert review of all medical records of deaths due to hematologic disorders
Findings: risk of death 1:524 000 in general population in 18-month period; in chloramphenicol-treated patients, risk of death assuming 4.5-g average dose to calculate population at risk was 1:36 118 and at 7.5-g dose 1:21 671. At 4.0-g total dose average risk increased 13 times with chloramphenicol

73:1   Livingston S, Berman W, Pauli LL. Anticonvulsant drugs and vitamin D metabolism. *JAMA* 1973;*224*:1634-5

Drug Name: phenobarbital, phenytoin, primidone; *Category:* anticonvulsants
Dosing Criteria: maximum dosing
Study Methodology: prospective, cohort
Population Selection Criteria: epilepsy patients referred to Johns Hopkins Hospital Epilepsy Clinic
Total Number of Subjects: 15 000 cases
Drug Event: abnormal vitamin D metabolism
Validation of Outcome: skull X-ray, calcium and phosphorus concentrations, phosphatase, liver function test
Findings: no increased risk

74:1   Heinonen OP, Shapiro S, Tuominen L, Turunen MI. Reserpine use in relation to breast cancer. *Lancet* 1974;*2*:675-7

Drug Name: reserpine; *Category:* antihypertensives, rauwolfia alkaloids

Validation of Exposure: hospital records, letters of referral, outpatient notes
Study Methodology: retrospective, case-control
Population Selection Criteria: cases of newly diagnosed controls admitted for elective surgery, 1960–72
Total Number of Subjects: 876; *Cases:* 438; *Control Subjects:* 438
Comparability of Controls: matched for year of surgery and age (within five years)
Drug Event: breast cancer
Findings: RR 2.0

74:2   Inman WHW, Mushing WW. Jaundice after repeated exposure to halothane: an analysis of reports to the Committee on Safety of Medicines. *Br Med J* 1974; 1:5-10
Drug Name: halothane; *Category:* anesthetics (inhalation)
Dosing Criteria: number of inhalations; *Treatment Duration:* one year
Validation of Exposure: exposed in hospital
Study Methodology: retrospective, cohort
Population Selection Criteria: patients exposed to halothane in hospital during a one-year period
Total Number of Subjects: 130; *Cases:* 130
Drug Event: jaundice, death
Validation of Outcome: diagnosis of jaundice or death from halothane
Findings: repeated exposure to halothane increases likelihood of jaundice or death

75:1   Greenblatt DJ. Retrospective case-control study of diseases associated with oral contraceptive use. *Am Heart J* 1975;89:677-8
Drug Name: oral contraceptives; *Category:* estrogens/progestins
Validation of Exposure: drug history from charts
Study Methodology: retrospective, case-control
Population Selection Criteria: Boston Collaborative Drug Surveillance Program: women 20–66 years of age
Total Number of Subjects: 1195; *Cases:* 353 (idiopathic venous thromboembolism n=43, gallbladder n=212, breast tumor n=98); *Control Subjects:* 842
Comparability of Controls: premenopausal women free of known chronic disease, hospitalized for acute illnesses
Drug Event: idiopathic venous thromboembolism, gallbladder disease, benign breast tumor
Validation of Outcome: hospital records
Findings: age standard, RR 11; gallbladder disease, RR 2.0; benign breast tumor, RR 0.47

75:2   Mann JI, Inman WHW. Oral contraceptives and death from myocardial infarction in young women. *Br Med J* 1975;2:245-8
Drug Name: oral contraceptives; *Category:* estrogens/progestins
Validation of Exposure: interview with practitioners
Study Methodology: retrospective, case-control
Population Selection Criteria: death certificates of women under age 50 in England and Wales
Total Number of Subjects: 349; *Cases:* 153; *Control Subjects:* 196
Comparability of Controls: matched for age, marital status, and medical practice
Drug Event: death from myocardial infarction
Validation of Outcome: pathology report and death certificate
Rule Out Alternative Explanations: hypertension, diabetes
Findings: <40 years of age, RR 2.8; 40–44 years of age, RR 4.7

75:3   Mann JI, Vessey MP, Thorogood M, Doll R. Myocardial infarction in young women with special reference to oral contraceptive practice. Br Med J 1975;2:241-5
Drug Name: oral contraceptives; *Category:* estrogens/progestins
Treatment Duration: varied
Validation of Exposure: interviews with patients and questionnaires completed by patients or physicians
Study Methodology: retrospective, case-control
Population Selection Criteria: married women under age 45 treated for myocardial infarction
Total Number of Subjects: 252; *Cases:* 63; *Control Subjects:* 189
Drug Event: myocardial infarction
Validation of Outcome: diagnosis and treatment by physician
Rule Out Alternative Explanations: heavy cigarette smoking, hypertension, diabetes, pre-eclamptic toxemia, and obesity
Findings: RR 4.5

75:4   Report of the committee for the assessment of biometric aspects of controlled trials of hypoglycemic agents. JAMA 1975;231:583-612
Drug Name: insulin, tolbutamide; *Category:* hypoglycemics
Dosing Criteria: varied; *Treatment Duration:* varied, up to 14 years
Validation of Exposure: clinical trial records
Study Methodology: balanced design, stratified for treatment allocation
Population Selection Criteria: adult-onset, nonketotic diabetic patients enrolled in 12 medical centers in the U.S.
Total Number of Subjects: 823; *Cases:* 204 tolbutamide, 205 placebo, 210 standard-dose insulin, 204 variable-dose insulin; *Control Subjects:* none, except patients in other drug groups
Drug Event: cardiovascular death
Validation of Outcome: clinical trial records
Findings: cardiovascular deaths in patient groups—tolbutamide 12.7 percent (p=0.008 compared with placebo), placebo 4.9 percent, standard insulin 6.2 percent, variable insulin 5.9 percent

76:1   Ory H, Cole P, MacMahon B, Hoover R. Oral contraceptives and reduced risk of benign breast diseases. N Engl J Med 1976;294:419-22
Drug Name: oral contraceptives; *Category:* estrogens/progestins
Treatment Duration: never used, used <25 months, used ≥25 months
Validation of Exposure: mail questionnaire
Study Methodology: prospective, cohort
Population Selection Criteria: 97 254 married women in Greater Boston
Total Number of Subjects: 97 769; *Cases:* 1072
Comparability of Controls: all nonusers in Greater Boston area eligible
Drug Event: fibrocystic breast disease
Validation of Outcome: hospitalization
Findings: long-term use, RR 0.4

76:2   Rosenberg L, Armstrong B, Phil D, Jick H. Myocardial infarction and estrogen therapy in postmenopausal women. N Engl J Med 1976;294:1256-9
Drug Category: estrogens
Validation of Exposure: patient interview by nurse
Study Methodology: retrospective, case-control

Population Selection Criteria: Boston Collaborative Drug Surveillance Program
Total Number of Subjects: 7066; *Cases:* 336; *Control Subjects:* 6730
Comparability of Controls: hospitalized for noncardiac reasons
Drug Event: myocardial infarction
Validation of Outcome: hospitalization
Rule Out Alternative Explanations: age, past history of myocardial infarction, angina, diabetes, hypertension, and cigarette smoking
Findings: RR 0.97

76:3   Shapiro S, Hartz SC, Siskind V, et al. Anticonvulsants and parental epilepsy in the development of birth defects. *Lancet* 1976; *1*:272-5
Drug Category: anticonvulsants
Validation of Exposure: patient records
Study Methodology: retrospective, cohort
Population Selection Criteria: 2784 children with craniofacial anomalies from Finnish Register of Congenital Malformation
Total Number of Subjects: 5568; *Cases:* 2784; *Control Subjects:* 2784
Comparability of Controls: normal children born immediately before case in same maternity welfare district
Drug Event: congenital malformation
Validation of Outcome: presence of major congenital malformation in records
Findings: no increased risk

76:4   Sibley WA, Bamford CR, Laguna JF. Influenza vaccination in patients with multiple sclerosis. *JAMA* 1976;*236*:1965-6
Drug Name: influenza virus vaccine; *Category:* immunizing agents, vaccines
Dosing Criteria: 209 doses/93 patients
Study Methodology: prospective, cohort
Population Selection Criteria: multiple sclerosis patients, enrolled 1962–1975
Total Number of Subjects: 93
Drug Event: worsening of multiple sclerosis symptoms, moderate temperature elevation, malaise, and aching
Validation of Outcome: medical assessment
Findings: toxic reactions by seven percent vaccinations, allergic reactions by five percent vaccinations

76:5   Slone D, Siskind V, Heinonen OP, Monson RR, Kaufman DW, Shapiro S. Aspirin and congenital malformations. *Lancet* 1976; *1*:1373-5
Drug Name: aspirin; *Category:* analgesics, nonsteroidal antiinflammatory drugs
Dosing Criteria: heavily exposed (≥ eight d/lunar mo), intermediately exposed, not exposed; *Treatment Duration:* ≥ eight d/lunar mo
Validation of Exposure: review of the hospital or clinic record
Study Methodology: prospective, cohort
Population Selection Criteria: patients in Collaborative Perinatal Project
Total Number of Subjects: 50 282 heavily exposed mother-child pairs; *Cases:* 3428 malformations
Comparability of Controls: matched for characteristics of child
Drug Event: congenital malformation
Validation of Outcome: presence of obvious congenital malformation
Findings: no increased risk

76:6 Sponzilli EE, Ramcharan S, Wingerd J. Rheumatoid factor antigamma-globulin in women: effects of oral contraceptives use on its prevalence. *Arthritis Rheum* 1976; *19*:602-6
Drug Name: oral contraceptives; *Category:* estrogens/progestins
Treatment Duration: never used, current use, past use (at least 30 d)
Validation of Exposure: patient questionnaire
Study Methodology: prospective, case-control
Population Selection Criteria: Kaiser Foundation Health Plan members, women presenting themselves for general check-up
Total Number of Subjects: 14 856; *Cases:* 4562; *Control Subjects:* 10 294
Drug Event: rheumatoid arthritis
Validation of Outcome: rheumatoid factor titer
Findings: no increased risk

77:1 Boyce JG, Lu T, Nelson JH, Fruchter RG. Oral contraceptives and cervical carcinoma. *Am J Obstet Gynecol* 1977; *128*:761-6
Drug Name: oral contraceptives; *Category:* estrogens/progestins
Treatment Duration: 1–15, 16–35, 36–55, 56–75, 76–95, >95 months of exposure
Validation of Exposure: patient interview
Study Methodology: retrospective, case-control
Population Selection Criteria: patients under 50 years of age with cervical carcinoma
Total Number of Subjects: 1989; *Cases:* 689; *Control Subjects:* 1300
Comparability of Controls: matched for age, ethnic origin, age at first pregnancy, age at first coitus, socioeconomic status
Drug Event: cervical cancer
Validation of Outcome: medical examination of criteria of diagnosis
Findings: no increased risk

77:2 Fisch IR, Frank J. Oral contraceptives and blood pressure. *JAMA* 1977; *237*:2499-503
Drug Name: oral contraceptives; *Category:* estrogens/progestins
Treatment Duration: nonusers, past users, current users
Validation of Exposure: medical records and patient questionnaire
Study Methodology: prospective, cohort
Population Selection Criteria: Kaiser-Permanente Medical Care Program, women neither pregnant nor postpartum, aged 15–60 years, enrolled 1969–72
Total Number of Subjects: 9511 (two or more examinations), 3847 (one examination)
Drug Event: hypertension
Validation of Outcome: blood pressure >140/90 mm Hg measured two hours after start of examination
Findings: statistically significant (p<0.05) rise in mean blood pressure (systolic 5–6 mm Hg, diastolic 1–2 mm Hg)

77:3 McDonald TW, Annegers JF, O'Fallon WM, et al. Exogenous estrogen and endometrial carcinoma: case-control and incidence study. *Am J Obstet Gynecol* 1977; *127*:572-80
Drug Category: estrogens
Dosing Criteria: none, 0.625 mg, 1.25 mg, >2.5 mg; *Treatment Duration:* < six months, ≥ six months, ≥ three years
Study Methodology: retrospective, case-control

Population Selection Criteria: women exposed to estrogen in Rochester, Minnesota area, 1945–74
Total Number of Subjects: 725; *Cases:* 145; *Control Subjects:* 580
Comparability of Controls: matched for age and residency
Drug Event: endometrial cancer
Validation of Outcome: cell pathology
Findings: ≥ six months, RR 4.9, ≥ three years, RR 7.9

77:4   Paffenbarger RS Jr, Fasal E, Simmons ME, Kampert JB. Cancer risk as related to use of oral contraceptives during fertile years. *Cancer* **1977;*39*: 1887-91**
Drug Name: oral contraceptives; *Category:* estrogens/progestins
Treatment Duration: 1–24, 25–48, 49–96, ≥97 months
Validation of Exposure: patient interviews
Study Methodology: retrospective, case-control
Population Selection Criteria: patients at San Francisco Bay Area Hospitals, aged <50 years
Total Number of Subjects: 850; *Cases:* 452; *Control Subjects:* 398
Comparability of Controls: matched for age, race, religion, education, menopause, history of
   breast disease, and age at first childbirth
Drug Event: cancer
Validation of Outcome: diagnosis and physical examination
Findings: breast cancer, RR 1.1

77:5   Peritz E, Ramcharan S, Frank J, Brown WL, Huang S, Ray R. The incidence of cervical cancer and duration of oral contraceptive use. *Am J Epidemiol* **1977;*106*:462-9**
Drug Name: oral contraceptives; *Category:* estrogens/progestins
Treatment Duration: zero exposure, <2, 2–4, >4 years
Validation of Exposure: patient questionnaires, medical records, and repeat examinations
Study Methodology: prospective, cohort
Population Selection Criteria: Kaiser Foundation Health Plan members, women living in suburban communities of San Francisco
Total Number of Subjects: 16 459; *Cases:* 35; *Control Subjects:* 16 424
Drug Event: cervical cancer
Validation of Outcome: cytologic studies
Findings: zero exposure, RR 1.0; <2 years, RR 2.0; 2–4 years, RR 1.8; >4 years, RR 4.0 (controlled for selected confounders)

77:6   Shapiro S, Heinonen OP, Siskind V, et al. Antenatal exposure to doxylamine succinate and dicyclomine hydrochloride (Bendectin) in relation to congenital malformations, perinatal mortality rate, birth weight, and intelligence quotient score. *Am J Obstet Gynecol* **1977:*128*:480-5**
Drug Name: dicyclomine; doxylamine and pyridoxine (Bendectin); *Category:* antiemetics
Dosing Criteria: none, other, heavy (heavy = ≥8 d/lunar mo)
Validation of Exposure: recorded upon antenatal visit and confirmed by attending physician
Study Methodology: prospective, cohort
Population Selection Criteria: patients from Collaborative Perinatal Project
Total Number of Subjects: 50 282; *Cases:* 2720 (doxylamine n=1403, dicyclomine n=1317)
Control Subjects: 47 562
Comparability of Controls: children matched for characteristics of mother and child, illnesses,
   complications, reproductive history

Drug Event: congenital malformations
Validation of Outcome: measured congenital malformation, perinatal mortality, birth weight, and IQ score
Rule Out Alternative Explanations: race and socioeconomic factors
Findings: no increased risk

77:7   Slone D, Siskind V, Heinonen OP, et al. Antenatal exposure to the pheno-thiazines in relation to congenital malformations, perinatal mortality rate, birth weight, and intelligence quotient score. *Am J Obstet Gynecol* **1977; 128:486-8**

Drug Category: antiemetics, antipsychotics, phenothiazines
Treatment Duration: no exposure, regular, other
Validation of Exposure: recorded at patient visit and confirmed by physician
Study Methodology: prospective, cohort
Population Selection Criteria: Collaborative Perinatal Project
Total Number of Subjects: 52 648; *Cases:* 3675; *Control Subjects:* 48 973
Comparability of Controls: randomized according to mother and child characteristics
Drug Event: congenital malformation
Validation of Outcome: measured congenital malformation, perinatal mortality
Rule Out Alternative Explanations: race and socioeconomic factors
Findings: no increased risk

78:1   Evans DA, Hennekens CH, Miao L, et al. Oral contraceptive use and bac-teriuria in a community-based study. *N Engl J Med* **1978;299:536-7**

Drug Name: oral contraceptives; *Drug Category:* estrogens/progestins
Treatment Duration: oral contraceptive use in 1973 or 1976, or use in both 1973 and 1976
Validation of Exposure: patient interview at home
Study Methodology: prospective, cohort
Population Selection Criteria: women aged 16–49 years in defined neighborhood
Total Number of Subjects: 2390; *Cases:* 482 (oral contraceptive users); *Control Subjects:* 1908
Drug Event: bacteriuria
Validation of Outcome: urine specimen and culture collected at home
Findings: positive relationship of oral contraceptive use with bacteriuria, positive 5.6 percent in users, 4.0 percent in nonusers

78:2   Nora JJ, Nora AH, Blu J, et al. Exogenous progestogen and estrogen im-plicated in birth defects. *JAMA* **1978;240:837-43**

Drug Category: estrogens, progestins
Treatment Duration: five years
Validation of Exposure: patient charts
Study Methodology: three retrospective, case-control (studies 1, 2, and 3); one prospective, cohort (study 4)
Population Selection Criteria: pediatric cardiology service
Total Number of Subjects: 868; *Cases:* study 1 n=32, study 2 n=60, study 3 n=176, study 4 n=118
Control Subjects: study 1 n=64, study 2 n=60, study 3 n=352, study 4 n=6
Comparability of Controls: matched for age, sex, race, gestational age, socioeconomic level, area of residence, maternal age, and parity
Drug Event: congenital malformations
Validation of Outcome: presence confirmed by physician
Findings: study 1 RR 8.41; study 2 RR 5.58; study 3 RR 3.35; controlled, single-blind, prospective study, RR 2.75

78:3 Pfeffer RI, Whipple GH, Kurosaki TT, Chapman JM. Coronary risk and estrogen use in postmenopausal women. *Am J Epidemiol* 1978;*1076*:479-97
Drug Category: estrogens
Treatment Duration: varied
Validation of Exposure: patient records
Study Methodology: retrospective, case-control
Population Selection Criteria: female residents (postmenopausal) of retirement community, 1964–79
Total Number of Subjects: 15 500; *Cases:* 162; *Control Subjects:* 15 338
Drug Event: myocardial infarction
Validation of Outcome: medical records, necropsy reports, and medical charts, including electrocardiograms
Findings: no increased risk

79:1 Antunes CMF, Stolley PD, Rosenshein NB, et al. Endometrial cancer and estrogen use. *N Engl J Med* 1979;*300*:9-13
Drug Category: estrogens
Treatment Duration: none, intermittent, cyclic, continuous
Validation of Exposure: patient interview, medical records
Study Methodology: retrospective, case-control
Population Selection Criteria: patients with primary cancer of the uterine body admitted to six Baltimore hospitals
Total Number of Subjects: 1339; *Cases:* 451; *Control Subjects:* 888
Comparability of Controls: matched for hospital, race, age (within five years), and date of admission (within six months)
Drug Event: endometrial cancer
Validation of Outcome: pathology specimens
Findings: all users, RR 6.0; long-term users (greater than five years), RR 15.0

79:2 Beg AA, Varma VK, Dash RJ. Effect of chlorpromazine on human growth hormone. *Am J Psychiatry* 1979;*136*:914-7
Drug Name: chlorpromazine; *Category:* antiemetics, antipsychotics, phenothiazines
Dosing Criteria: 200–400 mg/d; *Treatment Duration:* 13 weeks
Validation of Exposure: blood plasma samples
Study Methodology: cohort, prospective
Population Selection Criteria: subjects with human growth hormone concentrations <5 mg/mL
Sample Frame Limitations: children <11 years excluded from study protocol
Total Number of Subjects: 42; *Cases:* 15; *Control Subjects:* 27
Comparability of Controls: 12 schizophrenic patients, 15 normal patients
Drug Event: alteration of human growth hormone concentrations
Validation of Outcome: blood plasma concentrations measured
Findings: no increased risk

79:3 Coulam CB, Annegers JF, Abboud CF, Laws ER, Kurland LT. Pituitary adenoma and oral contraceptives: a case-control study. *Fertil Steril* 1979;*31*: 25-8
Drug Name: oral contraceptives; *Category:* estrogens/progestins
Treatment Duration: any duration, one to two years, greater than three years
Validation of Exposure: patient records and questionnaire

Study Methodology: retrospective, case-control
Population Selection Criteria: patients aged 15–44 years presenting to a hospital in Olmsted
  County, Minnesota
Total Number of Subjects: 45; *Cases:* 9; *Control Subjects:* 36
Comparability of Controls: matched for date of admission
Drug Event: pituitary adenoma
Validation of Outcome: surgery and angiogram
Rule Out Alternative Explanations: prior head injury, radiation therapy, seizures, smoking
Findings: RR 0.5

79:4   Horwitz RI, Feinstein AR. Intravaginal estrogen creams and endometrial cancer: no causal association found. JAMA 1979;241:1266-7
Drug Name: estrogen creams, intravaginal; *Category:* estrogens
Treatment Duration: any use of intravaginal estrogen creams
Validation of Exposure: telephone interview reports
Study Methodology: retrospective, case-control
Total Number of Subjects: 133; *Cases:* 83; *Control Subjects:* 50
Comparability of Controls: matched by age (within four years) and race
Drug Event: endometrial cancer
Validation of Outcome: diagnosis of endometrial cancer in chart
Findings: no increased risk

79:5   Hutchinson TA, Polansky SM, Feinstein AR. Postmenopausal estrogens protect against fractures of hip and distal radius. A case-control study. Lancet 1979;2:705-9
Drug Category: estrogens
Validation of Exposure: medical records, standardized interviews
Study Methodology: retrospective, case-control
Population Selection Criteria: 2609 female inpatients admitted to the orthopedic service of
  Yale–New Haven Hospital
Total Number of Subjects: 160; *Cases:* 80; *Control Subjects:* 80
Comparability of Controls: female inpatients admitted to same orthopedic service
Drug Event: fractures of hip and distal radius in postmenopausal women
Rule Out Alternative Explanations: race, age, height, weight, risk factors for bone diseases
  or fractures
Findings: RR 3.0

79:6   Inman WHW. Oral contraceptives and fatal subarachnoid haemorrhage. Br Med J 1979;2:1468-70
Drug Name: oral contraceptives; *Category:* estrogens/progestins
Validation of Exposure: patient records
Study Methodology: retrospective, case-control
Population Selection Criteria: deaths from subarachnoid hemorrhage in women aged 15–44
  years in England and Wales
Total Number of Subjects: 268; *Cases:* 156; *Control Subjects:* 112
Comparability of Controls: matched for time of use, hypertension, smoking habits, and medical practice
Drug Event: subarachnoid hemorrhage
Validation of Outcome: death certificate and records
Rule Out Alternative Explanations: hypertension, renal disease, preeclamptic toxiemia
Findings: no increased risk

79:7   Rooks JB, Ory HW, Ishak KG, et al. Epidemiology of hepatocellular adenoma: role of oral contraceptive use. *JAMA* 1979;242:644-8
Drug Name: oral contraceptives; *Category:* estrogens/progestins
Dosing Criteria: high hormonal potency; *Treatment Duration:* 0–12, 13–36, 37–60, 61–84, ≥85 months
Validation of Exposure: interview by trained interviewers
Study Methodology: retrospective, case-control
Population Selection Criteria: diagnosed by the Armed Forces Institute of Pathology, aged 16–61 years
Total Number of Subjects: 299; *Cases:* 79; *Control Subjects:* 220
Comparability of Controls: matched for age and neighborhood
Drug Event: hepatocellular adenoma
Validation of Outcome: histologic diagnosis
Findings: long-term users of oral contraceptives have an annual incidence of hepatocellular adenoma of 3.4/100 000 people; nonusers 1.0-1.3/million people

79:8   Vessey MP, Doll R, Jones K, McPherson K, Yeates D. Epidemiological study of oral contraceptives and breast cancer. *Br Med J* 1979;1:1757-60
Drug Name: oral contraceptives; *Category:* estrogens/progestins
Treatment Duration: according to time last used, interval first used, duration of use
Validation of Exposure: interviewed by trained medical social worker or nurse
Study Methodology: retrospective, case-control
Population Selection Criteria: women aged 16–50 years, diagnosed with breast cancer between 1968 and 1970 in London and Oxford
Total Number of Subjects: 1242; *Cases:* 621; *Control Subjects:* 621
Comparability of Controls: matched for age, marital status, age (within five years), parity, and hospital admitted
Drug Event: breast cancer
Validation of Outcome: physical examination and physician diagnosis
Findings: no increased risk

79:9   White SJ, McLean AEM, Howland C. Anticonvulsant drugs and cancer: cohort study in patients with severe epilepsy. *Lancet* 1979;2:458-60
Drug Category: anticonvulsants
Validation of Exposure: medical records
Study Methodology: prospective, cohort
Population Selection Criteria: epileptic patients admitted to the Chalfont Centre for Epilepsy, 1931–71
Total Number of Subjects: 1861 exposed cases
Drug Event: cancer
Validation of Outcome: presence of cancer diagnosis in chart
Rule Out Alternative Explanations: age and sex
Findings: higher mortality attributable to epilepsy, but population shows no higher incidence of cancer

80:1   Fineberg SE, Schneider SH. Glipizide versus tolbutamide, an open trial. Effects on insulin secretory patterns and glucose concentrations. *Diabetologia* 1980;18:49-54
Drug Name: glipizide, tolbutamide; *Category:* antidiabetic agents
Dosing Criteria: 40 mg or 3 mg; *Treatment Duration:* six months
Study Methodology: cohort, prospective

Population Selection Criteria: patients treated at a Boston, Massachusetts hospital
Total Number of Subjects: 29; *Cases:* 18; *Control Subjects:* 11
Comparability of Controls: matched for age, sex, and previous therapy
Drug Event: diabetes
Validation of Outcome: glucose concentrations
Findings: drugs were comparable with regard to efficacy and safety; however, only glipizide
   had chronic effects on insulin secretion

80:2   Greenspan AR, Hatcher RA, Moore M, Rosenberg MJ, Ory HW. The association of depo-medroxyprogesterone acetate and breast cancer. *Contraception* 1980;*216*:563-9

Drug Name: medroxyprogesterone acetate; *Category:* progestins
Dosing Criteria: 150 mg q3mo
Validation of Exposure: clinic records
Study Methodology: retrospective, case-control
Population Selection Criteria: women enrolled in the Grady Memorial Hospital's Family Planning Clinic in Atlanta Georgia, 1967–79
Total Number of Subjects: 209; *Cases:* 30; *Control Subjects:* 179
Comparability of Controls: matched for age (within two years), race, date of clinic visit (within six months)
Drug Event: breast cancer
Validation of Outcome: pathology studies
Rule Out Alternative Explanations: small number of patient cases, short drug exposure
Findings: no increased risk

80:3   Holm LE, Lundell G, Walinder G. Incidence of malignant thyroid tumors in humans after exposure to diagnostic doses of Iodine 131. Part 1. Retrospective cohort study. *J Natl Cancer Inst* 1980;*64*:1055-9

Drug Name: [131]iodine; *Category:* antithyroid agents
Dosing Criteria: 60 μCi; *Treatment Duration:* 84 percent of patients one-time dose, 16 percent of patients greater than one-time dose
Validation of Exposure: patient charts
Study Methodology: retrospective, cohort
Population Selection Criteria: patients with suspected thyroid carcinoma or dysfunction of the thyroid gland examination
Total Number of Subjects: 1133
Drug Event: thyroid cancer
Validation of Outcome: Swedish Cancer Registry records
Rule Out Alternative Explanations: patients diagnosed with carcinoma of the thyroid gland within five years excluded
Findings: no increased risk

80:4   Hulka BS, Fowler WC Jr, Kaufman DG, et al. Estrogen and endometrial cancer; cases and two control groups from North Carolina. *Am J Obstet Gynecol* 1980;*137*:92-101

Drug Category: estrogens
Dosing Criteria: <0.625 mg, ≥0.625 mg; *Treatment Duration:* considered latency, duration, recency, dose, cyclic or continuous dosing
Validation of Exposure: patient interviews, interviews with deceased patients' relatives, physician and hospital records
Study Methodology: retrospective, case-control

Population Selection Criteria: women who received therapy at North Carolina Memorial Hospital, 1970–76
Total Number of Subjects: 801; *Cases:* 256; *Control Subjects:* 224 gynecology controls, 321 community controls
Comparability of Controls: women admitted for gynecology or consultation on surgical or medical services of North Carolina Memorial Hospital, same frequency distribution for age and race
Drug Event: endometrial cancer
Rule Out Alternative Explanations: weight, ethnic, and health factors
Findings: <3.5 years of exposure, RR 0.8; ≥3.5 years of exposure, RR 4.1

80:5   Jick H, Walker AM, Watkins RN, et al. Oral contraceptives and breast cancer. Am J Epidemiol 1980;112:577-85
Drug Name: oral contraceptives; *Category:* estrogens/progestins
Treatment Duration: current users, 1–4, 5–9, ≥10 years of use
Validation of Exposure: prescriptions filled
Study Methodology: retrospective, case-control
Population Selection Criteria: diagnosis of breast cancer
Total Number of Subjects: 341; *Cases:* 132; *Control Subjects:* 209
Comparability of Controls: women in same age group, hospitalized with acute illnesses
Drug Event: breast cancer
Validation of Outcome: chart review
Findings: association dependent not on length of exposure, but on age

80:6   Labarthe DR, O'Fallon WM. Reserpine and breast cancer. A community-based longitudinal study of 2000 hypertensive women. JAMA 1980;243: 2304-10
Drug Name: reserpine; *Category:* antihypertensives, rauwolfia alkaloids
Treatment Duration: none, trivial, definite, <one year, ≥one year
Validation of Exposure: prescription records
Study Methodology: prospective, cohort
Population Selection Criteria: patients treated with reserpine at Mayo Clinic in Rochester, Minnesota
Total Number of Subjects: 1730; *Cases:* any exposure n=450, >1 year n=250; *Control Subjects:* 1030
Drug Event: breast cancer
Validation of Outcome: diagnosis from chart
Findings: no increased risk

80:7   Rosenberg L, Shapiro S, Slone D, et al. Thiazides and acute cholecystitis. N Engl J Med 1980;303:546-8
Drug Category: antihypertensives, diuretics, thiazide diuretics,
Treatment Duration: never used, <1, 1–4, ≥5 years, used for unknown time period
Validation of Exposure: hospital records and patient interview
Study Methodology: retrospective, case-control
Population Selection Criteria: patients aged 20–69 years with primary diagnosis of cholecystitis
Total Number of Subjects: 2095; *Cases:* 419; *Control Subjects:* 1676
Comparability of Controls: matched for age, 20–69 years of age, no diagnosis for cholecystitis, admitted for five other conditions
Drug Event: acute cholecystitis
Validation of Outcome: hospital admission diagnosis

Rule Out Alternative Explanations: hypertension, obesity
Findings: overall RR 2.0; greater than five years use RR 2.9

80:8   Rosenberg L, Slone D, Shapiro S, et al. Noncontraceptive estrogens and myocardial infarction in young women. *JAMA* 1980;*244*:339-42
Drug Name: conjugated estrogens, diethlystilbestrol; *Category:* estrogens
Dosing Criteria: 2.5 mg, 1.25 mg, 0.625 mg, 0.3 mg, dosage unspecified
Validation of Exposure: interviews
Study Methodology: retrospective, case-control
Population Selection Criteria: women aged 30–49 years
Total Number of Subjects: 2309; *Cases:* 477; *Control Subjects:* 1832
Comparability of Controls: selected from same wards, younger than age 50, diagnosis other than myocardial infarction
Drug Event: myocardial infarction
Validation of Outcome: medical records, validation with World Health Organization definition
Findings: RR 1.0

80:9   Ross RK, Paganini-Hill A, Gerkins VR, et al. A case-control study of menopausal estrogen therapy and breast cancer. *JAMA* 1980;*243*:1635-9
Drug Category: estrogens
Dosing Criteria: ≤0.625 mg, ≥1.25 mg, unknown dose
Validation of Exposure: interview, medical chart or pharmacy record
Study Methodology: retrospective, case-control
Population Selection Criteria: women taking menopausal estrogens in two Los Angeles area retirement communities
Total Number of Subjects: 276; *Cases:* 138; *Control Subjects:* 138
Comparability of Controls: matched for age, sex, and menstrual history
Drug Event: breast cancer
Validation of Outcome: pathology reports
Rule Out Alternative Explanations: age, height, weight, brassiere size, cup size, age at first full-term pregnancy
Findings: RR 2.5 for total cumulative dose >1500 mg in women with intact ovaries

81:1   Adam S, Williams V, Vessey MP. Cardiovascular disease and hormone replacement treatment: a pilot case-control study. *Br Med J* 1981;*282*:1277-8
Drug Category: estrogens
Validation of Exposure: questionnaires from practitioners
Study Methodology: retrospective, case-control
Population Selection Criteria: death certificates of women aged 50–59 years who died of acute myocardial infarction or subarachnoid hemorrhage
Total Number of Subjects: 295; *Cases:* 99 (myocardial infarction n=76, subarachnoid hemorrhage n=23); *Control Subjects:* 196
Comparability of Controls: matched for age and general practice
Drug Event: cardiovascular disease
Validation of Outcome: death reports and cause of death as reported by physicians
Findings: no increased risk

81:2   Brinton LA, Hoover RN, Szklo M, Fraumeni JF Jr. Menopausal estrogen use and risk of breast cancer. *Cancer* 1981;*47*:2517-22
Drug Category: estrogens
Dosing Criteria: 0.3 mg, 0.6 mg, 1.25 mg, 2.5 mg, unknown dose

Treatment Duration: never used, <5, 5–9, ≥10 years
Validation of Exposure: patient interview
Study Methodology: retrospective, case-control
Population Selection Criteria: patients from screening program, Breast Cancer Detection
  Demonstration Project
Total Number of Subjects: 1744; *Cases:* 863; *Control Subjects:* 881
Comparability of Controls: matched for age, race, family income, and history of breast surgery
Drug Event: breast cancer
Validation of Outcome: diagnosis and breast biopsy
Findings: RR 1.24; higher risks associated with high-dose preparations

**81:3   Horwitz RI, Feinstein AR. Improved observational method for studying
        therapeutic efficacy: suggestive evidence that lidocaine prophylaxis
        prevents death in acute myocardial infarction. JAMA 1981;*246*:2455-9**
Drug Name: lidocaine; *Category:* antiarrhythmics
Dosing Criteria: a bolus of intravenous lidocaine 50–100 mg followed by continuous intra-
  venous therapy (2–4 mg/min) for up to 48 hours; *Treatment Duration:* one week
Validation of Exposure: hospital records
Study Methodology: retrospective, case-control
Population Selection Criteria: patients hospitalized for myocardial infarction in a special care
  unit
Total Number of Subjects: 302; *Cases:* 151; *Control Subjects:* 151
Comparability of Controls: white men with similar symptoms
Drug Event: arrhythmia following myocardial infarction
Validation of Outcome: death or survival
Findings: lidocaine prophylaxis has no effect on death from pump failure or nonarrhythmic
  causes, but significantly protects against death from ventricular arrhythmias

**81:4   Johnson RE, Specht EE. The risk of hip fracture in postmenopausal females
        with or without estrogen drug exposure. Am J Public Health 1981;*71*:138-44**
Drug Category: estrogens
Treatment Duration: no exposure, <36 months, ≥36 months
Validation of Exposure: patient questionnaire, discharge summary, nurse interview, written
  drug order in medical chart
Study Methodology: retrospective, case-control
Population Selection Criteria: Kaiser-Permanente Medical Care Program of Oregon, women
  hospitalized during 1965–75, 52–80 years of age, discharged with hip fracture
Total Number of Subjects: 504; *Cases:* 168; *Control Subjects:* 336
Comparability of Controls: matched with two controls on age at date of fracture (within 12
  months), length of Health Plan membership (within 12 months), date of hospital dis-
  charge (within three years), type of menopause
Drug Event: hip fracture
Findings: RR 0.72

**81:5   Mitchell AA, Rosenberg L, Shapiro S, Slone D. Birth defects related to Ben-
        dectin use in pregnancy. I. Oral clefts and cardiac defects. JAMA 1981;
        245:2311-4**
Drug Name: doxylamine and pyridoxine (Bendectin); *Category:* antiemetics
Treatment Duration: first-trimester exposure
Validation of Exposure: mother interview
Study Methodology: retrospective, case-control

Population Selection Criteria: infants with isolated cleft palate (study 1), infants with cleft lip with or without cleft palate (study 2), and infants with selected heart defects (study 3)
Total Number of Subjects: 1411; *Cases:* 441; *Control Subjects:* 970
Comparability of Controls: malformed infants with none of the five outcomes
Drug Event: oral clefts and cardiac defects
Validation of Outcome: medical records
Rule Out Alternative Explanations: several social-demographic and health factors of infant and family considered
Findings: study 1 RR 0.9, study 2 RR 0.6, study 3 RR 1.0

81:6   Slone D, Shapiro S, Kaufman DW, Rosenberg L, Miettinen OS, Stolley PD. Risk of myocardial infarction in relation to current and discontinued use of oral contraceptives. N Engl J Med 1981;305:420-4
Drug Name: oral contraceptives; *Category:* estrogens/progestins
Treatment Duration: <5, 5–9, ≥10 years, unknown time
Validation of Exposure: telephone interview with patient
Study Methodology: retrospective, case-control
Population Selection Criteria: coronary care units of 155 hospitals in the northeastern U.S.
Total Number of Subjects: 2592; *Cases:* 556; *Control Subjects:* 2036
Comparability of Controls: admitted at similar time for reason unrelated to oral contraceptive use, aged 25–49 years
Drug Event: myocardial infarction
Findings: current user, rate ratio 3.5

81:7   Trapido EJ. Prospective cohort study of oral contraceptives and breast cancer. J Natl Cancer Inst 1981;67:1011-15
Drug Name: oral contraceptives; *Category:* estrogens/progestins
Treatment Duration: users versus nonusers
Validation of Exposure: patient questionnaires mailed out to residence
Study Methodology: prospective, cohort
Population Selection Criteria: resident of Boston, women born 1919–1944
Total Number of Subjects: 95 519; *Cases:* 622 (breast cancer)
Comparability of Controls: matched for age, parity, town, suburb, and age at completion of education
Drug Event: breast cancer
Validation of Outcome: physician's pathology reports of diagnosis of breast cancer from 34 hospitals serving the area
Findings: multiparous women, rate ratio 84; use of oral contraceptives, rate ratio 2.1

81:8   Vessey MP, Yeates D, Flavel R, McPherson K. Pelvic inflammatory disease and the intrauterine device: findings in a large cohort study. Br Med J 1981;282:855-7
Drug Name: intrauterine device; *Category:* contraceptive devices
Treatment Duration: varied, at least five months
Validation of Exposure: records and physician visits
Study Methodology: prospective, cohort
Population Selection Criteria: patients exposed to some form of birth control, using 1 of 17 family-planning clinics in England or Scotland
Total Number of Subjects: 17 032; *Cases:* 17 032
Drug Event: pelvic inflammatory disease
Validation of Outcome: hospital admissions

Findings: 1.51 hospital admissions per 1000 woman-years for users of intrauterine devices; 0.14 per 1000 woman-years for users of other methods

82:1   Bardhan KD, Cole DS, Hawkins BW, Franks CR. Does treatment with cimetidine extended beyond initial healing of duodenal ulcer reduce the subsequent relapse rate? *Br Med J* 1982;*284:*621-3

Drug Name: cimetidine; *Category:* histamine H_2-receptor antagonists
Dosing Criteria: 1 g/d; *Treatment Duration:* two to five months
Validation of Exposure: drug given in study
Study Methodology: prospective cohort
Population Selection Criteria: patients diagnosed in Rotherham (United Kingdom) 1977–1980
Total Number of Subjects: 194; *Cases:* 63 (two months), 66 (five months); *Control Subjects:* 65
Comparability of Controls: similar physical and clinical characteristics
Drug Event: duodenal ulcer
Validation of Outcome: endoscopy for duodenal ulcer
Findings: relapse rate 80 percent for two months of therapy, 90 percent for five months, 77 percent for placebo; prolonged treatment beyond time of healing does not increase risk of relapse

82:2   Bracken MB, Srisuphan W. Oral contraception as a risk factor for preeclampsia. *Am J Obstet Gynecol* 1982;*142:*191-6

Drug Name: oral contraceptives; *Category:* estrogens/progestins
Treatment Duration: 3–12 months before pregnancy, within two months of pregnancy
Validation of Exposure: patient interview and records
Study Methodology: retrospective, case-control
Population Selection Criteria: women giving birth to an infant with no congenital deformation
Sample Frame Limitations: women who used oral contraceptives within two months of pregnancy appeared to be younger
Total Number of Subjects: 341; *Cases:* 99; *Control Subjects:* 242
Drug Event: preeclampsia
Validation of Outcome: medical examination with diagnosis of preeclampsia
Rule Out Alternative Explanations: considered many maternal factors
Findings: no increased risk

82:3   Bulatao-Jayme J, Almero EM, Castro MC, Jardeleza MT, Salamat LA. A case-control dietary study of primary liver cancer risk from aflatoxin exposure. *Int J Epidemiol* 1982;*11:*112-9

Drug Name: aflatoxin; *Category:* toxin in food
Validation of Exposure: food analysis and urine samples
Study Methodology: retrospective, case-control
Population Selection Criteria: patients with primary liver cancer
Total Number of Subjects: 180; *Cases:* 90; *Control Subjects:* 90
Comparability of Controls: matched for economic status, age, and sex
Drug Event: primary liver cancer
Validation of Outcome: urinary sample and diagnosis
Rule Out Alternative Explanations: alcohol intake
Findings: low aflatoxin, high alcohol RR 3.9; high aflatoxin, low alcohol RR 17.5; high aflatoxin, high alcohol RR 35.0

82:4   Colin-Jones DG, Langman MJ, Lawson DH, Vessey MP. Cimetidine and gastric cancer: preliminary report from post-marketing surveillance study. *Br Med J (Clin Res)* 1982;*285:*1311-3

Drug Name: cimetidine; *Category:* histamine H_2-receptor antagonists
Validation of Exposure: physician interviews at practice site
Study Methodology: prospective, cohort
Population Selection Criteria: prescription-pricing behavior
Total Number of Subjects: 18 498; *Cases:* 8994; *Control Subjects:* 9504
Comparability of Controls: next patient in practice file matched for sex, age (in same decade), and physician visit in prior 12 months
Drug Event: gastric cancer
Validation of Outcome: diagnosis of gastric cancer by physician
Findings: no increased risk

82:5   Cramer DW, Hutchison GB, Welch WR, Scully RE, Knapp RC. Factors affecting the association of oral contraceptives and ovarian cancer. *N Engl J Med* 1982;307:1047-51

Drug Name: oral contraceptives; *Category:* estrogens/progestins
Treatment Duration: age at first use, duration of use, time since last use
Validation of Exposure: personal interviews
Study Methodology: retrospective, case-control
Population Selection Criteria: Massachusetts residents, aged 18–80 years, diagnosed ovarian cancer during 1978–81
Total Number of Subjects: 283; *Cases:* 144; *Control Subjects:* 139
Comparability of Controls: randomly selected from list of Massachusetts residents, matched for residence, age (within two years), and race
Drug Event: epithelian ovarian cancer
Validation of Outcome: diagnosis in medical record
Findings: adjusted for parity, RR 0.11; women aged <40 years, RR 1.98

82:6   Kaufman DW, Shapiro S, Slone D, et al. Diazepam and the risk of breast cancer. *Lancet* 1982;1:537-9

Drug Name: diazepam; *Category:* antianxiety agents, benzodiazepines
Treatment Duration: ≥four d/wk for more than six months
Validation of Exposure: patient questionnaire
Study Methodology: retrospective, case-control
Population Selection Criteria: hospital-based, case-control surveillance system located in several U.S. metropolitan areas
Total Number of Subjects: 1964; *Cases:* 1236; *Control Subjects:* 728
Comparability of Controls: other malignancies, matched for age and admission date
Drug Event: breast cancer
Validation of Outcome: record showing breast cancer
Rule Out Alternative Explanations: major risk factors for breast cancer
Findings: RR 0.9

82:7   Rosenberg L, Shapiro S, Slone D, et al. Epithelial ovarian cancer and combination oral contraceptives. *JAMA* 1982;247:3210-2

Drug Name: oral contraceptives; *Category:* estrogens/progestins
Treatment Duration: nonusers, <1, 1–4, ≥5 years, unknown use
Validation of Exposure: nurse interviewers administered questionnaires to ovarian cancer patients
Study Methodology: retrospective, case-control
Sample Frame Limitations: patient recollection of exposure
Total Number of Subjects: 690; *Cases:* 138; *Control Subjects:* 552

Comparability of Controls: admitted at same time, no history of cancer, aged <60 years, no history of bilateral oophorectomy
Drug Event: ovarian cancer
Validation of Outcome: pathology report
Findings: RR 0.6

82:8   Shapiro S, Slone D, Heinonen OP, et al. Birth defects and vaginal spermicides. JAMA 1982;247:2381-4
Drug Category: spermicides
Validation of Exposure: prescription database
Study Methodology: prospective, cohort
Population Selection Criteria: births between 1956 and 1965 in 12 Seattle hospitals
Total Number of Subjects: 50 282; *Cases:* 462; *Control Subjects:* 49 820
Comparability of Controls: similar birth factors
Drug Event: limb-reduction deformities, neoplasms, Down's syndrome, and hypospadias
Validation of Outcome: patient records for birth defects
Findings: estimated rate ratio 0.9

82:9   Vandenbroucke JP, Boersma JW, Festen JJM, et al. Oral contraceptives and rheumatoid arthritis: further evidence for a preventive effect. Lancet 1982;2:839-42
Drug Name: oral contraceptives; *Category:* estrogens/progestins
Treatment Duration: never used, previously used, currently used
Validation of Exposure: patient questionnaires
Study Methodology: retrospective, case-control
Population Selection Criteria: five rheumatology outpatient clinics in the Netherlands, cases and controls randomly selected meeting diagnostic and age criteria
Total Number of Subjects: 530; *Cases:* 228; *Control Subjects:* 302
Comparability of Controls: have same clinic population with diagnosis for soft tissue rheumatism
Drug Event: rheumatoid arthritis
Findings: rate ratio 0.42

83:1   Atukorala TM, Dickerson JW, Basu TK, McElwain TJ. Longitudinal studies of nutritional status in patients having chemotherapy for testicular teratomas. Clin Oncol 1983;91:3-10
Drug Name: bleomycin, cisplatin, vinblastine; *Category:* antineoplastics
Treatment Duration: four 21-day courses
Validation of Exposure: intravenous administration in hospital
Study Methodology: prospective, cohort
Population Selection Criteria: patients with testicular teratoma at Royal Marsden Hospital, Sutton, Great Britain
Total Number of Subjects: 22; *Cases:* 14; *Control Subjects:* 8
Comparability of Controls: cases, aged 19–52 years, controls 10–34 years
Drug Event: weight loss, decreased concentrations of retinol, vitamins E, B_1, B_6
Validation of Outcome: blood samples of drug and nutrients
Findings: weight loss, decreased levels of retinol and vitamins E, B_1, and B_6

83:2   Blazer DG, et al. Risk of anticholinergic toxicity in the elderly. J Gerontol 1983;38:31-5
Drug Category: anticholinergics
Treatment Duration: varied

Validation of Exposure: Medicaid claims data
Study Methodology: drug utilization
Population Selection Criteria: Medicaid patients in Tennessee
Total Number of Subjects: 10 063; *Cases* 5902 nursing home patients; *Control Subjects:* 4161 ambulatory patients
Drug Event: anticholinergic toxicity due to concomitant prescriptions with anticholinergic properties in elderly
Validation of Outcome: number of drugs taken with anticholinergic effects
Findings: 59 percent of nursing home patients used drugs with anticholinergic properties, 23 percent of ambulatory patients used drugs with anticholinergic properties

83:3   Colin-Jones DG, Langman MJS, Lawson DH, Vessey MP. Postmarketing surveillance of the safety of cimetidine: 12-month mortality report. *Br Med J* 1983;286:1713-6
Drug Name: cimetidine; *Category:* histamine H$_2$-receptor antagonist
Validation of Exposure: patient records and questionnaires
Study Methodology: prospective, cohort
Population Selection Criteria: pharmacists' reports in Glasgow, Nottingham, Oxford, and Portsmouth, United Kingdom
Total Number of Subjects: 19 279; *Cases:* 9928; *Control Subjects:* 9351
Comparability of Controls: matched for age, sex, and same medical center
Drug Event: mortality rate after cimetidine use for peptic ulcer disease
Validation of Outcome: deaths
Findings: no increased risk

83:4   Greene MH, Young RC, Merrill JM, DeVita VT. Evidence of a treatment dose response in acute nonlymphocytic leukemias which occur after therapy of non-Hodgkin's lymphoma. *Cancer Res* 1983;43:1891-8
Drug Category: antineoplastics
Treatment Duration: 18 months
Validation of Exposure: drugs administered in study
Study Methodology: prospective, cohort
Population Selection Criteria: patients treated at the National Cancer Institute for non-Hodgkin's lymphoma
Total Number of Subjects: 517; *Cases:* 21; *Control Subjects:* 496
Comparability of Controls: similar diagnosis
Drug Event: nonlymphocytic leukemia
Validation of Outcome: pathology studies
Findings: excess risk, 4.1 cases per 1000 patients per year

83:5   Herman RL, Lamdin E, Fischetti JL. Postmarketing evaluation of atenolol (Tenormin): a new cardioselective beta-blocker. *Curr Ther Res* 1983;33:165-71
Drug Name: atenolol; *Category:* beta-adrenergic receptor antagonists; *Dosing Criteria:* 50 mg/d
Treatment Duration: 28 days
Validation of Exposure: patient compliance
Study Methodology: prospective, cohort
Population Selection Criteria: newly diagnosed with essential hypertension, aged 40–100 years, based on voluntary reports by physicians
Total Number of Subjects: 34 120
Drug Event: hypertension, general adverse reactions

Validation of Outcome: blood pressure measurements, questionnaires to physician about adverse events
Findings: 15.4 percent of patients reported unintended drug effects, 1.6 percent rated as severe by physicians

83:6   Inman WHW, Rawson NSB. Erythromycin estolate and jaundice. *Br Med J* **1983;*286*:1954-5**
Drug Name: erythromycin estolate; *Category:* antibacterials
Validation of Exposure: diagnosis of jaundice
Study Methodology: cross-sectional
Population Selection Criteria: patients found through prescription-event monitoring
Total Number of Subjects: 9236; *Cases:* 3314; *Control Subjects:* 5922
Drug Event: jaundice
Validation of Outcome: reported jaundice
Findings: incidence <1:1000

83:7   Janerich DT, Polednak AP, Glebatis DM, Lawrence CE. Breast cancer and oral contraceptive use: case-control study. *J Chronic Dis* **1983;36:639-46**
Drug Name: oral contraceptives; *Category:* estrogens/progestins
Treatment Duration: never used, used prior to first delivery, used <2, 2–4, 4–6, >6 years
Validation of Exposure: telephone interview, mailed questionnaire
Study Methodology: retrospective, case-control
Population Selection Criteria: breast cancer cases ≤45 years of age, New York Cancer Registry, 1974–76
Total Number of Subjects: 798; *Cases:* 278 (within one year); *Control Subects:* 520
Comparability of Controls: selected from birth records and matched for year of birth, date of birth of first child (within one year), and county of residence
Drug Event: benign breast tumor
Findings: no increased risk

83:8   McCredie J, Kricker A, Elliott J, Forrest J. Congenital limb defects and the pill. *Lancet* **1983;2:623**
Drug Name: oral contraceptives; *Category:* estrogens/progestins
Dosing Criteria: during pregnancy; *Treatment Duration:* never used, used >12 months before conception, used 6–12 months before conception, used 2–6 months before conception, used <2 months before conception, used during early pregnancy
Study Methodology: retrospective, case-control
Population Selection Criteria: liveborn children with congenital limb-reduction deformities born in New South Wales, 1970-81
Total Number of Subjects: 429; *Cases:* 155; *Control Subjects:* 274
Comparability of Controls: matched for child's birthdate (within two months) and area of residence
Drug Event: congenital malformation
Validation of Outcome: clinical and radiologic confirmation
Findings: RR 23.9

83:9   Mitchell AA, Schwingl PJ, Rosenberg L, Louik C, Shapiro S. Birth defects in relation to Bendectin use in pregnancy. II. Pyloric stenosis. *Am J Obstet Gynecol* **1983;*147*:737-42**
Drug Name: doxylamine and pyridoxine (Bendectin); *Category:* antiemetics
Validation of Exposure: patient interview by practitioners

Study Methodology: retrospective, case-control
Population Selection Criteria: children born in Boston, 1976–82
Total Number of Subjects: 4202; *Cases:* 325; *Control Subjects:* 3153 with other conditions, 724 with congenital malformations
Drug Event: birth defects (pyloric stenosis)
Validation of Outcome: diagnosis of pyloric stenosis in hospital lists, surgical logs, and clinic or office records
Findings: no increased risk

83:10 Persson I, Adami HO, Johansson E, Lindberg B, Manell P, Westerholm B. Cohort study of estrogen treatment and the risk of endometrial cancer: evaluation of method and its applicability. *Eur J Clin Pharmacol* 1983;25: 625-32
Drug Category: estrogens
Validation of Exposure: patient questionnaires
Study Methodology: prospective, cohort
Population Selection Criteria: patients prescribed estrogens presenting at all 120 pharmacies in the geographic area
Total Number of Subjects: 23 233; *Cases:* 23 233
Drug Event: endometrial cancer
Validation of Outcome: pathology studies reported from physician examination
Findings: see abstract 86:11

83:11 Pike MC, Henderson BE, Krailo MD, Duke A, Roy S. Breast cancer in young women and use of oral contraceptives: possible modifying effect of formulation and age at use. *Lancet* 1983;2:926-30
Drug Name: oral contraceptives; *Category:* estrogens/progestins
Treatment Duration: 0, 1–24, 25–48, 49–72, ≥73 months
Validation of Exposure: patient interview
Study Methodology: retrospective, case-control
Population Selection Criteria: Los Angeles county residents, white women with breast cancer, aged <34 years at diagnosis
Total Number of Subjects: 628; *Cases:* 314; *Control Subjects:* 314
Comparability of Controls: matched for vital statistics
Drug Event: breast cancer
Validation of Outcome: histology studies, pathology studies, and physician diagnosis
Findings: long-term use of oral contraceptives with high progestogen component before age 25, RR 4.0

83:12 Rosenberg L, Mitchell AA, Parsells JL, Pashayan H, Louik C, Shapiro S. Lack of relation of oral clefts to diazepam use during pregnancy. *N Engl J Med* 1983;309:1282-5
Drug Name: diazepam; *Category:* antianxiety agents, benzodiazepines
Treatment Duration: first-trimester exposure
Validation of Exposure: patient interview by nurse
Study Methodology: retrospective, case-control
Population Selection Criteria: children with cleft lips (445) and cleft palate (166) in Boston, Philadelphia, and Toronto
Total Number of Subjects: 3109; *Cases:* 611; *Control Subjects:* 2498
Comparability of Controls: all other malformed infants of birth defect surveillance program

Drug Event: oral clefts
Validation of Outcome: diagnosis
Findings: RR 1.0

83:13 Ruegsegger P, Medici TC, Anliker M. Corticosteroid-induced bone loss. A longitudinal study of alternate-day therapy in patients with bronchial asthma using quantitative computed tomography. *Eur J Clin Pharmacol* 1983;25:615-20

Drug Name: prednisone; *Category:* corticosteroids
Dosing Criteria: <17 mg, 17–34 mg, 34–51 mg; *Treatment Duration:* one year
Study Methodology: controlled, clinical trial
Total Number of Subjects: 20; *Control Subjects:* 20
Population Selection Criteria: outpatients with chronic bronchial asthma treated at the Medical
   Policlinic of the University Hospital, Zurich, 1981–82
Drug Event: osteoporosis
Validation of Outcome: bone studies including bone density
Rule Out Alternative Explanations: one year
Findings: prednisone 25 mg on alternate days caused an average reduction in trabecular
   bone of 3.5 percent over one year; young patients on 50 mg q2d lost 17 percent of trabec-
   ular bone in one year; bone loss was dose-dependent

83:14 Smith DH, Scott DL, Zaphiropoulos GC. Eosinophilia in D-penicillamine therapy. *Ann Rheum Dis* 1983;42:408-10

Drug Name: penicillamine; *Category:* heavy-metal antagonists, immunosuppressants
Dosing Criteria: 125–750 mg/d in accordance with a flexible response-related regimen
Treatment Duration: 10–12 months
Study Methodology: longitudinal, cross-sectional
Population Selection Criteria: attending rheumatology outpatient clinics in Coventry, England
Total Number of Subjects: 204; *Cases:* 63; *Control Subjects:* 141 in various treatment groups
Comparability of Controls: matched for diagnosis of definite or classical rheumatoid arthritis
Drug Event: eosinophilia in treatment of rheumatoid arthritis
Validation of Outcome: white cell platelet counts with total eosinophilia
Findings: no significant association

84:1 Austin H, Louv WC, Alexander WJ. Case-control study of spermicides and gonorrhea. *JAMA* 1984;251:2822-4

Drug Category: spermicides
Treatment Duration: never, ever, relative to development of gonorrhea
Validation of Exposure: patient questionnaire
Study Methodology: retrospective, case-control
Population Selection Criteria: patients attending sexually transmitted disease clinic of Jefferson
   County, Alabama
Total Number of Subjects: 1693; *Cases:* 735; *Control Subjects:* 958
Comparability of Controls: attended clinic at same time with negative cervical culture for gon-
   orrhea
Drug Event: gonorrhea, relapse
Validation of Outcome: presence of gonorrhea in cervical culture
Rule Out Alternative Explanations: education, marital status, number of sexual partners, fre-
   quency of sexual intercourse, intrauterine device use, and history of tubal ligation
Findings: RR 0.67

84:2   Balter MB, Manheimer DI, Mellinger GD, Uhlenhuth EH. A cross-national comparison of antianxiety/sedative drug use. Curr Med Res Opin 1984;8(suppl 4):5-20
Drug Category: antianxiety agents, sedatives
Treatment Duration: 18 years of sampling
Validation of Exposure: patient questionnaire
Study Methodology: drug utilization
Population Selection Criteria: household study in nine western European countries
Total Number of Subjects: nine studies, ranging from 1486 to 2018 patients; *Cases:* 460–965 patients; *Control Subjects:* 521-1026
Findings: rates of prevalence of use for 1983 varied from 17.6 percent in Belgium to 7.4 percent in the Netherlands; prevalence rates were higher for women than for men in every country surveyed

84:3   Bridgman KM, Carr M, Tattersall AB. Postmarketing surveillance of the Transderm-Nitro patch in general practice. J Int Med Res 1984;12:40-5
Drug Name: nitroglycerin transdermal patch; *Category:* antianginals
Dosing Criteria: 5 mg/24 h; *Treatment Duration:* 1–180 days
Validation of Exposure: response from physician using record cards
Study Methodology: prospective, cohort
Population Selection Criteria: 790 general practitioners submitted data on 2475 patients during a six-month period following instruction
Total Number of Subjects: 2461
Drug Event: adverse effects and withdrawal symptoms
Validation of Outcome: nature and severity of unintended effects and withdrawal from drug
Findings: 80.6 percent treatment effective; 70.5 percent no unintended effects (headache, dizziness, giddiness, lightheadedness, faintness, 23.6 percent of unintended effect symptoms); 5.7 percent rate of discontinuation due to headaches, 3.6 percent due to unwanted effects, 3.1 percent due to ineffective treatment

84:4   Ellrodt AG, Murata GH, Riedinger MS, Stewart ME, Mochizuki C, Gray R. Severe neutropenia associated with sustained-release procainamide. Ann Intern Med 1984;100:197-201
Drug Name: procainamide hydrochloride; *Category:* antiarrhythmics
Treatment Duration: 20 months
Validation of Exposure: patient charts
Study Methodology: retrospective, case-control
Population Selection Criteria: patients with cardiovascular surgery from Cedars-Sinai Medical Center, New York
Total Number of Subjects: 114; *Cases:* 5; *Control Subjects:* 109
Comparability of Controls: matched for age, sex, and time of surgery
Drug Event: neutropenia
Validation of Outcome: neutrophils <100/mm^3
Findings: significant association between use of sustained-release procainamide and development of neutropenia

84:5   Greenberg ER, Barnes AB, Resseguie L, et al. Breast cancer in mothers given diethylstilbestrol in pregnancy. N Engl J Med 1984;311:1393-8
Drug Name: diethylstilbestrol; *Category:* estrogens
Validation of Exposure: patient questionnaire and prenatal records
Study Methodology: retrospective, cohort

Population Selection Criteria: women receiving diethlystilbestrol during pregnancy between 1940 and 1960

Total Number of Subjects: 6066; *Cases:* 3033; *Control Subjects:* 3033

Comparability of Controls: women who had had prenatal care and had delivered at least one live child between 1940 and 1960

Drug Event: breast cancer

Validation of Outcome: pathology studies

Findings: RR 1.4 (crude)

84:6   Hadjimichael OC, Meigs JW, Falcier FW, Thompson WD, Flannery JT. Cancer risk among women exposed to exogenous estrogens during pregnancy. *J Natl Cancer Inst* 1984;73:831-4

Drug Category: estrogens

Dosing Criteria: <1000 mg, 1000–4500 mg, >4500 mg

Validation of Exposure: patient records

Study Methodology: prospective, cohort

Population Selection Criteria: patients identified in 11 offices of obstetricians and gynecologists in Fairfield and New Haven counties, Connecticut

Total Number of Subjects: 3111; *Cases:* 1706; *Control Subjects:* 1405

Comparability of Controls: same physician, demographic data, pregnancy and drug-use histories

Drug Event: cancer

Validation of Outcome: records of pathology studies

Findings: all cancers, RR 1.46; breast cancer, RR 1.37; cervical cancer, RR 1.40; ovarian cancer, RR 2.83

84:7   Helmrich SP, Rosenberg L, Kaufman DW, et al. Lack of an elevated risk of malignant melanoma in relation to oral contraceptives use. *J Natl Cancer Inst* 1984;72:617-20

Drug Name: oral contraceptives; *Category:* estrogens/progestins

Treatment Duration: never used, <1, 1–4, 5–9, ≥10 years, unknown use

Validation of Exposure: chart and patient interviews

Study Methodology: retrospective, case-control

Population Selection Criteria: white females, aged 20–59 years, with diagnosis of malignant melanoma

Total Number of Subjects: 800; *Cases:* 160; *Control Subjects:* 640

Comparability of Controls: admitted to hospital during same period of time, admitted for nonmalignant causes, no history of previous cancer, and within same decade of age

Drug Event: malignant melanoma

Validation of Outcome: physician diagnosis

Findings: RR 0.9

84:8   Inman WHW. Prescription-event monitoring. A preliminary study of benoxaprofen and fenbufen. *Acta Med Scand* 1984;683(suppl):119-26

Drug Name: benoxaprofen, fenbufen; *Category:* analgesics, nonsteroidal antiinflammatory drugs

Treatment Duration: two to four years

Validation of Exposure: prescription filled

Study Methodology: prospective, cohort

Population Selection Criteria: cohort of patients identified by prescriptions filled

Total Number of Subjects: 7665; *Cases:* 7665

Drug Event: general identification of any event that may be attributable to benoxaprofen or fenbufen
Validation of Outcome: survey instrument sent to physician to record the event
Findings: similar pattern of events for both drugs

84:9 Kleinerman RA, Brinton LA, Hoover R, Fraumeni JF Jr. Diazepam use and progression of breast cancer. *Cancer Res* 1984;*44*:1223-5

Drug Name: diazepam; *Category:* antianxiety agents, benzodiazepines
Treatment Duration: never used, <1, 1–4, ≥5 years
Validation of Exposure: patient interviews and records
Study Methodology: retrospective, case-control
Population Selection Criteria: patients from Breast Cancer Detection Demonstration
Total Number of Subjects: 2221; *Cases:* 1075; *Control Subjects:* 1146
Comparability of Controls: matched for race, age at entry of project (within five years), and length of continuation as screening participant
Drug Event: breast cancer
Validation of Outcome: diagnosis and physical examination
Findings: no increased risk

84:10 Rosenberg L, Miller DR, Kaufman DW, et al. Breast cancer and oral contraceptive use. *Am J Epidemiol* 1984;*1192*:167-72

Drug Name: oral contraceptives; *Category:* estrogens/progestins
Treatment Duration: zero exposure, <1, 1–4, 5–9, ≥10 years
Validation of Exposure: patient questionnaires
Study Methodology: retrospective, case-control
Population Selection Criteria: women diagnosed with breast cancer
Total Number of Subjects: 6217; *Cases:* 1191; *Control Subjects:* 5026
Comparability of Controls: admission for nongynecologic and nonmalignant conditions
Drug Event: breast cancer
Validation of Outcome: diagnosis according to patient chart and from patient interviews by trained nurse interviewers
Findings: no increased risk

84:11 Shapiro S, Parsells JL, Rosenberg L, Kaufman DW, Stolley PD, Schottenfeld D. Risk of breast cancer in relation to the use of rauwolfia alkaloids. *Eur J Clin Pharmacol* 1984;*26*:143-6

Drug Name: reserpine; *Category:* antihypertensives, rauwolfia alkaloids
Treatment Duration: none, <1, 1–4, ≥5 years
Validation of Exposure: patient charts and patient interviews
Study Methodology: retrospective, case-control
Population Selection Criteria: patients presenting to several U.S. hospitals with a diagnosis of breast cancer
Total Number of Subjects: 3404; *Cases:* 1881; *Control Subjects:* 1523
Comparability of Controls: matched for age (ten-year age group), health status, and past health history
Drug Event: breast cancer
Validation of Outcome: pathology report from physician
Rule Out Alternative Explanations: ethnic group, religion, marital status, years of education, body mass, age at menarche, age at first pregnancy, parity, menopausal status, history of breast cancer, diabetes, treated hypertension, angina pectoris, history of myocardial infarction
Findings: no increased risk

85:1   Greco D. Case control study on encephalopathy associated with diphtheria tetanus immunization in Campania, Italy. *Bull WHO* 1985;*63*:919-25

Drug Name: diphtheria and tetanus toxoids adsorbed; *Category:* immunizing agents, vaccines
Treatment Duration: one-time immunization
Validation of Exposure: immunization register
Study Methodology: retrospective, case-control
Population Selection Criteria: children 3–48 mo in Campania region of Italy
Total Number of Subjects: 225; *Cases:* 45; *Control Subjects:* 180—hospital controls (n=90), residence controls (n=90)
Comparability of Controls: matched for age, sex, and date of admission
Drug Event: encephalopathy
Validation of Outcome: diagnosis by physical examination
Findings: patients immunized within previous month, RR 40.9; immunized within previous week, RR 92.6

85:2   Jenkins AC, Dreslinski GR, Tadros SS, Groel JT, Fand R, Herczeg SA. Captopril in hypertension; seven years later. *J Cardiovasc Pharmacol* 1985;*7*(suppl 1):96-101

Drug Name: captopril; *Category:* angiotensin-converting enzyme inhibitors, antihypertensives
Dosing Criteria: <150 mg, ≥150 mg; *Treatment Duration:* 3518 patients for less than one year and 3219 patients for greater than or equal to one year
Study Methodology: prospective, cohort
Population Selection Criteria: 3428 patients treatment-resistant, 1159 patients adverse reactions to prior antihypertensive agents, others severe hypertension
Total Number of Subjects: 6737
Drug Event: rash, dysgenesia, bone marrow depression
Validation of Outcome: blood counts, serum chemistry, and urinalysis
Findings: 5.8 percent rate of discontinuation because of unintended drug effects; similar safety profile as other commonly used antihypertensive agents

85:3   Lubin F, Ron E, Wax Y, et al. A case-control study of caffeine and methylxanthines in benign breast disease. *JAMA* 1985;*253*:2388-92

Drug Name: caffeine; *Category:* cerebral stimulants, methylxanthines, stimulants
Dosing Criteria: 0, 1, 2–3, ≥4 cups of coffee/d
Validation of Exposure: interview at home
Study Methodology: retrospective, case-control
Population Selection Criteria: types of histology, degree of ductal atypia, and age
Total Number of Subjects: 2332; *Cases:* 854; *Control Subjects:* 1478
Comparability of Controls: surgical and neighborhood control groups, age (within five years), country of origin, and length of residence
Drug Event: benign breast tumor
Validation of Outcome: two pathology specimens
Findings: no increased risk

85:4   Morrow GR. The effect of a susceptibility to motion sickness on the side effects of cancer chemotherapy. *Cancer* 1985;*55*:2766-70

Drug Category: antineoplastics
Treatment Duration: varied
Validation of Exposure: chemotherapy administered in hospital

Study Methodology: prospective, case-control
Population Selection Criteria: outpatients at University of Rochester Cancer Unit, cases selected as individuals prove for motion sickness
Total Number of Subjects: 972; *Cases:* 486; *Control Subjects:* 486
Comparability of Controls: matched for sex, age, type, and dose of antineoplastic agent and antiemetic taken
Drug Event: nausea, vomiting, and unintended effects
Validation of Outcome: patient questionnaire
Findings: susceptibility to motion sickness determines susceptibility to side effects of cancer chemotherapy

85:5   Resseguie LJ, Hick JF, Bruen JA, Noller KL, O'Fallon WM, Kurland LT. Congenital malformations among offspring exposed in utero to progestins, Olmsted County, Minnesota, 1936–1974. *Fertil Steril* 1985;43:514-9
Drug Category: progestins
Dosing Criteria: total exposure 125, 500, 1625, 3000, 11 250 mg; *Treatment Duration:* 0–9 months
Validation of Exposure: patient records
Study Methodology: prospective, cohort
Population Selection Criteria: infants exposed in utero to progestins, Olmsted County, Minnesota
Total Number of Subjects: 24 000; *Cases:* 988; *Control Subjects:* 23 012
Comparability of Controls: matched for sex of child, age of mother, number of previous liveborn children
Drug Event: congenital malformation
Validation of Outcome: presence of anomalies among infants
Rule Out Alternative Explanations: age of mother, prior live births, gravida, prior miscarriages
Findings: no increased risk

85:6   Shapiro S, Kelly JP, Rosenberg L, et al. Risk of localized and widespread endometrial cancer in relation to recent and discontinued use of conjugated estrogens. *N Engl J Med* 1985;313:969-72
Drug Name: estrogen, conjugated; *Category:* estrogens
Treatment Duration: none, <1, 1–4, 5–9, ≥10 years
Validation of Exposure: patient interview by trained nurse interviewers
Study Methodology: retrospective, case-control
Population Selection Criteria: Boston Collaborative Drug Surveillance Program
Total Number of Subjects: 1217; *Cases:* 425; *Control Subjects:* 792
Comparability of Controls: postmenopausal women aged 50–69 years, no hysterectomies, no cancer, and admitted for other causes
Drug Event: endometrial cancer
Validation of Outcome: adenocarcinoma of the endometrium
Findings: rate ratio 3.5

85:7   Strom BL, Hibberd PL, Stolley PD. No evidence of association between methyldopa and biliary carcinoma. *Int J Epidemiol* 1985;14:86-90
Drug Name: methyldopa; *Category:* antihypertensives
Validation of Exposure: per capita sales of methyldopa (kg/year)
Study Methodology: secular trend analysis, comparing the correlation between drug sales and disease states with two different time lags, three and ten years
Population Selection Criteria: U.S., Canada, Europe, and Asia populations covered by cancer registries for ≥1952

Cases: 128 for three-year lag; 70 for ten-year lag
Comparability of Controls: population controls
Drug Event: biliary cancer
Validation of Outcome: patient records in 11 cancer registries in the U.S., Canada, Europe, and Asia
Findings: no increased risk

85:8   Waller PC, Ramsay LE. Do beta-blockers cause arthropathy? A case-control study. Br Med J 1985;291:1684
Drug Category: beta-adrenergic receptor antagonists
Study Methodology: retrospective, case-control
Population Selection Criteria: patients in Sheffield Hypertension Clinic
Total Number of Subjects: 381; *Cases:* 127; *Control Subjects:* 254
Comparability of Controls: matched for age and sex
Drug Event: arthropathy and arthritis
Validation of Outcome: diagnosis of arthritis
Findings: RR 1.14

85:9   Wolfe MS, Cordero JF. Safety of chloroquine in chemosuppression of malaria during pregnancy. Br Med J (Clin Res) 1985;290:1466-7
Drug Name: chloroquine; *Category:* antimalarials, plasmodicides
Dosing Criteria: 300 mg once a week; *Treatment Duration:* throughout pregnancy
Validation of Exposure: administered in study
Study Methodology: prospective, cohort
Population Selection Criteria: reports of malaria to medical officers at U.S. embassies
Total Number of Subjects: 623; *Cases:* 169; *Control Subjects:* 454
Comparability of Controls: matched for birth and maternal factors
Drug Event: congenital malformations
Validation of Outcome: presence of birth defect diagnosed by physician
Findings: no increased risk

86:1   Avorn J, Everitt DE, Weiss S. Increased antidepressant use in patients prescribed beta-blockers. JAMA 1986;255:357-60
Drug Category: antidepressants, beta-adrenergic receptor antagonists
Treatment Duration: minimum two-year prevalence of use
Validation of Exposure: Medicaid prescribing records
Study Methodology: retrospective, cohort
Population Selection Criteria: patients in Medicaid database
Total Number of Subjects: sample of 143 253 from database of 1.6 million; Cohort I= 8235 treated with beta-blockers—concurrent 23 percent tricyclic antidepressant exposure; Cohort II = treated with insulin—concurrent 15 percent tricyclic antidepressant exposure; Cohort III = methyldopa- or reserpine-treated—concurrent 10 percent tricyclic antidepressant exposure
Comparability of Controls: Medicaid patients prescribed insulin, hypoglycemics, methlydopa, or reserpine
Drug Event: depression following beta-blockade
Validation of Outcome: use of antidepressants
Findings: risk using tricyclic antidepressants 1.5 (95 percent CI 1.4–1.7) for patients receiving beta-blockers relative to patients receiving hydralazine or hypoglycemics

86:2   Celotti F, Nudemberg F, Magni O, Piaia F. Efficacy and clinical tolerance of a new combination of trimethoprim with sulphonamide. A post-mar keting and a literature survey. *J Int Med Res* 1986; *14*:236-41

Drug Name: trimethoprim/sulfonamide; *Category:* antibacterials
Dosing Criteria: 500 mg/400 mg d; *Treatment Duration:* varied, 6–20 days (mean 8.8 d)
Study Methodology: prospective cohort
Population Selection Criteria: each physcian selected four to six patients
Total Number of Subjects: 5885; *Cases:* 1177; *Control Subjects:* 4708
Comparability of Controls: none mentioned
Drug Event: infection
Validation of Outcome: pathology studies following drug therapy
Findings: 91.2 percent cure rate, 4 percent incidence of unintended effects, 0.97 percent rate of discontinuation because of unintended effects

86.3   Herbst AL, Anderson S, Hubby MM, Haenszel WM, Kaufman RH, Noller KL. Risk factors for the development of diethylstilbestrol-associated clear cell adenocarcinoma: a case-control study. *Am J Obstet Gynecol* 1986;*154*:814-22

Drug Name: diethylstilbestrol; *Category:* estrogens
Dosing Criteria: 1.0, 10, 100, 1000, >1000 mg; *Treatment Duration:* exposure before week 7, week 7–8, week 9–12, week 13 or later
Validation of Exposure: prenatal, hospital, and pharmacy records
Study Methodology: retrospective, case-control
Population Selection Criteria: women exposed to diethylstilbestrol
Total Number of Subjects: 2004; *Cases:* 156; *Control Subjects:* 1848
Comparability of Controls: dosage patterns, use of other hormones, mother's age and pregnancy history, and daughter's birth weight
Drug Event: adenocarcinoma
Validation of Outcome: pathology and review of cases
Findings: before week 7, adjusted RR 3.65; weeks 7–8, RR 4.84, weeks 9–12, RR 3.48; during or after week 13, RR 1.00

86.4   Kakar F, Weiss NS, Strite SA. Thiazide use and the risk of cholecystectomy in women. *Am J Epidemiol* 1986;*1243*:428-33

Drug Category: antihypertensives, diuretics, thiazide diuretics
Validation of Exposure: patient interview
Study Methodology: retrospective, case-control
Population Selection Criteria: Group Health of Puget Sound members: women, black or white, aged 20–74 years, who underwent cholecystectomy
Total Number of Subjects: 309; *Cases:* 153; *Control Subjects:* 156
Comparability of Controls: matched for sex, year of birth (within two years), and zip code of residence
Drug Event: cholecystectomy
Validation of Outcome: chart review
Rule Out Alternative Explanations: overweight
Findings: not overweight RR 5.0; overweight RR 1.0

86.5   Lammer EJ, Cordero JF. Exogenous sex hormone exposure and the risk for major malformations. *JAMA* 1986;*255*:3128-32

Drug Category: progestins, estrogens
Treatment Duration: first-trimester, sex-hormone exposure

Validation of Exposure: physician interview, chart of patient interview
Study Methodology: retrospective, case-control
Population Selection Criteria: patients registered in Metropolitan Atlanta Congenital Defects program
Total Number of Subjects: 2146; *Cases:* 1091; *Control Subjects:* 1055
Drug Event: congenital malformations
Validation of Outcome: presence of significant birth malformation according to birth defect registry
Findings: esophageal atresia and any sex hormone exposure OR 2.84; progestins OR 2.87; nonspecific sex hormones OR 2.99; hormonal pregnancy test OR 2.81

86.6   Lesko SM, Mitchell AA, Epstein M, et al. Heparin use as a risk factor for in traventricular hemorrhage in low-birth-weight infants. *N Engl J Med* 1986; *314*:1156-60

Drug Name: heparin; *Category:* anticoagulants
Study Methodology: retrospective, case-control
Population Selection Criteria: newborn infants with germinal matrix-intraventricular hemorrhage, low birthweight
Total Number of Subjects: 320; *Cases:* 66; *Control Subjects:* 254
Comparability of Controls: selected from population of monitored newborns without matrix-intraventricular hemorrhage or malformation of central nervous system
Drug Event: intravascular hemorrhage
Validation of Outcome: computerized tomographic scanning, ultrasonography, or postmortem examination
Findings: OR 14.0; including confounding factors in analysis OR 3.9

86.7   Lipnick RJ, Buring JE, Hennekens CH, et al. Oral contraceptives and breast cancer: prospective cohort study. *JAMA* 1986;*255*:58-61

Drug Name: oral contraceptives; *Category:* estrogens/progestins
Treatment Duration: never used, 1–11, 12–35, 36–59, 60–119, ≥120 months
Validation of Exposure: patient questionnaire
Study Methodology: prospective, cohort
Population Selection Criteria: questionnaires mailed to members of American Nursing Association, aged 30–55 years
Total Number of Subjects: 51 585; *Cases:* 592 (breast cancer)
Drug Event: breast cancer
Validation of Outcome: diagnosis of breast cancer in chart
Rule Out Alternative Explanations: family history of breast cancer, age at first use, timing of first birth, or other breast cancer risk factors
Findings: RR 1.0

86.8   McGlynn KA, Lustbader ED, Sharrar RG, Murphy EC, London WT. Isoniazid prophylaxis in hepatitis B carriers. *Am Rev Respir Dis* 1986;*134*:666-8

Drug Name: isoniazid; *Category:* antibacterials, tuberculostatics
Treatment Duration: approximately eight weeks
Validation of Exposure: patient compliance verified
Study Methodology: prospective, cohort
Population Selection Criteria: southeast Asian immigrants
Total Number of Subjects: 1833; *Cases:* 1833
Drug Event: hepatitis

Validation of Outcome: determined blood levels of alanine aminotransferase
Findings: no increased risk

86.9   Meirik O, Lund E, Adami HO, et al. Oral contraceptive use and breast cancer in young women: a joint national case-control study in Sweden and Norway. *Lancet* 1986;2:650-2

Drug Name: oral contraceptives; *Category:* estrogens/progestins
Treatment Duration: ≤3, 4–7, 8–11, ≥12 years
Validation of Exposure: in-house interview using a recall aid prompting for life events
Study Methodology: population-based, retrospective, case-control
Population Selection Criteria: all newly diagnosed breast cancer cases, aged <45 years, reported to Swedish Cancer Registries
Total Number of Subjects: 1144; *Cases:* 422; *Control Subjects:* 722
Comparability of Controls: no history of previous malignant disease, resident of Sweden in 1960, born same year and month, resident of same county
Drug Event: breast cancer
Validation of Outcome: confirmed by histologic examination
Findings: ≥12 years' use RR 2.2

86.10   Miller DR, Rosenberg L, Kaufman DW, Schottenfeld D, Stolley PD, Shapiro S. Breast cancer risk in relation to early oral contraceptive use. *Obstet Gynecol* 1986;68:863-8

Drug Name: oral contraceptives; *Category:* estrogens/progestins
Treatment Duration: never used, <1, 1–2, 3–4, ≥5 years, used for unknown time period, used before or after age 25
Validation of Exposure: patient questionnaire
Study Methodology: retrospective, case-control
Population Selection Criteria: major hospital between 1977 and 1983 participating in Boston Collaborative Drug Surveillance Program
Total Number of Subjects: 1042; *Cases:* 521; *Control Subjects:* 521
Comparability of Controls: matched for age, time of interview, and geographic area
Drug Event: breast cancer
Validation of Outcome: hospital records and laboratory results
Rule Out Alternative Explanations: oral contraceptive use for first birth or use before age 25
Findings: RR 1.0

86.11   Persson IR, Adami HO, Eklund G, Johansson ED, Lindberg BS, Lindgren A. The risk of endometrial neoplasia and treatment with estrogens and estrogen/progestogen combinations. First results of a cohort study after one to four completed years of observation. *Acta Obstet Gynecol Scand* 1986;65:211-7

Drug Name: various estrogens and oral contraceptives; *Category:* estrogens, estrogens/progestins
Treatment Duration: ≤3 years of exposure, >3 years (89 000 person-years)
Validation of Exposure: prescriptions filled for estrogens and progestogens, questionnaire survey
Study Methodology: prospective, cohort (see 83:10)
Population Selection Criteria: (1) one or more prescriptions for estrogen; (2) >35 years at first prescription; (3) residence in defined geographic area
Total Number of Subjects: 23 233; *Cases:* 73 incidence of endometrial cancer in the study population; *Control Subjects:* 299 incidence of endometrial cancer in the total population

Drug Event: endometrial neoplasia
Validation of Outcome: presence of endometrial neoplasia of reported cases in cohort to Regional Cancer Registry
Rule Out Alternative Explanations: none
Findings: estrogens RR 1.3; estrogen/progesterone combined RR 0.6

86.12 Sattin RW, Rubin GL, Wingo PA, Webster LA, Ory HW. Oral contraceptive use and the risk of breast cancer. *N Engl J Med* **1986;315:405-11**

Drug Name: oral contraceptives; *Category:* estrogens/progestins
Treatment Duration: <1, 1–2, 3–5, 6–9, 10–14, ≥15 years
Validation of Exposure: patient interview
Study Methodology: prospective, cohort
Population Selection Criteria: aged 20–54 years with newly diagnosed brest cancer from the Cancer and Steroid Hormone Study of the Centers for Disease Control
Total Number of Subjects: 9387; *Cases:* 4711; *Control Subjects:* 4676
Comparability of Controls: random dialing of local women in each five-year age group
Drug Event: breast cancer
Validation of Outcome: surgery performed
Rule Out Alternative Explanations: parity, age at first birth, age at menarche, and menopausal status
Findings: RR 1.0

86.13 Schmidt LG, Grohmann R, Muller-Oerlinghausen B, Ochsenfahrt H, Schonhofer PS. Adverse drug reactions to first- and second-generation antidepressants: a critical evaluation of drug surveillance data. *Br J Psychiatry* **1986;148:38-43**

Drug Name: amitriptyline, clomipramine, dibenzepin, doxepin, mianserin, nomifensine, zimeldine; *Category:* antidepressants
Treatment Duration: varied
Validation of Exposure: patient charts and reports
Study Methodology: retrospective, cohort
Population Selection Criteria: recorded exposures in Berlin and Munich hospitals
Total Number of Subjects: 3181; *Cases:* first-generation antidepressants n=2666, second-generation n=515
Drug Event: unintended drug effects
Validation of Outcome: discontinuation of drug, adverse drug reaction reports
Findings: rate of discontinuation because of adverse reactions for tricyclics 7.4 percent; rate of discontinuation for the second-generation antidepressants 3.1 percent

86:14 Strom BL, Rankiran N, Tamragouri RN, et al. Oral contraceptives and other risk factors for gall bladder disease. *Clin Pharmacol Ther* **1986;39:335-41**

Drug Name: oral contraceptives; *Category:* estrogens/progestins
Dosing Criteria: none, <50 μg, 50 μg, >50 μg; *Treatment Duration:* varied
Validation of Exposure: pharmacy billing data
Study Methodology: retrospective, cohort
Population Selection Criteria: women in COMPASS database, 1980–81
Sample Frame Limitations: Medicaid Management Information System, created for fiscal and administrative control
Total Number of Subjects: 480 421; *Cases:* 138 943 users; *Control Subjects:* 341 478
Drug Event: gallbladder disease
Validation of Outcome: physical examination

Findings: RR 1.14; in women aged 15–19 years RR 3.1; in women aged 40–44 RR 1.2; clear dose response (p<0.001) relationship

86:15   Van Heyningen R, Harding JJ. Do aspirin-like analgesics protect against cataract? A case-control study. *Lancet* 1986; *1*:1111-3

Drug Name: aspirin; *Category:* analgesics, nonsteroidal antiinflammatory drugs
Treatment Duration: ≥4 months
Validation of Exposure: patient interview
Study Methodology: retrospective, case-control
Population Selection Criteria: Oxford Eye Hospital patients with cataract extraction, aged 50–79 years
Total Number of Subjects: 909; *Cases:* 300; *Control Subjects:* 609
Comparability of Controls: matched for age and sex distribution
Drug Event: cataract
Validation of Outcome: cataract diagnosis
Findings: RR 0.43

87.1   Baker GL, Kahl LE, Zee BC, Stolzer BL, Agarwal AK, Medsger TA Jr. Malignancy following treatment of rheumatoid arthritis with cyclophosphamide: long-term case-control follow-up study. *Am J Med* 1987;*83*:1-9

Drug Name: cyclophosphamide; *Category:* antineoplastics
Dosing Criteria: 50-150 mg/day; *Treatment Duration:* 43.8±31.8 months for cyclophosphamide-treated patients with malignancies, 28.1±21.0 months for cyclophosphamide-treated patients without malignancies
Validation of Exposure: practice records
Study Methodology: long-term retrospective, case-control
Population Selection Criteria: 119 cases selected from private rheumatology practice between 1968 and 1973. Controls matched for sex, age, disease duration, and ARA function class in same practice group
Total Number of Subjects: 238; *Cases:* 119; *Control Subjects:* 119
Drug Event: malignancies, including urinary bladder, skin, and hematologic malignancies
Validation of Outcome: none
Findings: no OR calculation but significant differences at the p<0.05 level were found in the development of malignancies between cyclophosphamide-treated subjects and others

87.2   Carson JL, Strom BL, Morse L, et al. The relative gastrointestinal toxicity of the nonsteroidal antiinflammatory drugs. *Arch Intern Med* 1987;*147*:1054-8

Drug Name: fenoprofen, ibuprofen, indomethacin, naproxen, phenylbutazone, sulindac, tolmetin; *Category:* analgesics, nonsteroidal antiinflammatory drugs
Dosing Criteria: none, the average daily dose as a percentage of the maximum recommended daily dose
Validation of Exposure: Medicaid billing data
Study Methodology: retrospective, cohort study
Population Selection Criteria: subjects exposed to one nonsteroidal antiinflammatory drug as identified in 1980 Medicaid billing data for the states of Michigan and Minnesota
Total Number of Subjects: sulindac 14 427, tolmetin 4646, naproxen 8478, ibuprofen 35 918, indomethacin 10 323, fenoprofen 4286, phenylbutazone 9770
Drug Event: upper gastrointestinal bleeding
Validation of Outcome: Medicaid billing data based on physician reporting of ICD9-CM codes
Findings: with ibuprofen as reference category: sulindac RR 1.7 (95 percent CI 1.3–2.3); tol-

metin RR 1.4 (95 percent CI 0.9–2.2); naproxen RR 1.2 (95 percent CI 0.8–1.8); ibuprofen RR 1.0 (reference); indomethacin RR 0.9 (95 percent CI 0.6–1.4); fenoprofen RR 0.7 (95 percent CI 0.3–1.3); phenylbutazone RR 0.6 (95 percent CI 0.4–1.0)

87.3   Carson JL, Strom BL, Soper KA, West SL, Morse ML. The Association of non-steroidal antiinflammatory drugs with upper gastrointestinal tract bleeding. Arch Intern Med 1987;147:85-8
Drug Category: analgesics, nonsteroidal antiinflammatory drugs
Dosing Criteria: low, medium, high, relative to recommended dose
Validation of Exposure: patient charts
Study Methodology: retrospective, cohort
Population Selection Criteria: Medicaid billing data from Michigan and Minnesota
Total Number of Subjects: 91 770; *Cases:* 47 136; *Control Subjects:* 44 634
Comparability of Controls: matched fo age (within ten-year age groups) and sex
Drug Event: upper gastrointestinal bleeding
Validation of Outcome: diagnosis of upper gastrointestinal bleeding in Medicaid database
Findings: unadjusted RR for developing upper gastrointestinal bleeding 1.5

87.4   Haas JF, Kittelmann B, Mehnert WH, et al. Risk of leukaemia in ovarian tumour and breast cancer patients following treatment by cyclophosphamide. Br J Cancer 1987;55:213-8
Drug Name: cyclophosphamide; *Category:* antineoplastics
Treatment Duration: 8–12 weeks
Validation of Exposure: National Cancer Registry records
Study Methodology: retrospective, case-control
Population Selection Criteria: patients identified in the National Cancer Registry of West Germany
Total Number of Subjects: 338; *Cases:* 105; *Control Subjects:* 233
Comparability of Controls: matched for site of first neoplasm, year of diagnosis, year of birth, and not having developed leukemia
Drug Event: development of leukemia
Validation of Outcome: diagnosis entered in record
Findings: ovarian tumor patients RR 14.6; breast cancer patients RR 2.7

87.5   Henry DA, Johnston A, Dobson A, Duggan J. Fatal peptic ulcer complications and the use of nonsteroidal antiinflammatory drugs, aspirin, and corticosteroids. Br Med J 1987;295:1227-9
Drug Name: aspirin, prednisone; *Category:* analgesics, corticosteroids, nonsteroidal antiinflammatory drugs
Dosing Criteria: none; *Treatment Duration:* none
Validation of Exposure: hospital notes, validation showed 97 percent agreement of data with interview
Study Methodology: retrospective, case-control
Population Selection Criteria: patients admitted to hospitals in the Hunter region of New South Wales (Australia); records reviewed from patients who died during hospital stay with history of peptic ulcer complications; cases matched with two controls who had survived a bleeding or perforated ulcer within two years of case
Total Number of Subjects: 242; *Cases:* 81; *Control Subjects:* 161
Comparability of Controls: matched for age ± five years, sex, size of ulcer, and hemorrhage or perforation

Drug Event: death from peptic ulcer complications
Validation of Outcome: hospital records
Findings: corticosteroids OR 4.2 (95 percent CI 0.9–25.6), not statistically significant; aspirin OR 1.2 (95 percent CI 0.5–1.9), not statistically significant; nonsteroidal antiinflammatory drugs OR 1.1 (95 percent CI 0.6–2.1), not statistically significant

87.6 Hoffman HJ, Hunter JC, Damus K, et al. Diphtheria-tetanus-pertussis immunization and sudden infant death: results of the National Institute of Child Health and Human Development Cooperative Epidemiological Study of Sudden Infant Death Syndrome risk factors. *Pediatrics* 1987;*79*: 598-611

Drug Name: diphtheria-tetanus-pertussis vaccine; *Category:* immunizing agents, vaccines
Validation of Exposure: mother interview
Study Methodology: population-based, retrospective, case-control
Population Selection Criteria: National Institute of Child Health and Human Development and Sudden Infant Death Syndrome Cooperative Epidemiological Study
Total Number of Subjects: 1200; *Cases:* 400; *Control Subjects:* 800
Comparability of Controls: selected from birth certificate-defined pool of infants born in study center region
Drug Event: sudden infant death syndrome
Validation of Outcome: pathology classification
Findings: no increased risk

87:7 Ray WA, Griffin MR, Schaffner W, Baugh DK, Melton LJ III. Psychotropic drug use and the risk of hip fracture. *N Engl J Med* 1987;*316*:363-9

Drug Category: psychotropics
Dosing Criteria: short elimination half-lives versus long half-lives
Validation of Exposure: Medicaid files
Study Methodology: retrospective, case-control
Population Selection Criteria: elderly Medicaid enrollees
Total Number of Subjects: 6627; *Cases:* 1021; *Control Subjects:* 5606
Drug Event: hip fracture
Validation of Outcome: hospital records
Findings: psychotropics with long elimination half-lives OR 1.8; tricyclic antidepressants OR 1.9; antipsychotics OR 2.0

87:8 Shu XO, Gao YT, Linet MS, et al. Chloramphenicol use and childhood leukemia in Shanghai. *Lancet* 1987;*2*:934-7

Drug Name: chloramphenicol; *Category:* antibiotics
Dosing Criteria: 30–50 mg/kg/d; *Treatment Duration:* none; 1–5 d; 6–10 d;> 10 d
Validation of Exposure: parents interview
Study Methodology: retrospective, case-control
Population Selection Criteria: all children under 15 years identified from the population-based Shanghai cancer registry with diagnosis of leukemia between July 1, 1977 and June 30, 1986
Total Number of Subjects: 927; *Cases:* 309 cases identified; *Control Subjects:* 618 matched for sex and calendar year of birth, selected from the Shanghai general population
Drug Event: acute lymphocytic leukemia and acute nonlymphocytic leukemia
Findings: 1–5 days of exposure OR 1.7 (95 percent CI 1.2–2.5); 6–10 days OR 2.8 (95 percent CI 1.5–5.1); >10 days OR 9.7 (95 percent CI 3.9–24.1)

87:9   Strom BL, Carson JL, Schinnar R, et al. Upper gastrointestinal tract bleeding from oral potassium chloride: comparative risk from microencapsulated versus wax-matrix formulations. *Arch Intern Med* 1987; *147*:954-7

Drug Name: Micro-K Extencaps, Slow-K; *Category:* potassium supplements
Dosing Criteria: none; *Treatment Duration:* recorded in months of use
Validation of Exposure: Medicaid billing data
Study Methodology: two-phase, retrospective, cohort
Population Selection Criteria: Medicaid billing data from the states of Michigan, Minnesota, Florida, and Ohio, 1980–89
Total Number of Subjects: 28 790 for 193 512 patient-months of exposure to microencapsulated formulation; 76 118 patients for 560 341 patient-months of exposure to wax-matrix formulation
Drug Event: upper gastrointestinal tract bleeding within 30 days after drug is dispensed
Validation of Outcome: billing data for physician visits based on ICD9-CM code
Findings: OR 0.67 (95 percent CI 0.52–0.85) for microencapsulated versus wax-matrix formulations

87:10   Tucker MA, Meadows AT, Boice JD Jr, et al. Leukemia after therapy with alkylating agents for childhood cancer. *J Natl Cancer Inst* 1987; *78*:459-64

Drug Category: antineoplastics
Dosing Criteria: agents with alkylator score ≤ 4, agents with alkylator score ≥ 5
Treatment Duration: ≥ 2 years
Validation of Exposure: patient chart
Study Methodology: retrospective, case-control
Population Selection Criteria: two-year survivor of primary cancer treatment
Total Number of Subjects: 9170; *Cases:* 2497; *Control Subjects:* 6673
Comparability of Controls: type of cancer, treatment, age, and responder factors
Drug Event: leukemia
Validation of Outcome: pathologic evidence of leukemia
Findings: RR 4.8

88:1   Charpin O, Benzarti M, Hemon Y, et al. Atopy and anaphylatic reactions to suxamethonium. *J Allergy Clin Immunol* 1988; *82*:356-60

Drug Name: succinylcholine chloride; *Category:* muscle relaxants
Dosing Criteria: none; *Treatment Duration:* none
Validation of Exposure: none
Study Methodology: prospective, case-control
Population Selection Criteria: positive skin test to succinylcholine chloride in patients referred to allergy clinic during six-year period, 1978–84. Controls selected in surgical wards from patients hospitalized at the same hospital for minor surgery unrelated to allergic condition.
Total Number of Subjects: 160; *Cases:* 32 atopic; *Control Subjects:* 128 subjects matched for age, sex, and socio-economic status
Drug Event: IgE-dependent anaphylactic reactions
Validation of Outcome: skin tests and IgE antibody fibers
Findings: Atopy is not a risk factor for anaphylactic reactions to muscle relaxants

88:2   Faulkner G, Prichard P, Somerville FM, Langman MJS. Aspirin and bleeding peptic ulcers in the elderly. *Fr Med J* 1988; *297*:1311-13

Drug Name: aspirin; *Category:* analgesics, nonsteroidal antiinflammatory drugs

Dosing Criteria: none; *Treatment Duration:* use within previous hours of bleeding incidence cases; if interview controls use within previous week regular use
Validation of Exposure: personal interview
Study Methodology: retrospective, case-control
Population Selection Criteria: all patients referred to Nottingham University and City Hospitals between April 1983 and March 1985, 230 patients > 60 years of age were included
Control Subjects: 207 community controls
Drug Event: gastric ulcers, duodenal ulcers (haematemesis or melaena)
Validation of Outcome: endoscopically confirmed
Findings: 2.6 (95percent CI 1.5–4.5) use within previous week of aspirin use; 2.4 (95 percent CI 1.3–5.2) use within 24 hours of aspirin use; RR 2.2 (95 percent CI 1.4–3.6) for aspirin; 1.4 (95 percent CI 0.6–3.1) regular use of aspirin; paracetamol not significant

88:3   Griffin MR, Ray WA, Schaffner W. Non-steroidal anti-inflammatory drug use and death from peptic ulcer in elderly persons. Ann Intern Med 1988; 109:359–63.

Drug Name: aspirin, diflunisal, fenoprofen, ibuprofen, indomethacin, meclofenamate sodium, naproxen, oxyphenbutazone, phenylbutazone, piroxicam, sulindac, tolmetin, zomepirac sodium; *Category:* analgesics, nonsteroidal antiinflammatory drugs
Dosing Criteria: none; *Treatment Duration:* four exposure criteria: current users—prescription filled within 30 days of death, indeterminate users—prescription filled 31–90 days before death, previous users—prescription filled 91–180 days before death, non-users—no prescription for nonsteroidal antiinflammatory drugs in 180 days before death
Validation of Exposure: pharmacy billing records
Study Methodology: retrospective, nested, case-control
Population Selection Criteria: Tennessee Medicaid enrollees aged >60 1976–84, death from peptic ulcer in hospital during the period 1976–84.
Total Number of Subjects: 4019; *Cases:* 122; *Control Subjects:* 3897 population controls; Random sample of non-case Medicaid enrollees stratified according to sex, race, and year of birth (± one year), Medicaid enrollment, and comparable nursing home status, excluding < 180 days' enrollment in Medicaid and the use of anticoagulants, antineoplastic agents, or systemic corticosteroids.
Drug Event: death
Validation of Outcome: death due to gastric or duodenal ulcer confirmed by surgery, endoscopy, X-ray, or autopsy
Findings: adjusted OR 1.9 (95 percent CI 0.7–4.7)

88:4   Guess HA, West R, Strand LM, et al. Fatal upper gastrointestinal hemorrhage or perforation among users and non-users of nonsteroidal antiinflammatory drugs in Saskatchewan, Canada 1988. J Clin Epidemiol 1988;41:35–45

Drug Category: analgesics, nonsteroidal antiinflammatory drugs
Dosing Criteria: none; *Treatment Duration:* number of prescriptions/year
Validation of Exposure: Saskatchewan Health Plan Pharmacy billing data
Study Methodology: retrospective, cohort
Population Selection Criteria: individuals who filled prescriptions for nonsteroidal antiinflammatory drugs in the Saskatchewan Health Plan in 1983
Total Number of Subjects: 134 000 users
Drug Event: upper gastrointestinal hemorrhage and/or upper gastrointestinal perforation

Validation of Outcome: Linkage of prescription records with hospital records; discharge summaries and autopsy records were reviewed.
Findings: A low risk for fatal gastrointestinal hemorrhage was found, except that patients >75 years of age with a previous history of upper gastrointestinal disease are at a higher risk

88:5   Harding JJ, Van Heyningen R. Drugs, including alcohol, that act as risk factors for cataract and possible protection against cataract by aspirin-like analgesics and cyclopenthiazide. *Br J Ophthalmol* 1988;72:809-14

Drug Name: acetaminophen, aspirin, cyclopenthiazide, ibuprofen, nifedipine, paracetamol, spironolactone; *Category:* analgesics, diuretics, nonsteroidal antiinflammatory drugs, steroids
Dosing Criteria: none; *Treatment Duration:* at least four months
Validation of Exposure: questionnaire interview
Study Methodology: retrospective, case-control
Population Selection Criteria: patients 50–79 having cataract extracted in the Oxford Eye Hospital; four groups of controls; patients in ear, nose, and throat, and patients in dermatology; three control groups; registers of local general practitioners; age and sex matched
Total Number of Subjects: 909; *Cases:* 300; *Control Subjects:* 609
Drug Event: cataract/drugs as contributing risk factors or protection
Findings: nifedipine RR 2.7 (95 percent CI 1.00–7.32); spironolactone RR 2.3 (95 percent CI 1.002–5.28); steroids longer than 4 months RR 1.79 (95 percent CI 1.09–2.93); diuretics RR 0.69 (95 percent CI 0.49–0.97); cyclopenthiazide RR 0.31 (95 percent CI 0.16–0.60)

88:6   Horn PL, Thompson WD. Exposure to chemotherapeutic agents and the risk of a second breast cancer: preliminary findings. *Yale J Biol Med* 1988;61:223-31

Drug Category: antineoplastics
Validation of Exposure: 1) hospital records; 2) outpatient records
Study Methodology: retrospective, case-control
Population Selection Criteria: Connecticut Tumor Registry
Total Number of Subjects: 300 incident cases of contralateral breast cancer, 300 randomly selected controls with unilateral breast cancer; *Cases:* (1) 292, (2) 305; *Control Subjects:* (1) 264, (2) 273
Drug Event: contralateral breast cancer
Validation of Outcome: (1) review of medical records at hospitals; (2) second study on same patients with in-person interviews, hospital records, and outpatient chemotherapy records
Findings: (1) OR 0.5 (95 percent CI 0.3–1.0), (2) OR 0.5 (95 percent CI 0.2–1.2) crude ratios; Woolf's method

88:7   Petitti DB, Sidney S, Perlman JA. Increased risk of cholecystectomy in users of supplemental estrogen. *Gastroenterology* 1988;94:91-5

Drug Category: estrogens
Dosing Criteria: none; *Treatment Duration:* never, current, past use, mixed oral contraceptive and estrogen users
Validation of Exposure: interview during physician office visit and follow-up mail survey
Study Methodology: prospective, cohort
Population Selection Criteria: women aged 18–54 years who were not pregnant or postpartum and enrolled in Kaiser-Permanente's Walnut Creek facility

Total Number of Subjects: 16 638
Drug Event: cholecystectomy
Validation of Outcome: computer-stored hospital discharge records
Findings: RR 2.1 (95 percent CI 1.5–3.0) for those who had used versus those who had never used

88:8   Retsagi G, Kelly JP, Kaufman DW. Risk of agranulocytosis and aplastic anaemia in relation to use of antithyroid drugs. International Agranulocytosis and Aplastic Anaemia Study. *Br Med J* 1988;*297*:262-5

Drug Name: carbimazole, methimazole, propylthiouracil; *Category:* antithyroid agents
Dosing Criteria: none; *Treatment Duration:* drug used daily, drug last used on day before onset, duration of use <1, 1–2, ≥3 months
Validation of Exposure: standard questionnaire by trained nurse interviewers prompting for drug use for the first seven days before admission, week by week before, anytime in five months before.
Study Methodology: retrospective, case-control (International Agranulocytosis and Aplastic Anaemia Study)
Population Selection Criteria: Patients identified through telephone networks were enrolled in seven regions of Europe and in Israel, 1980–86 (population area 23 000 000).
Total Number of Subjects: 4313; *Cases:* 262 agranulocytosis, 135 aplastic anemia
Control Subjects: 1771 agranulocytosis, 2145 aplastic anemia
Drug Event: agranulocytosis, aplastic anemia
Validation of Outcome: diagnosis confirmed by panel of hematologists; granulocyte count of ≤0.5 × 10⁹/L; a hemoglobin concentration of ≥100 g/L or a packed cell volume of ≥0.3, and a platelet count of ≥100 × 10⁹/L; criteria for diagnosis of aplastic anemia: white cell count of ≤ 10 g/L, a platelet count of ≤ 50 × 10 g/L and a hemoglobin of ≤100 g/L, or a packed cell volume of ≤0.3 with a reticulocyte count of <30 × 10 g/L.
Findings: agranulocytosis: 45 patients (17 percent) and 5 controls (0.3 percent) used antithyroid drugs; RR 102 (95 percent CI 38–275); aplastic anemia: 4 patients (3 percent) and 5 controls (0.2 percent); RR 9.2 (95 percent CI 1.8–47.0)

88:9   Strom BL, Carson JL, Schinnar R, Sim E, Morse ML. The effect of indication on the risk of hypersensitivity reactions associated with tolmetin sodium versus other nonsteroidal antiinflammatory drugs. *J Rheumatol* 1988;*15*: 695-9

Drug Name: fenoprofen, meclofenamate, naproxen, piroxicam, sulindac, tolmetin
Category: nonsteroidal antiinflammatory drugs
Dosing Criteria: none; *Treatment Duration:* person-year exposure
Validation of Exposure: pharmacy billing records
Study Methodology: retrospective, cohort
Population Selection Criteria: 1980–84 Medicaid claims data for Michigan, Minnesota, and Missouri; 1980–84 users of multiple nonsteroidal antiinflammatory drugs excluded
Total Number of Subjects: 128 344; *Control Subjects:* 16 900 tolmetin users, > 111 444 other nonsteroidal antiinflammatory drug users
Drug Event: hypersensitivity reactions
Validation of Outcome: measured on the day of and during the 30 days after each exposure
Findings: no statistically significant results

89:1   Bergkvist L, Adami HO, Persson I, Hoover R, Schairer C. The risk of breast cancer after estrogen and estrogen-progestin replacement. *N Engl J Med* 1989;*321*:293-7

Drug Category: estrogens, progestins
Dosing Criteria: none; *Treatment Duration:* ≤ 6, 7–36, 37–72, 73–108, ≥ 109 months of exposure and any treatment
Validation of Exposure: pharmacist prescription, patient mail questionnaire in 3.3 percent sample
Study Methodology: prospective, cohort
Population Selection Criteria: women > 35 years of age who had replacement estrogens prescribed were identified by pharmacies in the larger region of Uppsala, Sweden
Total Number of Subjects: 23 244; *Control Subjects:* The entire female population, except for the cohort, was defined as the reference population
Drug Event: breast cancer
Validation of Outcome: new cases of breast cancer reported to the National Cancer Registry in Sweden by primary physician as well as pathologist
Findings: estrogen cohort versus other women in region 1.1 (95 percent CI 1.0–1.3); estrogen cohort less than nine years of use 1.7 (95 percent CI 1.1–2.7); estradiol greater than six years of use 1.8 (95 percent CI 0.7–4.6); estrogen and progestin combination greater than six years of use 4.4 (95 percent CI 0 .9–22.4); no increase in risk after use of conjugated estrogens

89:2   Bloom BS. Risk and cost of gastrointestinal side effects associated with nonsteroidal antiinflammatory drugs. *Arch Intern Med* 1989; *149*:1019-22
Drug Category: analgesics, nonsteroidal antiinflammatory drugs (excluding aspirin)
Dosing Criteria: none; *Treatment Duration:* at least 30 days per one prescription
Validation of Exposure: none
Study Methodology: retrospective, cohort
Population Selection Criteria: Pennsylvania Medicaid-eligibles between July 1, 1984 and March 31, 1985; at least one nonsteroidal antiinflammatory drug prescription, excluding aspirin, between January 1, 1985 and March 31, 1985
Total Number of Subjects: 70 100; *Cases:* 33 800; *Control Subjects:* 36 200
Drug Event: duodenal ulcer, gastrointestinal bleeding, peptic ulcer, and disorders of stomach function
Validation of Outcome: Medicaid pharmacy claims data
Findings: RR 2.52 (95 percent CI 2.25–2.82); RR for duodenal ulcer 1.64 (95 percent CI 0.92–2.91); RR for gastrointestinal bleeding 3.27 (95 percent CI 1.40–7.66)

89:3   Caan BJ, Coldhaber MK. Caffeinated beverages and low birthweight: a case control study. *Am J Public Health* 1989; *79*:1299-300
Drug Name: caffeine; *Category:* cerebral stimulants
Dosing Criteria: none, < 300 mg/d, > 300 mg/d all sources; *Treatment Duration:* during first trimester of pregnancy
Validation of Exposure: postpregnancy interview
Study Methodology: retrospective, case-control
Population Selection Criteria: women pregnant in northern California between July 1, 1981 and June 30, 1982
Total Number of Subjects: 267; *Cases:* 131; *Control Subjects:* 136 women with normal birthweight babies randomly selected from >9000 normal-weight births
Comparability of Controls: yes, except for birthweight
Drug Event: low birthweight babies
Validation of Outcome: hospital records

Findings: >300 mg/d OR 2.94 (95 percent CI 0.89–9.65) caffeine has a small but measurable effect on fetal growth

89:4   Chavez GF, Mulinare J, Cordero J. Maternal cocaine use during early pregnancy as a risk factor for congenital urogenital anomalies. *JAMA* **1989;*262*:795-8**

Drug Name: cocaine
Dosing Criteria: none; *Treatment Duration:* anytime during first trimester of pregnancy
Validation of Exposure: telephone interview of mother
Study Methodology: retrospective, population-based, case-control
Population Selection Criteria: babies with urinary and genital anomalies noted in Atlanta Birth Defects Case-Control Study Registry
Total Number of Subjects: 6875; *Cases:* 276 urinary anomalies, 791 genital anomalies
Control Subjects: 2835 for urinary control, 2973 for genital control
Comparability of Controls: mothers with normal babies matched to mothers with abnormal babies
Drug Event: urogenital anomaly
Validation of Outcome: medical records at Atlanta area hospitals
Findings: urinary tract defects crude OR 4.39 (95 percent CI 1.21–17.24); genital defects crude OR 2.26 (95 percent CI 0.67–7.62); significant association for urinary defects but not for genital defects

89:5   Crane J, Pearce N, Flatt A, et al. Prescribed fenoterol and death from asthma in New Zealand, 1981–1983: case-control study. *Lancet* **1989; 1:917-22**

Drug Name: fenoterol; *Category:* bronchodilators
Dosing Criteria: metered dose inhaler, 200 mg/puff preparation; *Treatment Duration:* as needed, usually two puffs
Validation of Exposure: double data abstraction of hospital records and comparative analysis of hospital records and general practitioner records; general practitioner questionnaire, by personal interview, by telephone, and mail records
Study Methodology: retrospective, case-control
Population Selection Criteria: cases 5–45 years of age who died of asthma between August 1981 and July 1983; controls matched for age and ethnic group, selected from asthma admissions to same hospitals to which cases were admitted
Total Number of Subjects: 585; *Cases:* 117; *Control Subjects:* 468
Comparability of Controls: physician with each case (identified from the New Zealand National Asthma Mortality Survey) chose four matched controls who would have been treated at same hospital as the subject who died
Drug Event: death
Findings: RR 1.55 (95 percent CI 1.04–2.33); RR 2.21 (95 percent CI 1.26–3.88) in patients with or more asthma drugs; RR 2.16 (95 percent CI 1.14–4.11) in patients with a hospital admission for asthma during previous month, and RR 6.45 (95 percent CI 2.72–15.3) in patients prescribed oral corticosteroids at time of death or admission

89:6   Czeizel A, Kiss R, Rácz K, Mohori K, Gláz E. Case-control cytogenic study of offspring of mothers treated with bromocriptine during early pregnancy. *Mutat Res* **1989;*210*:23-7**

Drug Name: bromocriptine; *Category:* dopamine agonist
Dosing Criteria: any dose; *Treatment Duration:* anytime during early pregnancy
Validation of Exposure: medical records

Study Methodology: retrospective, case-control
Population Selection Criteria: women in Budapest clinic treated for hyperprolactinemia and who subsequently became pregnant during treatment
Total Number of Subjects: 94; *Cases:* 31 mothers, 32 children; *Control Subjects:* 31
Drug Event: cytogenic abnormalities
Validation of Outcome: cytogenetic studies
Findings: no effect of bromocriptine noted; distribution of mitosis similar

89:7   Giercksky KE, Huseby G, Rugstad HE. Epidemiology of NSAID-related gastrointestinal side effects. *Scand J Gastroenterol* 1989;24(suppl 163):3-8
Drug Name: naproxen, piroxicam; *Category:* nonsteroidal antiinflammatory drugs
Dosing Criteria: piroxicam 20 mg/d or naproxen 750 mg/d; *Treatment Duration:* 12 weeks
Validation of Exposure: interview
Study Methodology: prospective, cohort
Population Selection Criteria: men and women over 17 years of age with documented radiographic and symptomatic evidence of osteoarthritis of the hip or knee
Total Number of Subjects: 2035; *Cohort I:* piroxicam (n=1021), *Cohort II:* naproxen (n=1014)
Drug Event: gastrointestinal unintended effects
Validation of Outcome: patient visits by interviewer
Findings: gastrointestinal UDE - 31.4 percent piroxicam, 37.6 percent naproxen; serious gastrointestinal UDE - 0.8 percent piroxicam, 0.9 percent naproxen; central nervous system UDE - 7.7 percent piroxicam, 4.6 percent naproxen

89:8   Ginsberg JS, Kowalchuk G, Hirsh J, Brill-Edwards P, Burrows R. Heparin therapy during pregnancy. *Arch Intern Med* 1989;149:2233-6
Drug Name: heparin; *Category:* anticoagulants
Dosing Criteria: variable based on condition treated and various bleeding time test results
Treatment Duration: during pregnancy, duration varied
Validation of Exposure: medical records located by computer search
Study Methodology: historical cohort
Population Selection Criteria: three hospitals in Hamilton, Ontario, Canada; all pregnant women treated with heparin, taken consecutively
Total Number of Subjects: 100 pregnancies in 77 women; *Control Subjects:* Canadian and Ontario historical data
Comparability of Controls: uncertain, historical gross data used
Drug Event: maternal bleeding and thromboembolic complications; adverse fetal/neonatal outcomes
Validation of Outcome: medical records
Findings: maternal bleeding serious in two percent of patients; fetal/neonatal outcomes similar to historical controls

89:9   International Agranulocytosis and Aplastic Anemia Study. Antiinfective drug use in relation to the risk of agranulocytosis and aplastic anemia. *Arch Intern Med* 1989;149:1036-40
Drug Name: beta-lactams, macrolides, sulfamethoxazole, sulfonamides, tetracycline, trimethoprim; *Category:* antibiotics, antiinfectives
Dosing Criteria: none; *Treatment Duration:* two weeks before symptoms of agranulocytosis; 29–180-day period before hospitalization with aplastic anemia
Validation of Exposure: standard questionnaire and interview
Study Methodology: retrospective, population-based, case-control
Population Selection Criteria: hematologists in Europe and Israel representing 25 million people

Total Number of Subjects: 3067; *Cases:* 251 agranulocytosis, 135 aplastic anemia
Control Subjects: 1271 agranulocytosis, 1410 aplastic anemia
Comparability of Controls: admitted to hospital for reasons not related to aniinfective therapy
Drug Event: agranulocytosis, aplastic anemia
Validation of Outcome: pathology reports
Findings: trimethoprim/sulfamethoxazole RR 14.0 (95 percent CI 4.9–42.0); other sulfon-
amides RR 3.6 (95 percent CI 0.7–18,0); beta-lactams RR 1.9 (95 percent CI 0.9–4.0); tetra-
cycline RR 1.1 (95 percent CI 0.3–3.8); macrolides RR 50.0 (95 percent CI 5.1–500.0)

**89:10   Jick SS, Walker AM, Stergachis A, Jick H. Oral contraceptives and breast
cancer. Br J Cancer 1989;59:618-21**
Drug Name: oral contraceptives; *Category:* estrogens/progestins
Dosing Criteria: daily dose; *Treatment Duration:* less than one to greater than four years
Validation of Exposure: computerized drug-usage records
Study Methodology: retrospective, population-based, case-control
Population Selection Criteria: Group Health Cooperative of Puget Sound; hospital discharge
diagnoses, tumor registry; women < 43 years old using drug before first pregnancy
Total Number of Subjects: 231; *Cases:* 95 women with breast cancer; *Control Subjects:* 136
Comparability of Controls: matched controls not using oral contraceptives
Drug Event: breast cancer
Validation of Outcome: pathology reports
Findings: RR 0.9 (95 percent CI 0.4–2.1)

**89:11   Lashner BA, Heidenreich PA, Su GL, Kane SV, Hanauer SB. Effect of folate
supplementation on the incidence of dysplasia and cancer in chronic
ulcerative colitis. Gastroenterology 1989;97:255-9**
Drug Name: folic acid; *Category:* vitamin
Dosing Criteria: 1 mg/d; *Treatment Duration:* long-term
Validation of Exposure: hospital clinic records
Study Methodology: retrospective, case-control
Population Selection Criteria: patients with pancolitis enrolled in a surveillance program at
University of Chicago Medical Center
Total Number of Subjects: 99; *Cases:* 35 with dysplasia; *Control Subjects:* 64 without dysplasia
Comparability of Controls: patients with neoplasia were older and had disease longer
Drug Event: dysplasia of colon
Validation of Outcome: pathology reports
Findings: folate use OR 0.38 (95 percent CI 0.12–1.20); pending larger study, folate supple-
mentation recommended possibly to prevent dysplasia or cancer in ulcerative colitis

**89:12   McKendry RJ, Cyr M. Toxicity of methotrexate compared with azathio-
prine in the treatment of rheumatoid arthritis: a case-control study of 131
patients. Arch Intern Med 1989;149:685-9**
Drug Name: azathioprine, methotrexate; *Category:* antineoplastics, immunosuppressants
Dosing Criteria: azathioprine 102.7±32.9 mg/d, methotrexate 8.4±3.0 mg/wk
Treatment Duration: 38± 23.3 months
Validation of Exposure: based on prescriptions issued, compliance established through fre-
quency of return to clinic
Study Methodology: prospective, case-control
Population Selection Criteria: 131 classic or definite rheumatoid arthritis patients enrolled be-
tween 1977 and 1986 at the Ottowa General Hospital's Rheumatic Diseases Unit Clinic
Total Number of Subjects: 131 cases vs. controls: 94 methotrexate, 37 azathioprine

Drug Event: includes laboratory values: alkaline phosphatase, aspartate aminotransferase, lactic dehydrogenase, hemoglobin, white blood cells, platelets, blood urea nitrogen, serum creatinine, and others
Validation of Outcome: interview each three- or four-week return to hospital for drug-related toxic reactions
Findings: no statistically significant difference

89:13   Paul C. Skegg DCG, Spears GFS. Depot medroxyprogesterone (Depo Provera) and risk of breast cancer. *Br Med J* 1989;*299*:759-62
Drug Name: medroxyprogesterone acetate; *Category:* progestogens
Dosing Criteria: monthly injections for birth control; *Treatment Duration:* varied
Validation of Exposure: interviews and clinic records
Study Methodology: retrospective, population-based, case-control
Population Selection Criteria: women aged 25–54 years with newly diagnosed breast cancer in New Zealand
Total Number of Subjects: 2755; *Cases:* 891; *Control Subjects:* 1864
Drug Event: breast cancer
Validation of Outcome: hospital and clinic records
Findings: drug used by 110 patients and 252 controls; overall RR 1.0 (95 percent CI 0.8–1.3); women aged 25–34 years RR 2.0 (95 percent CI 1.0–3.8); despite overall finding, drug may increase risk of breast cancer in young women

89:14   Persson I, Adami HO, Bergkvist L, et al. Risk of endometrial cancer after treatment with oestrogens alone or in conjunction with progestogens: results of a prospective study. *Br Med J* 1989;*298*:147-51
Drug Category: estrogens, progestins
Dosing Criteria: none; *Treatment Duration:* compiled as person-year of exposure, the following categories are used: ≤ 6 months, 7–36 months, 37–72 months, ≥ 73 months of exposure
Validation of Exposure: 95 percent of prescriptions processed by pharmacists included 3.3 percent of sample verified by questionnaire
Study Methodology: prospective, cohort
Population Selection Criteria: women >35 years of age who had replacement estrogens prescribed were identified by pharmacists
Total Number of Subjects: 23 244 cases (133 373 person-years); *Control Subjects:* entire female population of Uppsala healthcare region
Drug Event: endometrial neoplasia
Validation of Outcome: primary clinical and pathology report to Cancer Registry of the Uppsala healthcare region
Findings: RR 1.8 (95 percent CI 1.1–3.2) for any estrogen compound without progestogen six or more years; RR 2.2 for conjugated estrogens without progestogen; RR 2.7 (95 percent CI 1.4–5.1) three or more years for estradiol compounds without progestogen

89:15   Pommer W, Bronder E, Greiser E, et al. Regular analgesic intake and the risk of end-stage renal failure. *Am J Nephrol* 1989;*9*:403-12
Drug Name: acetaminophen, caffeine, phenacetin; *Category:* analgesics, nonsteroidal anti-inflammatory drugs
Dosing Criteria: ≥15 analgesic doses/mo; *Treatment Duration:* at least one year
Validation of Exposure: standardized questionnaire administered through interview
Study Methodology: retrospective, case-control
Population Selection Criteria: all patients ≥20 years in West Berlin with endstage renal disease undergoing therapy

Total Number of Subjects: 1034; *Cases:* 517; *Control Subjects:* 517
Drug Event: endstage renal failure
Validation of Outcome: medical records
Findings: RR 2.44 (95 percent CI 1.77–3.39) for any analgesic; RR 2.65 (95 percent CI 1.91–3.67) for combination drugs; no increase in RR for single analgesic use

89:16   Psaty BM, Koepsell TD, LoGerfo JP, Wagner EH, Inni TS. Beta-blockers and primary prevention of coronary heart disease in patients with high blood pressure. JAMA 1989;261:2087-94

Drug Name: atenolol, metoprolol, nadolol, propranolol; *Category:* beta-adrenergic receptor antagonists
Dosing Criteria: none, but at least 80 percent compliance based on prescirption records
Treatment Duration: those treated during 1982–84
Validation of Exposure: computerized pharmacy records
Study Methodology: retrospective, population-based, case-control
Population Selection Criteria: patients with hypertension treated with drugs and presenting with angina or myocardial infarction
Total Number of Subjects: 985; *Cases:* 248; *Control Subjects:* 737
Comparability of Controls: similar except for beta-blocker use
Drug Event: myocardial infarction
Validation of Outcome: hospital records
Findings: fewer cases than controls were taking beta-blockers; RR 0.62 (95 percent CI 0.39–0.99); higher doses conferred greater protection

89:17   Ray WA, Griffin MR, Downey W. Benzodiazepines of long and short elimination half-life and the risk of hip fracture. JAMA 1989;262:3303-7

Drug Name: alprazolam, bromazepam, chlorazepate, chlordiazepoxide, diazepam, flurazepam, lorazepam, oxazepam, triazolam; *Category:* benzodiazepines
Dosing Criteria: none; *Treatment Duration:* prescription within 30 days of drug event
Validation of Exposure: computerized prescription records
Study Methodology: retrospective, nested, case-control
Population Selection Criteria: hip fractures in Saskatchewan in elderly between 1977 and 1985
Total Number of Subjects: 28 542; *Cases:* 4501; *Control Subjects:* 24 041
Comparability of Controls: matched for age; small sample matched for dementia, ambulatory status, functional status, and body mass
Drug Event: hip fracture
Validation of Outcome: random review of hospital records sample
Findings: hip fracture in patients taking drug with long half-life RR 1.7 (95 percent CI 1.5–2.0); hip fracture in patients taking drug with short half-life RR 1.1 (95 percent CI 0.9–1.3)

89:18   Ray WA, Griffin MR, Downey W, Melton J III. Long-term use of thiazide diuretics and risk of hip fracture. Lancet 1989;1:687-90

Drug Category: diuretics
Dosing Criteria: none, adjusted for compliance using refill rate; *Treatment Duration:* < 2, 2–5 , and ≥ 6 years; calculated as summation of estimated duration of all prescriptions filled in the 8-year period preceding hospital admission date.
Validation of Exposure: computerized pharmacy records of patients who had a prescription filled in the six months prior to hospital admission
Study Methodology: retrospective, nested, case-control

Population Selection Criteria: residents of Saskatchewan ≥ 65 years; cases with concurrent use of corticosteroids, anticonvulsants, thyroid hormone, calcium supplements, and replacement estrogens were excluded.
Total Number of Subjects: 6042; *Cases:* 905 hip fractures; *Control Subjects:* 5137 population controls, matched for age and sex
Comparability of Controls: similar except for hip fracture
Drug Event: fracture of the proximal femur; outcome protective effect of thiazide
Validation of Outcome: hip fractures identified by hospital discharge records
Findings: RR 1.2 (95 percent CI) less than two years of use; RR 0.8 (95 percent CI 0.7–1.0) for use two to five years; RR 0.5 (0.3–0.7) for six or more years

89:19   Ross RK, Paganini-Hill A, Landolph J, Gerbins V, Henderson BE. Analgesics, cigarette smoking, and other risk factors for cancer of the renal pelvis and ureter. Cancer Res 1989;49:1045-8

Drug Name: acetaminophen, aspirin, caffeine, phenacetin; *Category:* analgesics, nonsteroidal antiinflammatory drugs
Dosing Criteria: number of person-months of use of all analgesics
Treatment Duration: use of over-the-counter analgesics for 30 days per year or 30 consecutive days
Validation of Exposure: telephone interviews using structured questionnaire
Study Methodology: retrospective, case-control
Population Selection Criteria: residents of Orange County, California diagnosed with cancer of renal pelvis and ureter cancer over a four-year period ending December 31, 1982; sex-, age-, race-matched neighborhood controls, date of birth (± five years)
Total Number of Subjects: 374; *Cases:* 121 primary tumors of the renal pelvis, 66 primary tumors of the ureter; *Control Subjects:* 121 primary tumors of the renal pelvis, 66 primary tumors of the ureter
Drug Event: cancer of the renal pelvis and ureter
Validation of Outcome: through the Cancer Surveillance Program, a population-based tumor registry of Los Angeles County
Findings: RR 1.6 (p < 0.04) for more than 30 days per year; RR 2.1 (p < 0.0003) for more than 30 consecutive days

89:20   Sandler DP, Smith JC, Weinberg CR, et al. Analgesic use and chronic renal disease. N Engl J Med 1989;320:1238-43

Drug Name: acetaminophen, aspirin, phenacetin; *Category:* analgesics, nonsteroidal antiinflammatory drugs
Dosing Criteria: daily use with any drug or combination thereof; *Treatment Duration:* long-term
Validation of Exposure: telephone interviews
Study Methodology: retrospective, multicenter, case-control
Population Selection Criteria: newly diagnosed cases of renal disease in four North Carolina hospitals; $S_{cr} \geq 130$ μmol/L or ≥ 1.5 mg/100 mL
Total Number of Subjects: 1070; *Cases:* 554; *Control Subjects:* 516
Comparability of Controls: matched for age, sex, race, and proximity to study hospitals
Drug Event: chronic renal failure
Validation of Outcome: hospital medical records
Findings: frequent users versus infrequent users OR 2.79 (95 percent CI 1.85–4.21); phenacetin users OR 5.11 (95 percent CI 1.76–14.9); acetaminophen users OR 3.21 (95 percent CI 1.05–9.80); aspirin users OR 1.32 (95 percent CI 0.69–2.51)

89:21 Strom BL, West SL, Sim E, Carson JL. The epidemiology of the acute flank pain syndrome from suprofen. *Clin Pharmacol Ther* 1989;46:693-9

Drug Name: suprofen; *Category:* analgesics, nonsteroidal antiinflammatory drugs
Dosing Criteria: none; *Treatment Duration:* varied
Validation of Exposure: cases reported to manufacturer, follow-up with reporting physicians
Study Methodology: retrospective, case-control
Population Selection Criteria: cases spontaneously reported to manufacturer
Total Number of Subjects: 247; *Cases:* 62 (163 cases reported); *Control Subjects:* 185 suprofen-treated patients without drug event
Drug Event: flank pain syndrome
Validation of Outcome: local physician records
Findings: participate in regular exercise OR 5.9 (95 percent CI 1.1–30.7); use alcohol OR 4.4 (95 percent CI 1.1–17.5); more men than women OR 3.8 (95 percent CI 1.2–12.1); suffer from hay fever, asthma OR 3.4 (95 percent CI 1.0–11.9)

89:22 Thomas DB, Molina R, Cuevas HR, et al. Monthly injectable steroid contraceptives and cervical carcinoma. *Am J Epidemiol* 1989;130:237-47

Drug Name: dihydroxyprogesterone, estradiol enanthate; *Category:* estrogens/progestins
Dosing Criteria: monthly injections; *Treatment Duration:* varied, any length of time
Validation of Exposure: Spanish-language standard questionnaire
Study Methodology: retrospective, binational, hospital-based, case-control
Population Selection Criteria: cases of cervical cancer admitted to selected hospitals in Mexico and Chili
Total Number of Subjects: Mexico 1036, Chili 342; *Cases:* Mexico 155 (13 used drug), Chili 118 (13 used drug); *Control Subjects:* Mexico 881 subjects, (100 used drug), Chili 224 subjects, (20 used drug)
Comparability of Controls: yes, except for drug use
Drug Event: cervical carcinoma
Validation of Outcome: pathology reports
Findings: Mexico RR 0.7 (95 percent CI 0.3–1.3); Chili RR 0.8 (95 percent CI 0.4–1.9); these data refute smaller study done previously by authors (*Br Med J* 1985;290:961-5)

89:23 UK National Case-Control Study Group. Oral contraceptive use and breast cancer risk in young women. *Lancet* 1989;1:973-82

Drug Name: oral contraceptives; *Category:* estrogens/progestins
Dosing Criteria: daily, any product; *Treatment Duration:* 49–96, ≥97 months
Validation of Exposure: interviews inhome by trained personnel
Study Methodology: retrospective, case-control
Population Selection Criteria: all women, <36 years with breast cancer in 11 areas of Britain
Total Number of Subjects: 1510; *Cases:* 755; *Control Subjects:* 755
Comparability of Controls: control selected from physician's clinic reporting the case; matched for age; methods varied for selection from clinic to clinic
Drug Event: breast cancer
Validation of Outcome: hospital and clinic records
Findings: 49–96 months use RR 1.43 (95 percent CI 0.97–2.12); ≥97 months use RR 1.74 (95 percent CI 1.15–2.62); oral contraceptive <50 µg of estrogen may have less effect; no support for these findings in national breast cancer registration rates which are not increasing

89:24 Vessey MP, McPherson K, Villard-Mackintosh L, Yeates O. Oral contraceptives and breast cancer: latest findings in a large cohort study. *Br J Cancer* 1989;59:613-7

Drug Name: oral contraceptives; *Category:* estrogens/progestins
Dosing Criteria: daily dose, various products; *Treatment Duration:* ≤23 to ≥120 months
Validation of Exposure: medical records
Study Methodology: retrospective, cohort, case-control
Population Selection Criteria: women in Oxford Family Planning Association contraceptive study with breast cancer (17 032 total patients), aged 25–39 years
Total Number of Subjects: 567; *Cases:* 189; *Control Subjects:* 378
Comparability of Controls: yes
Drug Event: breast cancer
Validation of Outcome: hospital records
Findings: no evidence of association between breast cancer and oral contraceptive use

89:25   Werler MM, Mitchell AA, Shapiro S. The relation of aspirin use during the first trimester of pregnancy to congenital cardiac effects. *N Engl J Med* 1989;321:1639-42

Drug Name: aspirin; *Category:* analgesics, nonsteroidal antiinflammatory drugs
Dosing Criteria: any dose; *Treatment Duration:* anytime in first trimester of pregnancy
Validation of Exposure: mother interview to determine total drug use
Study Methodology: retrospective, population-based, case-control
Population Selection Criteria: all mothers with cardiac defect babies in Slone Epidemiology Unit Birth Defect Study
Total Number of Subjects: 8347; *Cases:* 1381; *Control Subjects:* 6966
Comparability of Controls: mothers of babies who had congenital defects other than cardiac defects
Drug Event: congenital cardiac defects
Validation of Outcome: hospital records
Findings: any cardiac defect RR 0.9 (95 percent CI 0.8–1.1); for aortic stenosis RR 1.2 (95 percent CI 0.6–2.3); for coarctation RR 1.0 (95 percent CI 0.6–1.4); for hypoplastic left ventricle RR 0.9 (95 percent CI 0.6–1.4); for transposition of great arteries RR 0.9 (95 percent CI 0.6–1.2)

90:1   DeWood MA, Wolbach RA. Randomized double-blind comparison of side effects of nicardipine and nifedipine in angina pectoris. The Nicardipine Investigation Group. *Am Heart J* 1990;119:468-78

Drug Name: nicardipine hydrochloride, nifedipine; *Category:* calcium-channel blockers
Dosing Criteria: nicardipine 30 mg tid, nifedipine 20 mg tid; *Treatment Duration:* 8 weeks
Study Methodology: prospective, randomized trial, two cohorts: (I) with nifedipine unintended effects; (II) without nifedipine unintended effects
Population Selection Criteria: patients 21 years or older with a primary diagnosis of angina pectoris
Total Number of Subjects: 250; *Cases:* (I) 140, (II) 110; *Control Subjects:* in both cohorts, groups randomly assigned to nicardipine or nifedipine therapy
Drug Event: dizziness, pedal edema, flushing, headaches, and palpitations
Findings: dizziness: nifedipine 18 percent, nicardipine 6 percent; p=0.02

90:2   Kaldor JM, Day NE, Petterson F, Clarke A, et al. Leukemia following chemotherapy for ovarian cancer. *N Engl J Med* 1990;322:1-6

Drug Name: chlorambucil, cyclophosphamide, melphalan, thiotepa, treosulfan
Category: antineoplastics
Dosing Criteria: low versus high dose defined with respect to median dose
Treatment Duration: none

Validation of Exposure: medical records
Study Methodology: retrospective, case-control
Population Selection Criteria: 114 cases of leukemia following ovarian cancer identified in cancer registries and hospital internationally
Total Number of Subjects: 456; *Cases:* 114; *Control Subjects:* 342
Drug Event: leukemia
Validation of Outcome: leukemia histologically confirmed
Findings: chemotherapy RR 12 (95 percent CI 4.4–32.0)

	low dose	high dose
chlorambucil	RR 14.0 (p <0.05)	23.0 (p <0.01)
cyclophosphamide	RR 2.2	4.1
melphalan	RR 12.0 (p <0.05)	23.0 (p <0.01)
thiotepa	RR 8.3 (p <0.05)	9.7
treosulfan	RR 3.6	33.0 (p <0.01)

90:3   McKinney PA, Roberts BE, Brien CO, et al. Chronic myeloid leukemia in Yorkshire: a case-control study. *Acta Haematol (Basel)*1990;*83*:35-8

Drug Name: digoxin, methyldopa, nifedipine; *Category:* beta-adrenergic receptor atagonists, diuretics
Dosing Criteria: none; *Treatment Duration:* none
Validation of Exposure: patient interview by trained interviewers with medical confirmation if available
Study Methodology: retrospective, case-control
Population Selection Criteria: cases included with hematologic finding of chronic myeloid leukemia in people aged ≥15 years and residents of Yorkshire Health Region between January 10, 1979 and September 27, 1986
Total Number of Subjects: 363; *Cases:* 122; *Control Subjects:* 241
Comparability of Controls: hospital controls matched for age (± three years) and sex
Drug Event: chronic myeloid leukemia
Validation of Outcome: hospital and general practitioner records
Findings: methylodopa OR 9.8 (95 % CI 0.9–483.0) p < 0.06; nifedipine OR 7.3 (95 % CI 1.3–75.1) p < 0.02; diuretics OR 4.0 (95 % CI 1.9–8.8) p < 0.001; digoxin OR 2.4 (95 % CI 0.6–10.9) p < 0.28; beta-blockers OR 2.2 (95 % CI 1.1–4.5) p < 0.02

Pharmacoepidemiology Glossary

Adulterants: Chemical impurities or substances that by law do not belong in a food, drug, plant, animal, or pesticide formulation.

Adverse drug event: Any undesirable effect associated with the use of a drug. The effect may be an extension of the drug's pharmacologic action or of an idiosyncratic nature. An undesirable effect presumably related in a causal way to the use of a drug. See also **unintended drug effect.**

Adverse drug reaction: See **adverse drug event, unintended drug effect.**

Adverse drug reaction—type A: Reactions consistent with the agent's pharmacology, commonly occurring, usually dose-dependent, and fairly predictable.

Adverse drug reaction—type B: Reactions that represent allergic and idiosyncratic reactions to the drug and are independent of the drug's pharmacologic action. These occurrences are rare, not dose-related, and cannot be predicted.

Agent: Factor whose presence is essential for the occurrence of an *unintended drug effect.* See also **signal.**

Algorithm: Any systematic process that consists of an ordered sequence of steps, each step depending on the *outcome* of the previous one; a systematic problem-solving strategy.

Allergic reaction: Reaction to a drug characterized by antigen-antibody formation and interaction.

Ambispective study: Study design in which a part of the data is collected retrospectively and a part of the data is collected prospectively. Used in connection with *cohort studies.*

Anamnesis: History of a particular case of disease.

Association: Degree of statistical dependence between two or more events or *variables.* Events are said to be associated when they occur more frequently together than one would expect by chance.

Attack rate: A case rate that is a *cumulative incidence* rate often used for particular groups, observed for limited periods and under special circumstances, as in an epidemic.

Attribution: Process of deducing the causative role of the suspect drug in the production of an *unintended drug effect.*

Automated database: Computerized information file that allows for fast and cost-effective studies on drug effects, both short-term and delayed, often in very large populations. See also **database.**

Note: Words appearing in italic type are defined elsewhere in the glossary.

415

Bayes' theorem: Theorem in probability theory used in *epidemiology* to obtain the probability of disease in a group of people with some characteristic, on the basis of overall rate of the disease and of the likelihood of that characteristic in healthy and diseased individuals.

Bayesian statistics: Branch of *biostatistics* that incorporates the use of *Bayes' theorem* in arriving at patient-specific predictive parameters.

Bias: Any systematic distortion of the true value of an *association* or difference, e.g., treating patients with mild disease with drug A and patients with severe disease with drug B generally biases the comparison in favor of drug A. The opposite of a biased study is a valid study.

Bioavailability: Degree to which a drug becomes available in the blood after administration.

Biologic markers: *Pharmacogenetic* variants with the potential to be useful in the diagnosis and prediction of drug toxicity *risk*.

Biostatistics: Application of statistical methods to biologic problems.

Biotechnology: Technology associated with the use of microorganisms to produce certain drug entities in mass quantities, e.g., through the use of recombinant DNA procedures.

Case-control study: Study that identifies a group of persons with the *unintended drug effect* of interest and a suitable comparison group of people without the unintended drug effect. The relationship of a drug to the drug event is examined by comparing the groups exhibiting and not exhibiting the drug event with regard to how frequently the drug is present. See also **prospective study, retrospective study.**

Case report: Reporting of a unique clinical *outcome*, procedure, or *unintended drug effect* associated with an individual patient.

Causality: In *pharmacoepidemiology*, causality concerns the relationship between the drug and its *unintended drug effect*. Criteria applied to establish causality are strength, *specificity*, and consistency of the *association*; dose response; biologic plausibility; and *concordance* among investigators.

Cause: Drug or therapeutic entity or drug event that brings about any condition or produces any side effect of which the *causality* is established. See also **determinant.**

Center for Drug Evaluation and Research: Division of the *FDA* responsible for regulating the review and approval of drug products intended for human use.

Center for Drugs and Biologics: See **Center for Drug Evaluation and Research.**

Centers for Disease Control (CDC): Government-operated research center responsible for maintaining the safety of the public through epidemiologic monitoring of disease processes in the U.S. and issuing public health safety warnings when necessary to prevent disease spread.

Chemotherapy: Use of a chemical to treat a clinically recognizable disease or to limit its further progress.

Clinical decision analysis: Application of decision analysis in a clinical setting with the aims of applying epidemiologic and other data on probability of outcomes when alternative decisions can be made, e.g., surgical intervention or drug treatment for myocardial ischemia.

Clinical epidemiology: Application of the epidemiologic knowledge, methods, and reasoning to the problems of patient care.

Clinical trial: An experiment on humans to determine the safety or effectiveness of a preventive or therapeutic agent or procedure.

Cohort study: Method of pharmacoepidemiologic study in which subsets of a defined *population* who vary with respect to exposure to a particular drug are followed over time, with the purpose of comparing the groups so defined in terms of subsequent *unintended drug effect incidence* or *mortality rates*. Cohort studies can be *retrospective, prospective,* or *ambispective* in design.

Comorbidity: Presence of more than one disease state at a given time in a patient, which may have an effect on the condition of interest.

Comparative proportional analysis: Analytical approach that assesses the strengths of an *association* between a particular drug and event relative to the strength of association between comparable drugs and the same event.

Compliance: Degree to which a patient adheres to the recommendations of a health professional.

Concomitant exposure: State in which a *population* has exposure to more than one variable during the same observation period (e.g., a patient on a drug regimen consisting of more than one drug).

Concurrent therapy: Therapy administered to a patient already undergoing another therapy for a disease state. Concurrent therapy may be of the same or a different modality.

Confidence interval: Range of values determined by the degree of presumed random variability in the data, within which the value of a parameter is thought to lie, with the specified level of confidence.

Confounder: Risk factor for a particular *outcome* that is unequally distributed among the exposed and the unexposed, thus distorting the true effect of the exposure on the outcome. To estimate the true effect, the confounder needs to be controlled for, either in the study design or the statistical analysis.

Confounding: Situation in which the effect of one *variable* over another (e.g., the effect of exposure of interest on the *outcome* of interest) is mixed together with the effects of other variables. Confounding is said to be present in a set of data when the crude measure of effect (e.g., risk ratio) differs from the measure of effect obtained after taking into account potential confounding variables.

Confounding by the indication: Type of *bias* that may occur when a symptom or sign, perceived and judged (by a health professional or a patient) as an *indication* for treatment with a drug, is associated both with the intake of the drug and higher probability of the event.

Contraindication: Any condition, especially any condition of disease, that renders a particular treatment modality improper or undesirable.

Contributory cause: A drug that plays a role in the *etiology* of an *adverse event* along with other causative factors.

Controlled trial: Experimental trial in which numerous patient *variables* are taken into account via the study design for both a treated and a control group in order to assess more accurately true differences in a therapeutic regimen.

Correlation: Measure of *association* that indicates the degree to which two or more *variables* fit a linear relationship.

Cost-benefit analysis: An economic analysis in which the costs of drug therapy, medical care costs, and the patient's loss of net earnings due to death or disability are considered. The marginal benefit of improved *health status* to marginal cost (i.e., the cost of treatment) provides the cost/benefit ratio for a treatment modality.

Cost-effectiveness analysis: An economic approach to analyzing the cost and effectiveness of drug therapy or alternative drug therapies and medical care interventions to determine if they will result in the desired objectives and *outcomes*. The preferred drug therapy requires the least cost to attain a certain patient outcome, or has the most effect on patient outcome for a defined cost.

Cost-utility analysis: An economic analysis in which therapeutic *outcomes* are measured in terms of their social value.

Covariant: Condition in which the value of a *variable* changes in accordance with changes in an associated variable.

Crossover study: Study in which subjects, upon completion of the course of one study arm, are switched to another study arm, one of which is usually a *placebo*. The order of treatment arms are allocated at random.

Cross-sectional study: Study that examines the relationship between an *unintended drug effect* and other variables of interest as they exist in a defined *population* at one particular time.

Cumulative incidence: Proportion of a group initially showing no *unintended drug effects* developing drug events upon exposure to a drug over a fixed time interval.

Database: File system in which vast amounts of data concerning specific patient, disease, or drug characteristics can be stored, e.g., medical records, pharmacy files. See also **automated database.**

Dechallenge: Process of removing the drug from a patient thought to have suffered from a drug-induced *adverse drug event*. Cessation of toxicity upon removal increases the likelihood that the reaction was drug-induced. See also **rechallenge.**

Defined daily dose (DDD): Unit of analysis used in *drug utilization studies*. It is the average adult maintenance dose when used for the major *indication* for a particular drug. In order to promote international comparisons of drug utilization patterns, the World Health Organization has defined the DDD for most marketed drugs.

Demography: Study of *populations*, especially with reference to size and density, fertility, mortality, growth, size distribution, migration, and the interaction of all these factors with social and economic conditions.

Determinant: Any factor, whether *unintended drug effect*, patient characteristic, or other attribute, that brings about change in a health condition or other defined characteristic. See also **cause.**

Diagnostic suspicion bias: Distortion that occurs when knowledge of the subject's prior exposure to a putative cause influences both the intensity and *outcome* of the diagnostic process.

Distribution: Complete summary of the frequencies of the values or categories of a measurement made on a group of people. The distribution tells either how many or what proportion of the group were found to have each value out of all possible values.

Division of Epidemiology and Surveillance: Division within the *Center for Drug Evaluation and Research* of the *FDA* that performs pharmacoepidemiologic functions and serves as the postmarketing risk assessors for pharmaceutical products.

Dose-response relationship: Relationship in which a change in amount, intensity, or duration of exposure is associated with a change—either an increase or a decrease—in risk of a specified *outcome*.

Double-blind clinical study: An experiment where assignment of study subjects to randomized treatment and control groups and assessment of *outcome* are designed to ensure that ascertainment of outcome is not biased by knowledge of the groups to which an individual was assigned. "Double" refers to both parties, i.e., the observer(s) in contact with the subjects, and the subjects in the treatment and control groups; neither are informed about the assignment. See also **triple-blind clinical study.**

Double-masked: Synonym for "double-blind"; a preferred term, especially in ophthalmologic trials.

Drug exposure vector: Defines the characteristics of drug exposure, such as the strength and length.

Drug use: The prescribing, dispensing, administering, and ingesting of drugs. The marketing, distribution, prescription, and use of drugs in society. See also **drug utilization study.**

Drug utilization study: Study designed to describe use patterns of a drug by specific *population* groups in a specified clinical or social setting. See also **drug use.**

Dyskinesia: Abnormal body movements, commonly drug-induced.

Ecologic studies: See **secular trend analyses.**

Effectiveness: Extent to which an intervention, procedure, regimen, or service (e.g., a drug), when used under the usual clinical circumstances, does what it is intended to do for a defined *population*.

Efficacy: Extent to which a specific intervention, procedure, regimen, or service produces a beneficial result under ideal conditions. Preferably the determination of efficacy is based on the results of a randomized controlled trial.

Efficiency: Results achieved in relation to the resources invested. In *biostatistics*, the relative *precision* with which a particular design or estimator will estimate a clinical or biological *outcome*.

Endpoint: Primary *outcome* or *variable* of interest in an epidemiologic study.

Epidemiology: Study of the *frequency* and *distribution* of disease and health in *populations*.

Ethical drugs: Drugs that can be obtained only with a prescription.

Etiology: Cause or collection of causes of a condition.

Event monitoring: The documentation and collection of data on any new diagnosis, unexpected deterioration, or improvement in a preexisting condition, and any *unintended drug effect* or any complaint of symptoms that were not present before the treatment was started.

Expectancy effect bias: *Bias* that results in members of an experimental group developing preconceived ideas about the *outcome* of a therapy.

Explanatory study: Observational or experimental study whose emphasis is on isolating the effects of specific *variables* and understanding the mechanisms of action. Study conditions include strict selection criteria. Use of *multivariate* analysis is common.

Exposed group: Group whose members have been exposed to a drug or factor or possess a characteristic that is a supposed cause of a disease or health state of interest.

False negative: A negative test result in a subject who possesses the attribute for which the test is conducted. The labeling of a diseased person as healthy when screening in the detection of disease.

False positive: A positive test result in a subject who does not possess the attribute for which the test is conducted. The labeling of a healthy person as diseased when screening in the detection of disease.

Fixed-dose regimen: Procedure of taking a specified amount of a drug at specified time intervals.

Follow-up study: See cohort study.

Food and Drug Administration (FDA): Government regulatory agency responsible for the public's safety through approval or disapproval of drug and food products.

Frequency: General term describing the quantitative occurrence of an *unintended drug effect*, disease, or other attribute in a *population*.

Global introspection: An expert's opinion or judgment regarding the causality between drug exposure and *unintended drug effect*.

Health maintenance organization (HMO): A prepaid healthcare delivery system having the potential to create and maintain large computerized *databases* useful in *record linkage* studies.

Health status index: Set of measurements designed to assess the health of members of a *population*. They generally include indications for physical and social functioning, emotional well-being, activities, and feelings.

Heterogeneous: Consisting of dissimilar elements; having no uniform quality throughout.

Historical controls: Patients used for comparison with a current treatment group who had the condition or treatment under study at a different time, generally at an earlier period than the study group.

Homogeneous: Composed of similar elements; of a uniform quality throughout.

Hypothesis: A supposition, arrived at from observation or reflection, that leads to refutable predictions via the experimental method.

Iatrogenic morbidity: Any adverse condition in a patient *population* as a result of medical treatment, e.g., the adverse consequences of pharmacotherapy prescribed by a health professional.

Idiosyncratic reaction: An abnormal susceptibility to a drug that is unpredictable, patient-specific, and usually very rare.

Incidence: Number of new instances of an *unintended drug effect* during a given period in a specified *population*. Specifically, the number of new cases of *unintended drug effects* in a defined population within a specified period of time for a selected drug.

Index time: Point in time from which drug exposure is measured.

Indication: Presence of specific disease states for which a drug has demonstrated *efficacy*, via controlled clinical trials.

Indicator variable: *Variable* used as a sign or signal for a larger entity.

Induction period: In *pharmacoepidemiology*, the period required for a specific drug to initiate pathologic changes or induce *unintended drug effects*.

Inequalities: Uneven *distribution* of health and health-related factors (e.g., drug use) among different *population subgroups*.

Institutional review board (IRB): A panel of healthcare providers and laypersons at a specific institution who must decide the appropriateness (ethicality) of proposed human research.

International Classification of Diseases (ICD): Classification of specific conditions and groups of conditions determined by an internationally representative group of experts who advise the World Health Organization, which publishes the complete list in a periodically revised book, the *Manual of the International Statistical Classification of Diseases, Injuries and Causes of Death*. Every disease entity (and procedure) is assigned a number.

Investigational new drug (IND) application: A very complete and thorough document a manufacturer presents to the *FDA* in support of a new drug the manufacturer wishes to study scientifically in humans.

Joint Commission on the Accreditation of Healthcare Organizations (JCAHO): Panel of healthcare practitioners responsible for ensuring high standards of patient care in hospitals and other medical care settings.

Labeling: Complete prescribing information required by the *FDA* to accompany every drug package. It provides information to the clinician about indications, preferred dosing regimens, toxicity, and so on for prescription drugs.

Latent period: In *pharmacoepidemiology*, the period of delay between exposure to a drug and the appearance of an *unintended drug effect*.

Liability: Degree to which someone is legally responsible for a given *outcome*.

Markers: Agents that allow one to observe unobtrusively the interactions of physical and chemical components in the human body.

Marketing: Process a drug manufacturer goes through to bring a drug product to the general public. All drug products must obtain *FDA* approval before they may be sold to the public.

Masking: Set of measures intended to keep one or more groups of study participants from knowing some facts or observations, the most common of which is the treatment assignment.

Medical audit: Method of analysis in *drug utilization studies* that evaluates differences in prescribing among individuals or groups, identifies problems associated with drug prescribing, and provides recommendations to solve the identified problems.

Meta-analysis: Analytical method that critically reviews and statistically combines the results of previous research to increase *statistical power.*

Methodology: Scientific use of study methods. In a research paper, this section details how the study was conducted regarding both data gathering and data analysis.

Misclassification: Erroneous classification of an individual, a value, or an attribute into a category other than that to which it should be assigned. The probability of misclassification may be the same in all study groups (nondifferential misclassification) or may vary among groups (differential misclassification).

Moiety: Any part or portion of a molecule.

Morbidity rate: Term used to refer to *incidence* rates of disease.

Mortality rate: *Rate* expressing the proportion of a *population* that dies within a specified period of time.

Multivariate: Statistical analysis involving relations among more than one *variable.*

N of 1 randomized clinical trial: The subject serves as his/her own control in a *crossover-*design, clinical trial.

National Prescription Audit: A continual cross-sectional survey of 1200 computerized pharmacies in the U.S. used to yield data estimates concerning drug prescribing volume.

Natural history: Well-defined stages of a disease through which it logically progresses if outside forces do not intervene.

NDA Rewrite: Revised new drug regulations effective in 1985 intended to facilitate the approval of drugs shown to be safe and effective and to ensure the disapproval of drugs not shown to be safe and effective. It also established an improved flow of communications between the applicant and the *FDA* and improved the FDA's surveillance of marketed drugs.

NDA supplement: Additions that must be made to an already-submitted *NDA* when significant changes are necessary. They may reflect changes made in dosage, formulation, or indications of the drug.

New drug application (NDA): Application by a manufacturer to the *FDA* for approval to market a drug. This is submitted to the FDA once Phase III trials are completed and the sponsor believes the drug is safe and effective for specific indications.

New molecular entity: A pharmacologically active molecule that has not been previously marketed (either as the parent compound or as a salt, ester, or derivative of the parent compound) in the U.S. for use in a drug product either as a single ingredient or part of a combination.

Nonrepresentative sample: A sample chosen such that it does not truly resemble the population from which it is taken with regard to *variables* of interest.

Numerator analysis: Analytical approach used in ascertaining drug-associated *outcomes*, either by drug category (across events) or by event category. It does not use denominators, i.e., total number of people at risk of developing the outcome, or a control group.

Observational study: A research methodology that does not include intervention by the investigator; one observes changes in one characteristic in relationship to changes in other *variables* in a naturalistic environment.

Odds: Probability that an individual will develop *unintended drug effects*, assuming the exposure status is known.

Odds ratio: the odds of developing the *unintended drug effects* in the drug-exposed group over the odds of developing the unintended effects in the nonexposed groups. The odds ratio is commonly reported for *case-control studies*. It approaches the *relative risk* estimator when the odds of the unintended drug effect are low in the *population* studied. See **relative risk.**

Office of Biologics Research and Review: See Offices of Drug Evaluation I and II.

Office of Drug Research and Review: See Offices of Drug Evaluation I and II.

Office of Epidemiology and Biometrics: One of the six main offices of the *Center for Drug Evaluation and Research*, directly responsible for statistical review of new drug applications and for assembling postmarketing *adverse drug event* and epidemiologic information.

Offices of Drug Evaluation I and II: The offices within the *Center for Drug Evaluation and Research* directly responsible for drug regulation.

Orphan drug: Drugs defined by the Orphan Drug Act (1983); indicated for small patient groups, and often approved for marketing after an abbreviated drug approval process.

Outcome: Any one of all possible results or endpoints that may stem from exposure to a causal factor, or from preventive or therapeutic interventions (e.g., disease, death, cure).

Overreporting: Tendency to falsely identify and therefore errantly include cases of interest, leading to a false increase of numerator in a *rate*.

Over-the-counter (OTC) product: A medication that is considered safe when properly labeled to be used directly by the consumer.

Pathogenesis: Events leading to the development of a disease state.

Patient identifier: Any one of a set of unique numbers assigned to a patient in a *database* that ensures the correct identification of the patient (e.g., Social Security number, registry assigned number).

Period prevalence: Total number of persons known to have had a disease or to have shown an *unintended drug effect* at any time during a specified time period.

Pharmacodynamics: Study of the biochemical and physiological effects of drugs and the mechanisms of their actions, including the correlation of effects of drugs with their chemical structure.

Pharmacoepidemiology: Application of the methods of *epidemiology* to the study of the effects (beneficial and adverse) and uses of drugs in human *populations*.

Pharmacogenetics: Discipline that researches inborn errors of metabolism that affect the pharmacokinetics and dynamics of drugs in *subgroups* of the *population*.

Pharmacokinetics: Study of the properties and disposition of drugs in the body, including their absorption, distribution, localization in tissues, biotransformation, and excretion.

Phase I clinical trial: First phase of human testing for a drug. It is directed at determining the safe dosage range for a drug, how it is absorbed into the body, and possible levels of toxicity. These tests are usually conducted on 20–80 normal healthy volunteers.

Phase II clinical trial: Second phase of human testing for a drug. This phase is mainly directed at learning more about safety and *effectiveness* of the drug for a specific indication or disease state. Seldom are more than 200 patients involved.

Phase III clinical trial: Phase involving the most extensive testing of the drug, intending to more accurately assess safety and *efficacy* and monitor for drug-related adverse effects. This phase contains the largest number of patients, ranging up to several thousand.

Phase IV clinical trial: Synonymous with experimental postmarketing study, any clinical trial conducted after a drug has been approved for marketing. Not all postmarketing studies are Phase IV clinical trials; some are observational (i.e., without *random allocation* of treatments).

Phase IV studies: A structured postmarketing program. They include experimental studies (phase IV clinical trials) and observational epidemiologic studies, such as *cohort, case-control,* and *cross-sectional studies.*

***Physicians' Desk Reference*:** General reference for healthcare providers that includes reprints of the approved product labeling on drugs marketed in the U.S. The monographs are provided by the manufacturers and include major indications, dosing information, and *adverse drug events.*

Placebo: Inert formulation devoid of any beneficial pharmacologic effects on a disease state.

Point prevalence: Number of persons with a disease or showing an *unintended drug effect* at a specified point in time. See also **prevalence.**

Population: Entire collection of units from which a sample may be drawn.

Population-based: Pertaining to a general *population* defined by geopolitical boundaries; this population is the denominator and/or the sampling frame.

Postmarketing surveillance: Process of continual monitoring for drug effects after the drug has been approved by the *FDA* and marketed to the public subject to FDA rules and regulations. During this period new indications as well as *adverse drug events* of very low *incidence* may be uncovered.

Pragmatic study: *Observational* or experimental epidemiologic study whose main objective is to test alternative clinical or public health decisions. Emphasis is on making the study conditions as close as possible to real life. Assessment criteria include considering the overall benefit of the interventions (as judged by both the health professionals and the recipients).

Precision (statistical): Inverse of the variance of a measurement or estimator (e.g., the higher the precision, the smaller will be the *confidence interval* of the relative *risk*).

Premarketing surveillance: Process of active and intense monitoring for drug effects from the clinical trials before the drug has been approved for marketing by the *FDA*. Adverse reactions of very low *incidence* are usually not discovered because the number of patients in whom the drug is tested is relatively small.

Prescribing pattern: Frequency, indications, refills, quantity, and directions of drug prescribing by a licensed clinician.

Prescription event monitoring: System created to monitor for *adverse drug events* in a population. Prescribers are requested to report all events, regardless of whether they are suspected adverse events, for identified patients receiving a specified drug.

Prevalence: Number of instances of a given disease or other condition in a given *population* at a designated time. See also **point prevalence.**

Primary efficacy: Extent to which a drug is able to effect immediate changes in the body associated with its indicated use, i.e., a hypoglycemic agent's ability to lower blood glucose concentrations.

Procedures selection bias: See **susceptibility bias.**

Professional review organization (PRO): Panel of peers that reviews the use of services, quality assurance activities, and credentialing of physicians.

Prognosis: Likely *outcome* of a disease. A prediction based on what is known about the natural history of the disease and the effectiveness of the treatment.

Prospective study: Study design by which the *population* is enrolled in the study and followed over time. The *incidence* of *unintended drug effects* and/or disease *outcomes* is recorded during the study period. The term is often used in connection with *cohort studies*. See also **case-control study, observational study.**

Proxy variable: *Variable* that measures by indirect means another variable that is of interest but cannot be directly measured.

Random allocation (randomization): Process of assigning individuals to study groups by chance in order to increase the probability of obtaining comparable groups that should be free of *bias*.

Rate: *Ratio* whose essential characteristic is that time is an element of the denominator and in which there is a distinct relationship between numerator and denominator.

Rate ratio: See **relative risk.**

Ratio: Relationship between any two magnitudes expressed as a quotient or the product of a division.

Rational drug prescribing: Optimal regimen of drug prescribing by health professionals based on known kinetic, dynamic, and toxic parameters to achieve greatest benefit with the least degree of toxicity.

Recall bias: Systematic error due to differences in accuracy or completeness of recall to memory of prior events among patients with different exposures.

Rechallenge: Process of readministering a drug to a patient thought to have suffered an *unintended drug effect* upon previous exposure. Reemergence of the toxicity is strong evidence of a drug-induced adverse reaction. See also **dechallenge.**

Record linkage: Method of assembling information contained in two or more records, e.g., in different sets of medical charts, and in vital records such as birth and death certificates. This makes it possible to relate significant health events that are remote from one another in time and place.

Registry: File of data concerning all cases of a particular disease or other health-relevant condition in a defined population such that the cases can be related to a *population* base.

Regression to the mean: Tendency of unusually low or high values to become less extreme on subsequent readings.

Regulatory review period: Begins when a new drug is filed with the *FDA*. The FDA is required by law to review the application within 180 days, during which time the FDA determines whether the benefits of the drug outweigh the risks for a specific indication.

Relapse rate: *Rate* at which a disease returns after its apparent cessation.

Relative risk: *Ratio* of the *risk* of a particular *unintended drug effect* between people exposed to the drug and those unexposed to the drug.

Reliability: Degree to which the results obtained by a measurement procedure can be replicated. See also **validity.**

Representative sample: Sample chosen such that it truly resembles the *population* from which it is taken.

Retrospective study: A *case-control study* in which a hypothesis is tested with data derived from characteristics or *unintended drug effects* occurring in the past. The essential feature is that the past drug exposures of people who show the drug event are compared with a group who do not show the drug event in question. Secondary data sources are often used in retrospective study designs. Sometimes also used in connection with *cohort studies*. See also **case-control study, prospective study.**

Risk: Probability that an event will occur, e.g., that an individual will develop an *unintended drug effect* within a stated period of time or age.

Risk factor: Attribute or drug exposure associated with an increased probability of a specified *outcome*, such as the occurrence of an *unintended drug effect*.

Safety profile: Description of the toxic effects of a drug; it also yields expected frequencies of *unintended drug effects*.

Sample: Selected subset of a population. A sample may be random or nonrandom, representative or nonrepresentative.

Secondary efficacy: Ability of a drug to prevent the complications of a disorder for which it is an indicated treatment.

Secular trend analysis: Examines trends in drug exposure and trends in *unintended drug effects* over time or geographic areas, and statistically tests for *association* among the trends.

Selection bias: Error due to systematic differences in characteristics between those who are selected for study and those who are not.

Sensitivity: Proportion of truly diseased persons in the screened *population* who are identified as diseased by the screening test. The probability that any given case will be identified by the test.

Sick role: Role played by those who have assumed the status of sick. Term originated from the sociology of Talcott Parsons.

Side effect: Effect consistently associated with the use of a drug that is not a primary indication or targeted *outcome* of the drug intervention; includes both desirable and undesirable events.

Signal: Reporting of an *unintended drug effect* pair that alerts health professionals that a causal relationship may exist and should be explored further. See also **agent.**

Single drug-event analysis: Analytical approach that can examine the context in which a specific *adverse drug event* occurred through analysis of all available patient-specific data.

Specificity: Proportion of truly nondiseased people who are so identified by the screening test. The probability of correctly identifying a nondiseased person with a screening test.

Spontaneous Reporting System: System maintained by the U.S. FDA and other national drug regulatory agencies in which case reports of *adverse drug events* are voluntarily submitted from health professionals and pharmaceutical manufacturers. This system may serve as an early warning system for serious drug events.

Standardized assessment method (SAM): Flowchart of factors and other considerations that provide an assessment of the likelihood of *causality* between drug exposure and *unintended drug effect.*

Standardized event rate: Form of *comparative proportional analysis* that examines whether the observed reporting *rate* for a specific *unintended drug effect* pair is greater than would be expected in a set of comparable drugs.

Statistical power: Probability that a study will detect a true difference between the study groups, if such difference exists.

Subgroup: That portion of a *population* that shares a common element of interest.

Susceptibility bias: *Bias* incurred from an initial lack of comparability in the prognostic expectations of treated and nontreated patients.

Synergy: Situation in which the combined effect of two or more factors is greater than the sum of their solitary effects.

Target behavior: Any observed behavior for which corrective treatment is initiated, e.g., psychosis in the schizophrenic patient.

Target population: Group of people for whom an intervention is planned, or a *population* to which study results can be generalized.

Therapeutic failure: Inability of a therapeutic regimen to produce the desired results either because of inefficacy or intolerable toxicity.

Therapeutic index: *Ratio* of the toxic to the effective dose of a drug.

Therapeutics: Treatment of disease by any of several modalities.

Third-party payer: Usually an insurance company; a party responsible for direct reimbursement of the health professional for services rendered to the patient.

Treatment investigational new drug (IND): *FDA* regulation allowing limited distribution of a promising drug.

Triple-blind clinical study: Study in which neither the investigator, patient, nor the epidemiologist/statistician knows the patient's therapy. See also **double-blind clinical study.**

Underreporting: Failure to have all identified cases of interest reported, leading to a reduction of numerator in a *rate.*

Unintended drug effect: Any desirable or undesirable effect associated with the use of a drug that is not an intended pharmacologic outcome of the therapy. See also **adverse drug event.**

Univariate: Pertaining to analysis involving only one independent *variable.* See also **multivariate.**

Valid database: *Database* in which all of the individuals in the database with documentation of a given characteristic truly have that attribute.

Validity, external: Degree that a specific study result can be generalized or applied to subjects other than those included in the study. It is generally a subjective assessment. See also **reliability.**

Validity, internal: Degree that an assessment measures what it purports to measure; the absence of *bias* or systematic errors. See also **reliability.**

Validity, measurement: Expression of the degree to which a measurement instrument measures what it purports to measure.

Variable: Any quantity that varies; any attribute that can have different values.

Vital statistic: Systematically tabulated information concerning births, marriages, divorces, separations, migrations, and deaths based on registrations of these vital events.

Wash-out phase: An intermediate phase during a study (usually a *crossover study*) in which treatment is withdrawn so that its effects disappear and the subject's characteristics return to their baseline state.

The editors thank Charles Adcock for his assistance in compiling the glossary.

Index